PATIENT ASSESSMENT IN PHARMACY

PATIENT ASSESSMENT IN PHARMACY

Richard N. Herrier, Pharm. D., FAPhA, CAPT., USPHS (Ret.)

Professor, Department of Pharmacy Practice and Science
College of Pharmacy, University of Arizona
Tucson, Arizona

David A. Apgar, Pharm. D., PA-C (1976-78), CAPT., USPHS (Ret.)

Assistant Professor, Department of Pharmacy Practice and Science
College of Pharmacy, University of Arizona
Tucson, Arizona

Robert W. Boyce, RPh, FASHP, CAPT., USPHS (Ret.)

Director of Pharmacy
Plageman Student Health Center, College of Pharmacy
Oregon State University
Corvallis, Oregon

Stephan L. Foster, Pharm. D., FAPhA, FNAP, CAPT., USPHS (Ret.)

Professor and Vice Chair, Department of Clinical Pharmacy
College of Pharmacy, University of Tennessee Health Sciences Center
Memphis, Tennessee

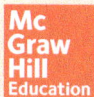

Mc Graw Hill Education | Medical

New York   Chicago   San Francisco   Athens   London   Madrid
Mexico City   Milan   New Delhi   Singapore   Sydney   Toronto

1 2 3 4 5 6 7 8 9 0 CTP/CTP 18 17 16 15 14

ISBN 978-0-07-175194-0
MHID 0-07-175194-7

This book was set in Utopia Std by MPS Limited.
The editors were Michael Weitz and Christie Naglieri.
The production supervisor was Catherine Saggese.
Project management was provided by Asheesh Ratra of MPS Limited.
The text was designed by Diana Andrews.
China Translation & Printing Services, Ltd. was printer and binder.

This book is printed on acid-free paper.

Library of Congress Cataloging-in-Publication Data

Herrier, Richard N., author.
    Patient assessment in pharmacy / Richard N. Herrier, David A. Apgar,
Robert W. Boyce, Stephan L. Foster.
        p. ; cm.
    Includes bibliographical references and index.
    ISBN 978-0-07-175194-0 (pbk. : alk. paper)—ISBN 0-07-175194-7 (pbk. : alk. paper)
    I. Apgar, David A., author. II. Boyce, Robert W., author. III. Foster,
Stephan L., author. IV. Title.
    [DNLM: 1. Pharmaceutical Services. 2. Diagnostic Techniques and
Procedures. 3. Pharmacists. 4. Professional-Patient Relations. QV 737.1]
    RM300
    615.1—dc23
                                                                2014009412

This textbook is dedicated to those Indian Health Service (IHS) pharmacists and other health professionals who from the 1960s through the 1970s pioneered the development of the first pharmacy practice model that focused on the PATIENT rather than on the dispensing process. These patient-centered practice innovations included (1) verifying patient understanding on proper use of prescription medications through patient counseling in private consultation rooms; (2) review of prescription orders for appropriateness; and (3) rectifying problems prior to dispensing; and (4) using pharmacists as primary care providers with prescriptive authority. This pharmacist-based management of patients with common chronic diseases and the diagnosis and treatment of common minor acute illnesses was supported by the IHS Pharmacist Practitioner Training Program (IHS PPTP). This program, initiated as an HRSA grant-funded program in 1973, expanded to an IHS-wide program in 1976. The principles of the training for the IHS PPTP serve as the foundation for this textbook. Successor to the IHS PPTP, the IHS Clinical Pharmacy Training Program (IHS CPTP) provided postgraduate training to enable pharmacists to practice in this unique patient-centered pharmacy practice model. All of these patient-centered pharmacy practice innovations were made possible by the farsighted leadership of Admiral Allen J Brands, who directed the pharmacy programs of the Indian Health Service and the U.S. Public Health Service. His dedication and persistence in developing and sharing these innovations with the pharmacy profession eventually became the basis for today's ambulatory clinical pharmacy practice.

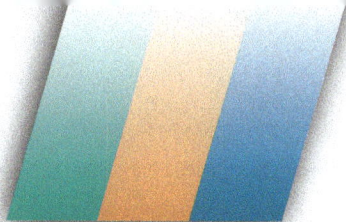

CONTENTS

Dedication   v
Preface   ix

Introduction to Patient Assessment for Pharmacists   1

PART ONE
PRINCIPLES OF PATIENT ASSESSMENT   5

1. Approach to Differential Diagnosis   7
2. Obtaining a Patient History   15
3. Documentation   31
4. Dealing With Patients and Health Care Professionals   41
5. Dealing With Patient Adherence Issues   47
6. Organizing Patient Visits   59

PART TWO
ASSESSMENT OF SYMPTOMS   67

7. Symptoms Related to the Ears, Nose, and Throat   69
8. Cough   89
9. Chest Pain   105
10. Heartburn and Abdominal Pain   115
11. Nausea and Vomiting   127
12. Diarrhea and Constipation   135
13. Headache   147
14. Inflamed (Red) Eye   159
15. Musculoskeletal Symptoms and Disorders   175
16. Dysuria and Vaginal Discharge   185
17. Common Skin Disorders   197

PART THREE
ASSESSMENT IN THE DIAGNOSIS AND MANAGEMENT OF CHRONIC DISEASES AND THEIR COMPLICATIONS   227

18. Essential Hypertension   229
19. Dyslipidemia   243
20. Diabetes Mellitus   259

21. Asthma and Chronic Obstructive Pulmonary Disease (COPD)   273
22. Heart Failure   287
23. Seizure Disorders   293

PART FOUR
ASSESSMENT OF POTENTIAL DRUG-RELATED PROBLEMS   303

24. Liver and Renal Disease   305
25. Anemia, Bleeding, and Infection   325

Answer Keys   339
Index   388

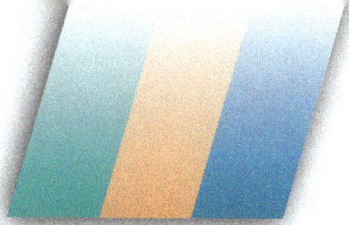

PREFACE

This textbook is intended to fill the significant resource gaps in patient assessment needed by pharmacists to provide optimal patient-centered pharmacy services including primary care. Existing pharmacy materials do not include the necessary breadth and depth in these areas. This textbook is intended to help pharmacists integrate the pathophysiology, findings from history taking, physical examination, and laboratory test interpretation to make accurate assessments in two areas. The first helps the pharmacist make a more accurate diagnosis and thus enables them to better advise patients regarding appropriate use of products intended for self-care or accurately refer patients to higher levels of care if indicated. The second area is to enhance the pharmacist's ability to assist patients in the management of their chronic diseases, outlining monitoring parameters for disease control, early detection of disease-based complications, and drug therapy–based adverse effects. In addition, the textbook will enhance pharmacist's ability to counsel patients about both prescription and nonprescription medications, enhance their ability to communicate with other health care professionals, and assist in identification of potential drug-related problems.

Richard N. Herrier, Pharm. D., FAPhA, CAPT., USPHS (Ret.)

David A. Apgar, Pharm. D., PA-C (1976-78), CAPT., USPHS (Ret.)

Robert W. Boyce, RPh, FASHP, CAPT., USPHS (Ret.)

Stephan L. Foster, Pharm. D., FAPhA, FNAP, CAPT., USPHS (Ret.)

Introduction
to Patient Assessment
for Pharmacists

As pharmacy continues its rapid transition to a more patient-centered profession, patient assessment is one of the most important skill sets a pharmacist will use in daily clinical practice. Patient assessment has five important roles in providing pharmaceutical care. First, it is essential to identify drug-related problems. Many times the pharmacist is required to determine whether a problem is caused by a drug or the patient's illness. Second, patient assessment skills are needed to monitor or manage patients requiring chronic drug therapy. Third, they enable the pharmacist to diagnose and treat common minor acute illnesses and/or appropriately refer patients who require a higher level of care. Fourth, they enhance the pharmacist's ability to educate patients about their disease, its presentation, complications, and management. Finally, since the foundation of communication among health professionals is based on the patient assessment process, it enables the pharmacist to more effectively communicate with other providers (Table 1).

This textbook is intended to fill the significant resource gaps in patient assessment that are needed by pharmacists to provide optimal patient-centered pharmacy services, including primary care. Existing pharmacy materials do not include the necessary breadth and depth in this area. There are several areas that are intentionally not covered in detail, as other sources exist for this information. This is not a therapeutics text, but it will provide skills needed to monitor a patient's drug therapy or assist in controlling their chronic disease. It is not a physical examination textbook, but shows the reader how to integrate physical findings into the overall assessment process. While it does cover chief complaint history taking, it is not a textbook on patient communication. While there is some pathophysiology content in the textbook, in-depth coverage of this material is not the primary intent. Instead, it shows the reader how to integrate pathophysiology, medical history, physical findings, and laboratory tests to accurately assess and monitor patient problems. The focus of this textbook is on two major practice areas for pharmacists. The first is the management of patients with chronic diseases in the ambulatory care. The second is the community pharmacy setting, where pharmacists advise patients on self-care and counsel patients regarding their prescription medication for both acute and chronic diseases. While the content

TABLE 1	Pharmacist Roles That Require Patient Assessment Skills

Identifying potential drug-related problems—*Pharmacist may have to differentiate cause of patient's problem regarding drug induced versus disease induced*

Monitoring/managing patient drug therapy for chronic diseases—*Must evaluate response to therapy and for the presence of adverse drug effects or complications due the chronic disease*

Assessing patients for appropriateness for self-care treatment or referral to higher levels of medical care—*More accurately assess patients for self-care or referral*

Counseling/educating patients about disease and drug therapy

Communicating effectively with other health professionals—*The protocol for "presenting" patients among providers generally follows the format used in chief complaint history taking or history of present illness (HPI)*

emphasizes the ambulatory care setting, the same processes and information apply to most pharmacists practicing in the inpatient setting. This textbook is intended as a primary text in a patient assessment course and would be best used in conjunction with a physical assessment textbook. In addition, it will serve as a useful text in both prescription and nonprescription pharmacotherapeutics courses, as well as in pharmacy practice laboratories, where assessment skills may be taught.

The textbook is organized to provide needed assessment and practice skills for pharmacists working in an ambulatory care environment. Part One, entitled Principles of Patient Assessment covers skills needed to practice in both a chronic disease management role and a community pharmacy setting as a self-care advisor. Chapters One and Two, Approach to Differential Diagnosis and Obtaining a Patient History are focused on the pharmacist's role as a self-care advisor in the community pharmacy setting, but also have applications for those assisting patients in managing their chronic illnesses. Both those chapters, plus the remaining Chapters in Part One, Documentation, Dealing with Patients and Health Care Professionals, Dealing with Patient Adherence Issues, and Organizing Patient Visits are focused on pharmacists involved in assisting patients to optimize treatment of their chronic diseases. However, this information will also have applications to community pharmacists, as chronic care management roles move from health care systems to the community setting. Part Two entitled Assessment of Symptoms is focused on the community pharmacist's role as a self-care advisor. The information in those chapters is intended to assist the community pharmacist to optimize their role in this service they are already frequently called upon to perform. For those patients not candidates for self-care, these chapters will provide knowledge so that the pharmacist will be better able to explain the reasons why the patient needs to see their primary care provider or immediately proceed to urgent or emergent care. Also, it will enable the community pharmacist to more accurately counsel the patient on medications for acute illnesses, including what symptoms to observe to assess the efficacy of therapy and/or indications of potential adverse effects. However, these chapters are also of value to pharmacists practicing in the ambulatory care clinic or inpatient setting since many of these signs or symptoms can also be caused by adverse effects of medication. Part Three entitled Assessment in the Diagnosis and Management of Chronic Diseases and Their Complications focuses on information for pharmacists who assist patients in the management of their chronic illnesses. Part Four entitled Assessment of Potential Drug-Related Problems, is intended for all pharmacists, regardless of practice setting. These chapters cover interpretation of laboratory tests that help detect adverse medication effects on the hepatic, renal, and hematopoietic systems or monitor patients with impaired function of these systems.

The reader should realize that this textbook is *not a comprehensive patient assessment textbook*. It does not cover *all* potential diagnostic possibilities and health problems. Rather, it focuses on those *common* symptom complexes and ambulatory diseases that pharmacists frequently encounter in an ambulatory care setting, including community pharmacies. This textbook is not intended to make the pharmacist a comprehensive diagnostician, but to augment existing knowledge and skills to enable them do a better job at what they already do. Most of the terminology used in the textbook should be familiar to pharmacists. Care has been taken to include other common names used for various diseases. However, some terms and information unfamiliar to the reader may still require the use of other resources.

PART
ONE

Principles of Patient Assessment

Approach to Differential Diagnosis

• INTRODUCTION

Whether it is called problem identification, diagnosis, differential diagnosis, or identifying potential drug-related problems, this universal process to identify patient problems is complex and multifaceted. Much effort and debate have gone into studying exactly how health professionals identify clinical problems (differential diagnosis) with limited success. Regardless of profession, the processes taught and used for identification of clinical problems are almost identical, with small differences in terminology, focus, and structure doing their best to disguise the commonalities among the processes. This chapter seeks to introduce the medical process of differential diagnosis for use by pharmacists in the self-care advisor and chronic disease management roles. It is effective and used by all health professionals who diagnose illness in humans, e.g., primarily physicians, nurse practitioners, and physician assistants. It is also the basis for communication among members of health care teams, envisioned as the future practice modality of choice by the Institute of Medicine. In addition, it will help pharmacists recognize the similarities between the medical process and the pharmacy problem identification processes, plus introduce some practical application of the medical process to the pharmacist's assessment repertoire.

• ELEMENTS NEEDED TO ASSESS PATIENT ILLNESS

There are four major elements required to accurately assess patient illnesses and health problems (Table 1.1). The first is the knowledge of the characteristic patterns of signs and symptoms associated with each disorder, whether acute symptoms or illnesses, chronic diseases, or potential drug-related problems. The second is some type of evaluative or diagnostic criteria. For example, these can be a comprehensive list of all conditions that can cause sore throats or a shorter list that focuses on the most common conditions that cause a sore throat (diagnostic schemata). For chronic diseases and some acute diseases, those evaluative criteria could be national guidelines for the diagnosis/diagnostic workup of that disorder. The third and most important element is the patient history. The published medical literature supports the old adage, "with just the patient history, an accurate diagnosis can be made in 70-90% of patients. Physical examination just confirms the impression formed by the history." What the adage and the literature really show is that the first three elements together yield an accurate diagnosis in 70% to 90% of adult patients who are capable of providing a history. Infants, children, unconscious, mechanically ventilated, or demented adults cannot provide an accurate history, so the adage does not apply to those situations. However, for pharmacists practicing in the self-care arena or disease management in an ambulatory setting, the adage and supporting literature are quite applicable. Therefore, the emphasis of this textbook is on the first three elements. The fourth element, data obtained from the physical examination, laboratory test results, and medical imaging (objective data), is also important. For those patients who are unable to provide an accurate history, objective parameters may be the only data available for accurate assessment. Regarding the fourth element, this textbook does not describe how to do a physical examination, how to conduct a laboratory test, or how to interpret a medical imaging procedure, but it does discuss interpretation of commonly used laboratory tests and how to integrate all objective findings into the assessment process, to improve the accuracy of the diagnosis.

TABLE 1.1	Elements Needed to Assess Patient Health Problems

KNOWLEDGE

Characteristic patterns of signs and symptoms associated with each disorder
Characteristic presentation of potential drug-related problems
Chronic disease guidelines for diagnosis and treatment of specific disorder

DIAGNOSTIC/EVALUATIVE CRITERIA (E.G., DIAGNOSTIC SCHEMATA)

Sore Throat Causes	*Ibuprofen Side Effects*
Allergic rhinitis	Gastrointestinal irritation/upset
Viral URI	Ulcerogenic
Streptococcal pharyngitis	Platelet effects
Viral pharyngitis	Induces asthma
Infectious mononucleosis	CNS effects
	Renal effects
	Interferes with β-blockers, ACEI, diuretics antihypertensive effects

SUBJECTIVE DATA

Patient history

OBJECTIVE DATA

Physical examination
　Observation
　Auscultation
　Palpation
　Percussion
Laboratory test results
Diagnostic imaging

• ANALYTIC VERSUS NONANAYLTIC APPROACHES TO DIFFERENTIAL DIAGNOSIS

The analytic approach is very comprehensive, logical, stepwise in nature, and is used to look for *all of the possible diagnoses* for the patient's primary symptom complex, ranging from common disorders to rare diseases. An analogy frequently used for this comprehensive approach depicts a herd of horses, and the physician is the detective who needs to identify each specific type and breed of horse (more common diseases) in the herd, as well as look for any "zebras" hidden among the herd of horses (rare/uncommon diseases). This approach is very time consuming, but is an essential educational approach for physicians and other health professionals for complex medical problems. This comprehensive analytical approach includes a complete medical history, a complete and thorough physical examination, plus a broad range of laboratory studies. The complete medical history includes history of present illness, past medical history, medication history, social history, and review of systems. The equivalent comprehensive workup in pharmacy is the patient workup of drug therapy (PWDT) developed by Linda Strand and colleagues at the University of Utah, College of Pharmacy, and includes a classification of types of potential drug-related problems. An updated version was developed by the American Society of Health-System Pharmacists (ASHP) and is used in most colleges of pharmacy to teach identification of potential drug-related problems and their solutions in pharmacotherapeutics.

Do clinical pharmacy faculty or experienced physician specialists use this comprehensive analytical approach frequently? The surprising answer from the research literature is no. With their extensive knowledge and experience, they use an efficient nonanalytic approach. Many times expert health care providers of all professions cannot explain the process they use, but research has identified and labeled their approach with a variety of terms, from heuristics to pattern recognition as the primary nonanalytic method used to approach diagnosis and clinical problem identification. Experts develop diagnostic schemata that usually represent 80% to 90% of all causes of a specific symptom by frequency of occurrence. Usually, these schemata are limited to five to eight disorders (Table 1.2). For each disorder in the symptom-specific schemata, there is a "pull-down menu" that includes the major subjective and objective characteristics of that disease. As they begin the history of the primary symptom or chief complaint, the pattern of characteristics usually begins to match one or more of the disorders in their pull down menu. Objective data from the focused physical examination and laboratory studies are then used to confirm the diagnosis or differentiate between two or more possibilities. If the history, physical and lab results are inconsistent with any of the items in the symptom-specific diagnostic schemata and its individual pull-down menus, then the physician reverts to the more comprehensive analytical approach or refers the patient to a higher level of care. Experts have innumerable well-developed diagnostic schemata, which are highly integrated. With these integrated schemata, experts process available information, which allows them to quickly recognize the pattern of subjective and objective information to arrive at the correct diagnosis. With more experience comes a larger number of schemata and subschemata, which are more intimately interconnected and integrated, resulting in better pattern recognition. One interesting note is when experts in one area attempt diagnosis in an area outside their specialty, they revert to the more rudimentary schemata developed prior to specialization, and when they do not help, they tend to revert to the more comprehensive analytical process.

TABLE 1.2	Analytic Versus Nonanalytic Diagnostic Processes	
Analytic	**Nonanalytic**
Comprehensive	Short process
Logical, stepwise look for all the diagnostic possibilities	Use heuristics/pattern recognition and diagnostic schemata of five to eight disorders representing 80% to 90% of the common causes for each symptom (most frequently encountered)
Knowledge of characteristic presentation patterns for every disease	Pull-down menus of characteristic presentations of five to eight disorders in the diagnostic schemata
COMPLETE MEDICAL HISTORY	
History of present illness (HPI)	Chief complaint history (HPI)
Past medical history (PMH)	
Social history	
Review of systems (ROS)	
Medication history	
COMPLETE PHYSICAL EXAMINATION	Focused symptom-based physical examination
COMPLETE LAB AND IMAGING	Focused laboratory testing
Takes hours	Takes minutes
Also known as System 2 process or "zebra hunt"	Also known as System 1 process or heuristics

Pharmacists assisting patients with self-care primarily use the nonanalytical process. If the data fit a specific diagnosis that precludes self-care, e.g., otitis externa, or if the data are inconsistent with all the diseases in a symptom-specific diagnostic schemata and its pull-down menus, then the pharmacist refers the patients to an appropriate higher level of care. Similarly, pharmacists working in a primary care role for patients with chronic diseases when faced with a complicated situation or a problem outside the scope of their clinical privileges refer patients to the appropriate higher level of care. Finally, like their medical counterparts, clinical pharmacy experts also possess groups of highly integrated schemata based on specific classes of medications and use them to quickly identify potential drug-related problems. If that process fails to identify the problem, then they revert to a more comprehensive approach such as the Strand/ASHP process mentioned previously.

• TEXTBOOK ORGANIZATION BY DIAGNOSTIC PROCESS

The Symptom section in this textbook is organized around the nonanalytical heuristic/pattern recognition approach. In those chapters, for every major symptom there is a table. Located at the top of each table is the diagnostic schemata for that symptom. The remainder of the table contains the pull-down menus describing the subjective and objective characteristics of each disease within the diagnostic schemata for that symptom, organized side by side to facilitate pattern recognition (Table 1.3). The Chronic Diseases section is organized around another schemata (the 3 Cs), designed to help organize gathering subjective and objective data, evaluating disease control and the presence of complications due to the chronic disease itself or the drugs used to treat that disorder (Table 1.4). There are only three major categories of information needed to evaluate the quality of care for *any* chronic disease. The first category is control of the disease. Each disease has different subjective and objective parameters that are indicators of disease control. In diabetes, nocturia and the presence of candidal skin rashes or vaginitis are subjective criteria for poor disease control. Objective parameters include A1C and fasting or postprandial plasma glucose. The second category is compliance. In diabetes, compliance includes not only medicines but also diet, exercise, and home blood glucose testing. Pharmacy medication profiles and changes in the patient's weight are objective parameters of compliance with various aspects of the therapeutic regimen. The last category is complications. This category has two parts, complications caused by the chronic disease and adverse effects of medications used to manage the disease. Subjective parameters for diabetes would include symptoms of urinary tract infections, chest pain, and symptoms that might indicate a stroke. Objective parameters for disease complications in diabetes complications would include testing for microalbuminuria, for early stages of nephropathy, and dilated ophthalmoscopic examination for early signs of retinopathy. Subjective parameters for complications due to medication will be drug specific. Nausea, diarrhea, and changes in taste are subjective parameters for common side effects of metformin, while a serum creatinine and respiratory rate would be objective examples to monitor for metformin-induced lactic acidosis. The Follow-up Visit section of each of the chronic disease chapters is organized using the 3 Cs schemata including a table that lists all the objective and subjective parameters to be gathered to evaluate the chronic disease at follow-up visits. These parameters could be used to develop a disease-specific flow sheet to display key findings longitudinally for a quick reference for the progress of each patient and to remind the primary care provider, regardless of profession what items need to be covered every visit. Lastly, at the end of many chapters are cases that students can use to practice these assessment skills for both acute and chronic symptoms and/or diseases. Answer Keys to these case are found in the back of the book.

TABLE 1.3   EAR Pain/Discharge

A. DIAGNOSTIC SCHEMATA FOR EAR PAIN/DISCHARGE

Acute Otitis Media
Otitis Externa aka Swimmer's Ear
Otitis Media With Effusion aka Serous Otitis Media
TMJ Pain Dysfunction Syndrome
Chronic Suppurative Otitis Media

B. DIFFERENTIAL DIAGNOSIS OF EAR PAIN/DISCHARGE

SUBJECTIVE	Acute Otitis Media	Otitis Media with Effusion (Serous Otitis Media)	Chronic Suppurative Otitis Media	Otitis Externa (Swimmer's ear)	TMJ Pain Dysfunction Syndrome
Location	N/A	N/A	N/A	N/A	N/A
Onset	Typically get URI for 2 to 3 days, then notice ear symptoms or allergic rhinitis symptoms for several days	Usually occurs post-AOM or when allergic rhinitis symptoms prominent	None	Occurs after periods of excessive moisture and/or trauma to the external canals	Variable with severity of TMJ disorder and presence of modifying factors
Quantity	Severe discomfort, although infants may just be fussy or irritable and toddlers, young children may just pull at ear; Pain disappears if TM ruptures	Painless unless changes in atmospheric pressure	Severity varies from significant to none		Severity of discomfort varies depending on severity of TMJ disorder and other modifying factors
Quality	Varies	Fullness in ear	Varies	Varies	Ache to muscle spasm
Setting	Requires Eustachian tube dysfunction and the passage of viruses or bacteria from the nasopharynx	Requires Eustachian tube dysfunction	None	Lots of moisture in the ear due to head sets, earphones, swimming Picks at ear with foreign object, e.g., Q-tip, bobby pin	None
Associated symptoms	Purulent discharge on the pillow if TM ruptures; Decreased hearing	Ear popping when yawns; Decreased hearing; May have perennial allergic rhinitis and its symptoms	Purulent discharge on the pillow; Decreased hearing	Purulent discharge on the pillow; Potentially decreased hearing if canal mostly occluded	Headache, grinding, or popping noise when open mouth. Jaw may temporarily lock when opening mouth wide
Modifying factors	None	None	None	Yawning, laying on the ear may worsen pain	Grinding teeth at night, chewing gum makes it worse

TABLE 1.4	Follow-Up Visit Checklist for Hyperlipidemia

CONTROL

S None since there are no symptoms of poor control other than atherosclerotic complications

O Lipid profile as indicated by level of control (at least annually in stable patients)

COMPLIANCE

S How have things been going with your diet? exercise?
What kind of problems have you been having following your diet? exercise plan?
What kind of problems have you been having remembering to take your medication?

O Weight
Medication refill record

COMPLICATIONS (DISEASE)

S What other changes or problems have you noticed since your last visit?
What kind of problems have you noticed when you exercise? **(CHF, PAD)**
What kind of problems have you been having sleeping? **(CHF)**
Have you had any of the following since your last visit?

Chest pain? **(angina)**   Shortness of breath? **(angina, CHF)**
Headache? **(TIA/CVA)**   Dizziness (unsteadiness)? **(TIA/CVA)**
Forgetfulness? **(TIA/CVA)**   Numbness/tingling in extremity? **(TIA/CVA)**
Ankle swelling? **(CHF)**   Number of pillows for sleep? **(CHF)**
Decreased ability to move extremities? **(TIA/CVA)**   Leg cramps/pain while exercising? **(PAD)**
Other unusual symptoms?

O Observational neurological examination (i.e., watch the patient while interviewing for facial and other movements and for coherency of speech and understanding of conversation, and while exiting and entering examination room for ease of mobility and balance **(CVA/TIA)**
Annual complete history and physical including dilated eye examination
Other physical examinations as indicated by history
Electrocardiogram as indicated

COMPLICATIONS (DRUG)

S What other changes or problems have you noticed since your last visit?
Have you had any of the following since your last visit?
Muscle pain, or weakness? **(myotoxicity)**
Fatigue, anorexia, malaise, nausea, vomiting, dark urine? **(hepatotoxicity)**
Difficulty concentrating or remembering things? **(cognitive effects)**

O Examinations/laboratory tests to f/u-specific symptoms
A1C annually   Creatine kinase, urine myoglobin (as indicated)
Folstein minimental status examination (as indicated)   LFTs (as indicated)

• KEY REFERENCES

1. Peterson MC, Holbrook JH, Hales D, Smith NL, Staker LV. Contributions of the history, physical examination and laboratory investigation in making medical diagnoses. *West J Med.* 1992;156:163-165.
2. Bowen JL. Educational strategies to promote clinical diagnostic reasoning. *N Engl J Med.* 2006;355:2217-2225.
3. Norman G. Building on experience—the development of clinical reasoning. *N Engl J Med.* 2006;355:2251-2252.
4. Ark TK, Brooks LR, Eva KW. The benefits of flexibility: the pedagogical value of instructions to adopt multifaceted diagnostic reasoning strategies. *Med Educ.* 2007;41:281-287.
5. Sinclair D, Croskerry P. Patient safety and diagnostic error. tips for your next shift. *Can Fam Physician.* 2010;56:28-30.

6. Rikers R, Te Winkel W, Loyens S, Schmidt H. Clinical case processing by medical experts and subexperts. *J Psychol.* 2003;137:213-223.
7. Tabak N, Bar-Tal Y, Cohen-Mansfield J. Clinical decision making of experienced and novice nurses. *West J Nurs Res.* 1996;18:534-548.
8. Audetat MC, Laurin S. Supervision of clinical reasoning. Methods and a tool to support and promote clinical reasoning. *Can Fam Physician.* 2010;56:e127-e129.
9. Mamede S, van Gog T, van den Berge K, et al. Effect of ovailability bias and reflective reasoning on diagnostic accuracy among internal medicine residents. *JAMA.* 2010;304:1198-1203.

TWO

Obtaining a Patient History

1. Describe the different types of patient histories.

2. Conduct a chief complaint history using LOQQSAM to assess patient's suitability for self-care or need for referral to a higher level of care.

3. Conduct a chief complaint history using LOQQSAM to assess the presence of an adverse reaction to medications.

4. Conduct the interview used in a follow-up visit for patients with a chronic disease such as diabetes mellitus.

• INTRODUCTION

Much of the information needed to accurately assess a patient's symptom complex is obtained from the patient's history, acquired by interviewing the patient in a structured method. Because the patient is telling their story, patient histories are referred to as subjective data, whereas laboratory tests, medical imaging test results and the physical examination, are called objective data. The general process to obtain a patient history by the pharmacist starts with broad open-ended questions to begin the interview, followed by more focused open-ended questions to obtain more specific information. Finally, closed-ended questions are used to assess key issues that may be important to the differential diagnosis, but not mentioned earlier in the interview by the patient, or to further clarify information previously obtained. Next, the pharmacist summarizes the information in the history, which allows the patient to verify the accuracy of the pharmacist's comprehension of the answers they have provided. Closed-ended questions are those that can be answered with a yes or a no and open-ended questions require a more detailed answer in the patient's own words. Open-ended questions are preferred because their use provides more extensive information than do closed-ended questions. Psychologically, closed-ended questions are generally perceived as a notice that the conversation will be coming to an end soon.

• TYPES OF HISTORIES (Table 2.1)

Patient histories can be patient-oriented or provider-oriented. Patient-oriented histories explore the patient's feelings regarding the physical aspects of the symptoms, personal or social components of the symptoms, and the patient's emotional reactions to the symptoms or disease, with the interviewer liberally using empathy, plus verbal and nonverbal cues such as silence and nodding to get the patient to tell their story. A skilled interviewer using both listening skills and observing nonverbal clues can obtain much of the same information that is obtained using a provider-centered process, plus key elements about other aspects of the illness. However, the interview is controlled mostly by the patient and their agenda and can take more time than other approaches. Provider-centered patient histories are designed to get specific types of information from the patient to use to make a diagnosis, with less attention paid to personal, social, and emotional aspects. Fortunately, the two are not mutually exclusive and elements of both can be easily combined. While this textbook focuses mostly on provider-centered techniques, the reader will recognize the integration of some patient-centered elements.

TABLE 2.1	Types of Patient Histories

PROVIDER CENTERED VERSUS PATIENT CENTERED
COMPLETE MEDICAL HISTORY
    HISTORY OF PRESENT ILLNESS (HPI)
        (aka Chief Complaint History Taking)
    PAST MEDICAL HISTORY (PMH)
        Includes Complete Medication History
    FAMILY HISTORY
    PERSONAL AND SOCIAL HISTORY
    REVIEW OF SYSTEMS (ROS)
CHIEF COMPLAINT HISTORY
CHRONIC DISEASE FOLLOW-UP VISIT HISTORY

The *complete medical history* is used in patients admitted to an inpatient facility, new patients to a provider's practice, or when the patient's symptoms do not fit the pattern of a recognizable common disease. Many times, much of this information can be found in the health record especially in an organized health care delivery system (e.g., Group Health, Kaiser, Veterans Administration, Indian Health Service) with integrated inpatient and outpatient health records. Problem lists and one- or two-page health summaries provide much of the information found in a complete medical history. A complete medical history consist of five components: *history of present illness (HPI), past medical history, family history, personal/social history, and a review of systems.* The HPI, also known as a chief complaint history, focuses on the present symptoms and by itself is the history used in most ambulatory situations, involving acute symptoms. Past medical history includes general health status, infectious diseases and immunizations, adverse reactions to medications, and hospitalizations. It contains both active and inactive problems in a problem list. Personal history includes occupation, marital status, personal habits such as alcohol or smoking, financial status, and current living arrangements. Family history asks about significant health events in the lives of parents, siblings, and offspring, looking for patterns of disease and common causes of death. A review of systems uses open-ended and closed-ended questions to probe for other symptoms or conditions, <u>not</u> found during the HPI; past, family, personal, and social histories; or a review of the health record. It tends to start at the top of the body (head, eyes, ears, nose and throat) and move down, e.g., respiratory, cardiovascular, gastrointestinal, genitourinary tract, etc.

The *chief complaint history* also known as the HPI is the most commonly used form of medical history. All patient histories begin with this type of history. In the ambulatory setting, many times that is all that is needed to accurately diagnose, with physical examination, laboratory tests, and medical imaging confirming the suspected diagnosis. Table 2.2 outlines the typical step-by-step process of the chief complaint history, and Table 2.3 outlines LOQQSAM, the pneumonic used to remember the structure and content of chief complaint history taking. The focus of the interview should be to characterize the problems as completely as possible, so that when you relate it to another member of the health care team or the patient's health care provider, they will have all or most of the information they need to assist the patient. That approach prevents the interviewer from jumping to conclusions based on the first few phrases from the patient. Also, it will help obtain enough information to decide whether this patient's illness can be treated with nonprescription medication or they need

TABLE 2.2	Structure of the Chief Complaint History
INTRODUCTION	
"Hi, I'm _____ your pharmacist and you are?"	
GENERAL BROAD OPEN-ENDED QUESTIONS	
"What can I help you with today?"	
"Tell me more about your _____."	
FOCUSED OPEN-ENDED QUESTIONS	
LOQQSAM	
CLOSED-ENDED QUESTIONS	
SUMMARIZATION	
"So you've had a _____ that started 3 days ago," etc.	
CLOSURE	
"Is there anything else we need to discuss today?"	

TABLE 2.3	Chief Complaint History Taking

FIRST OPEN-ENDED QUESTION
   What can I help you with today?
SECOND OPEN-ENDED PROBE\QUESTION
   Tell me more about it.
PARTIAL SUMMARY

LOQQSAM
   LOCATION
      Where is the symptom located?
      Where does it move to?
   ONSET
      When did it start?
      How long have you had it?
   QUALITY
      What does it feel like?
      Describe the feeling in your own words.
      f/u if not specific answer, e.g., pain. Is it dull, sharp, crushing, aching, or burning?
   QUANTITY
      How frequently does it happen?
      How bad is it? Pain rated on 1-10 scale
      How much does it interfere with your usual daily activities?
   SETTING
      How did it happen?
      When do you notice it?
      In what circumstances does/did it occur?
      What happened just before it started?
   ASSOCIATED SYMPTOMS
      What other symptoms do you have?
      What else happens?
      How else do you feel bad or different around the time it happened?
   MODIFYING FACTORS
      What makes it better?
      What makes it worse?
      What have you tried for this? How did it work?
   IMPORTANT ANCILLARY QUESTIONS
      What do you think caused this problem?
      What medications are you currently taking?
   SUMMARIZE/CLOSE——regarding patient problems/complaints

to be referred. Normally, the interview starts with introductions including verification of patient identity. "Good morning, I'm Dr. Smith and you are?" After confirming patient identity, address the patient by their name and ascertain the reason for the visit, "Mrs. Jones, what can I help you with today?" If you know the patient, then such formal identification procedures can be dispensed with other than the reason for the visit. A second open-ended statement encourages the patient to begin talking, "Tell me more about your_____." Patients vary in the amount of information they volunteer from as little as "it's just a bad cold" to a complete recitation of LOQQSAM. Next, use the appropriate remaining LOQQSAM questions to complete the history. Location questions attempt to find the anatomical location of the symptom and where it may move (radiation). For some symptoms you can omit this question, e.g., a runny nose, cough, sore throat. It is mostly used for pain of any type, or dermatological symptoms. Onset questions are used to assess date/time the symptoms began. Quality questions probe for a detailed description of as many aspects of the symptom as possible. It should be in the patient's own words if possible. For example, the nature of the patient's pain can be important to assessing the cause of the pain. If the patient is unable to provide more details, ask, "Exactly how does it feel?" Sometimes, asking "choice" questions will help. "Which of the following would you say best describes your pain: crushing, squeezing, burning, sharp, or cramping?" Quantity questions attempt to measure the severity and/or frequency of the problem. Several approaches can be used, e.g., "How bad is it?" or "How much does this affect your daily routine/work schedule/activities?" For frequency ask, "How often does this happen?" or "How many times a day/hour does it happen?" Setting refers to the circumstances in which the symptom occurs. For example, if the patient complains of crushing, squeezing chest pain, the setting can be very important to determine the next appropriate action step. Consider the difference between the following answers to the question "When does your chest pain occur?" "Oh, only when I'm outside shoveling snow during the winter" would likely indicate chronic stable angina pectoris, while "Well, last night it started while I was just sitting in my recliner watching my favorite TV show" might indicate acute coronary syndrome, which ranges from unstable angina pectoris to the beginning of a myocardial infarction. Associated symptoms looks for other symptoms that may help characterize the symptom pattern to help identify the specific cause. Ask: "What else happens when this occurs?" or "What else do you notice when your symptom starts?" Modifying factors questions are used to find out what makes the symptom better and what makes it worse. Each question should be asked separately. Note that the modifying factors are not always medications. Sometimes certain movements worsen or improve some types of back pain. Avoiding certain foods may improve some gastrointestinal problems. Ask questions such as: "What have you tried to make it better?" or "What seems to make it better?" and "What makes it worse?" Finally, there are two additional questions that can be used to further clarify the situation. The first is to ask the patient what they think caused this problem. "So, what do you think may have caused this?" Sometimes the patient has a good idea of the cause of a given symptom. Sometimes asking a question of this type stimulates the patient to add more information that was not already given. Also, asking the patient their thoughts gives them the idea that their opinion is valued and even implies that they have a role in their own care. The second question is asked whenever you are contemplating recommending a nonprescription product for self-care. "What medications are you currently taking?" This question is intended for patients who are not regular prescription customers. If it is a regular customer you can say, "Let me double-check your medication profile to make sure that what I'm going to suggest won't cause any problems with your existing therapy." Finally, you should summarize what the patient has told you. "Just to make sure I got it all, let me summarize what you have told me." This has several benefits. First, it allows the patient to verify the accuracy and correct any errors. Second, it may prompt the patient to remember something else they forgot to tell you. Finally, it may allow you to detect questions you have not asked or forgot to ask, that may be important in clarifying the diagnosis.

The *chronic disease follow-up visit history* is the second major type of medical history used by pharmacists to assess patient problems. It is structured around the "3 Cs" schemata of evaluating the quality of care in the patient with chronic diseases. For all chronic diseases, there are three things that need to be evaluated. *Control* of the disease, *compliance* with the therapeutic regimen, and *complications* due to the disease

TABLE 2.4	General Approach to Interviewing Patients Returning for Chronic Disease Follow-Up

HOW HAVE THINGS BEEN GOING WITH YOUR _____ SINCE YOUR LAST VISIT? (Control)

How have your home blood glucose readings been?

How many times do you get up from bed to go to the bathroom at night?

WHAT KIND OF PROBLEMS HAVE YOU HAD REMEMBERING TO TAKE YOUR MEDICATION OR HOW ARE THINGS GOING WITH YOUR DIET/EXERCISE? (Compliance)

Tell me about the last time it happened.

How many times has it happened since your last visit?

WHAT KIND OF CHANGES HAVE YOU NOTICED SINCE YOUR LAST VISIT? (Complications)

What kind of problems have you been having with your medication?

I WANT TO DOUBLE-CHECK AND MAKE SURE YOU ARE NOT HAVING ANY OF THE FOLLOWING PROBLEMS (Complications):

USE CLOSED-ENDED QUESTIONS COVERING MAJOR POTENTIAL DISEASE OR DRUG-SPECIFIC PROBLEMS/COMPLICATIONS

Chest pain? **(Angina)**	Shortness of breath? **(Angina, CHF)**
Headache? **(TIA/CVA)**	Dizziness (unsteadiness)? **(TIA/CVA)**
Forgetfulness? **(TIA/CVA)**	Numbness/tingling in extremity **(TIA/CVA)**
Ankle swelling? **(CHF)**	Number of pillows for sleep? **(CHF)**

Decreased ability to move extremities? **(TIA/CVA)**

Leg cramps/pain while exercising? **(PAD)**

Muscle pain, or weakness? **(Myotoxicity)**

Fatigue, anorexia, malaise, nausea, vomiting, dark urine? **(Hepatotoxicity)**

Difficulty concentrating or remembering things? **(Cognitive effects)**

If any problems are noted, shift gears to Chief Complaint Medical History Taking and begin with

TELL ME MORE ABOUT IT followed by LOQQSAM as needed.

and the drugs used to treat it. In this model, there is a general open-ended question to introduce each of the three areas of interest, plus disease-specific open-ended question for probing more specific issues (Table 2.4). "How have things been going with your diabetes since your last visit?" More specific questions probe other aspects that reflect the nature of control of the disease. "How have your home blood glucose readings been going?" "How many times do you get up to go to the bathroom after you go to bed at night?" Compliance questions such as "What kind of problems have you had remembering to take your medication?" "When was the last time it happened?" and "What do you think caused it to happen?" are questions used to probe for details of missed doses. "How have things been going with your exercise (or diet)?" probes for adherence to other therapeutic modalities. Objective data from the patient's pharmacy profile, weight, and resting pulse are objective indicators of diet and exercise. Discrepancies between objective and subject parameters require further probing. "What kind of problems or changes have you noticed since your last visit?" opens the discussion regarding complications from the disease and adverse effects from the medication regimen. Any positive response requires further probing most likely using LOQQSAM. If the patient does not volunteer any problems or changes, then a series of disease and drug-specific, closed-ended questions can be used to double-check for the presence of symptoms that might represent the presence of any complications due to the disease or medication used to treat it. Begin with "I just want to make sure you are not having any of the following: chest pain, breathing problems, etc." Any yes answers will require probing with LOQQSAM beginning with "Tell me more about your chest pain." Using multiple closed-ended questions also signals to the patients that the visit is nearing its end. Going over these lists of complications also educates the patient what to look for. When you routinely ask the open-ended question about problems or changes, you may get a rewarding answer, e.g., "Well you always ask about chest pain and I have had several episodes since I saw you last" or they may call you the first time it happens and ask what to do. Finally, the pharmacist can periodically ask about a fourth C, *concern*. "What kind of concerns do you have about your diabetes or its treatment?" This is a patient-centered question that can be used frequently at the beginning of their treatment and anytime the conversation or nonverbal clues potentially hint at some issue. This reminds them that the pharmacist wants to know about their concerns and it encourages them to ask even though it is not asked about at every visit.

• OTHER SKILLS USED IN HISTORY TAKING

As discussed previously, verification of patient identity and the introduction are important to beginning the history. Also important to a successful history is a *private environment*. Patients will be more open and forthcoming in a private environment. A private room, like an exam room, office, or counseling room would be best. Semi-private consultation booths or areas can be used effectively. However, many times the design of the community pharmacy precludes optimal privacy. If the patient is the only one in the pharmacy or near the pharmacy, then conducting the history anywhere would be private. If a private or semiprivate area in or immediately around the pharmacy is unavailable, take the patient to a quiet aisle containing nonprescription medications. *Patient comfort* is also important. In a private room the patient should be seated in a backed, comfortable chair. In many situations, especially follow-up visits for chronic diseases have the patient remain dressed while you take the history. Sitting in a cold room, in a thin paper gown is not very conducive to accurate and complete patient responses. Even if you are sure that some disrobing will be required, take the history first, while the patient is dressed. Then step outside and begin documentation of the history in the patient's record, while the patient disrobes in preparation for the physical examination. The use of *verbal and nonverbal encouragement* helps the patient provide more complete information, plus they demonstrate that the provider/pharmacist is very interested in what the patient is saying. Examples of verbal encouragement include: "Mm-hmmm, I see, Tell me more, Go on, Oh?, And?, What else?" Clarification of a patient's statement and further discussion can be done with more directed verbal encouragers such as "For instance?" or "Give me an example." Silence is a powerful nonverbal encouragement technique because in many cultures silence during a conversation causes psychological discomfort, encouraging one party to end the discomfort by speaking. Nodding, a surprised facial expression, direct eye contact (when appropriate), and interested facial expressions are all effective nonverbal ways to encourage further discussion by the patient. Patients may express emotion during the history. In these instances, *reflecting or empathetic responses* are used to explore and acknowledge those feelings, help them calm down and demonstrate a caring attitude by the interviewer. *Summarization* has also been discussed previously in this chapter. It usually occurs at the end of the history, but is also appropriate at other parts of the interview, especially if the interview is lengthy or the patient's response is complex or confusing. Finally, the visit should be ended with a *closure* statement in the form of a closed-ended question such as "Is there anything else we need to discuss today?"

There are patient scripts at the end of this chapter so students can practice both types of patient histories that are frequently used by pharmacists. Chief complaint history taking cases can be used concurrently with the symptom-specific diagnostic schemata tables to also practice differential diagnosis. Similarly, chronic disease follow-up visits require concurrent use of the disease-specific tables, which contain subjective parameters used to evaluate disease control, adherence (compliance) to the therapeutic regimen, and complications due to the disease and drug therapy.

• KEY REFERENCES

1. Henderson MC, Tierney LM, Smetana GW. *The Patient History: Evidence-Based Approach to Differential Diagnosis.* New York: McGraw-Hill; 2012.
2. Boyce RW, Herrier RN. Obtaining and using patient data. *Am Pharm.* 1991;NS31:65-70.
3. Haidet P, Paterniti DA. Building a patient history rather than taking one. *Arch Intern Med.* 2003;163: 1134-1140.
4. Platt FW, Gaspar DL, Coulehan JL, et al. Tell me about yourself: the patient-centered interview. *Ann Intern Med.* 2001;134:1079-1085.

CASE 2.1
PATIENT SCRIPT TO PRACTICE CHIEF COMPLAINT HISTORY-TAKING

WHAT CAN I DO FOR YOU TODAY?
What do you have that's good for a cold and runny nose?

TELL ME MORE ABOUT YOUR COLD.
I've had it for a while and just can't seem to get rid of it.

LOCATION
N/A.

ONSET
Started about 2 weeks ago, seemed to get better, and now it's back with a vengeance.

QUALITY
Now the discharge is thick and yellow-brown all the time. When it started it was clear most of the time except when I woke up it was thick and yellow.

QUANTITY
Not bad, just annoying.

SETTING
I caught it from the guys at work.

ASSOCIATED SYMPTOMS
Not sneezing, a slight fever, mild headache centered just below my eyes, mucous tastes and smells terrible.

MODIFYING FACTORS
Pseudoephederine hasn't helped much.
Bending over makes the facial discomfort worse.

MEDICATIONS/WHAT CAUSED IT
I don't take any medicines and I don't know why it got worse.

CASE 2.2
PATIENT SCRIPT TO PRACTICE CHIEF COMPLAINT HISTORY-TAKING

WHAT CAN I DO FOR YOU TODAY?
What do you have that's good for a cough?

TELL ME MORE ABOUT YOUR COUGH.
It's just a nagging cough that doesn't seem to go away.

LOCATION
N/A.

ONSET
Started about 1 month ago.

QUALITY
Nagging, dry, no sputum.

QUALITY
Not too bad, just annoying. I cough two to three times/hour.

SETTING
Had the flu that went to my chest and was left with this cough.

ASSOCIATED SYMPTOMS
I'm tired because I'm not getting much sleep. Without exposure to dust or TB. No allergy history. 3 packs/day; smoker up until 9 years ago.

MODIFYING FACTORS
Exercising makes worse, also worse at night.
Cough drops don't help.

WHAT DO YOU THINK CAUSED IT?
I don't have any idea what caused it.

WHAT MEDICATIONS DO YOU TAKE?
I take some omeprazole for my heartburn.

CASE 2.3
PATIENT SCRIPT TO PRACTICE CHIEF COMPLAINT HISTORY-TAKING

WHAT CAN I DO FOR YOU TODAY?
What do you have that's good for heartburn?

TELL ME MORE ABOUT YOUR HEARTBURN.
I've just got this pain that at times makes my stomach seem like it's on fire.

LOCATION
Just above my belly button.

ONSET
Started about 1 month ago.

QUALITY
Burning pain.

QUANTITY
Not too bad, but is getting worse.

SETTING
Get it about 1 to 2 hours after I eat and lately it's been waking me up at night.

ASSOCIATED SYMPTOMS
A lot of belching and gas, have had loose dark bowel movements the last few days.

MODIFYING FACTORS
Eating makes it better, Tums have helped a little, margaritas make it worse.

CASE 2.4
PATIENT SCRIPT TO PRACTICE CHIEF COMPLAINT HISTORY-TAKING

WHAT CAN I DO FOR YOU TODAY?
Do you have something that's good for the flu?

TELL ME MORE ABOUT YOUR FLU.
It's just the flu. My throat bothers me the most.

LOCATION
Pain is worst in the back of my throat and just under my left ear.

ONSET
Started about 3 days ago.

QUALITY
Just hurts.

QUANTITY
Sometimes it's so bad I can hardly swallow.
Is there 24 hours a day.

SETTING
It's been going around at work.

ASSOCIATED SYMPTOMS
Headache, feverish, aches all over, afraid to eat because my stomach seems real sensitive. No cold symptoms or dental problems.

MODIFYING FACTORS
Orange juice makes it hurt like the devil.

CASE 2.5
PATIENT SCRIPT TO PRACTICE CHRONIC VISIT HISTORY-TAKING

WHAT CAN I DO FOR YOU TODAY?
I'm here for a follow-up visit for my blood pressure.

SO HOW HAVE THINGS BEEN GOING WITH YOUR BLOOD PRESSURE SINCE YOUR LAST VISIT?
Fine, I had my blood pressure checked at a health fair and it was 130/80 and my home blood pressure readings are 120-138/78-88.

WHAT KIND OF PROBLEMS HAVE YOU HAD REMEMBERING TO TAKE YOUR MEDICATION?
None, the chlorthalidone is working well.

HOW ARE THINGS GOING WITH YOUR DIET AND EXERCISE?
I've lost another 2 lb and I'm still walking my dog for about 30 minutes every morning.

WHAT KIND OF CHANGES HAVE YOU NOTICED SINCE YOUR LAST VISIT?
None really.

SOUNDS LIKE THINGS ARE GOING REALLY WELL.

BEFORE YOU GO I WANT TO DOUBLE-CHECK AND MAKE SURE THAT YOU ARE NOT HAVING ANY OF THE FOLLOWING PROBLEMS:

CHEST PAIN? *No*

DIZZINESS? *No*

SHORTNESS OF BREATH? *No*

MUSCLE WEAKNESS? *No*

CHANGES IN VISION? *No*

HEADACHES? *No*

DIFFICULTY BREATHING? *No*

CHANGES IN ABILITY TO WALK OR DO REGULAR ACTIVITIES? *No*

DIFFICULTY SLEEPING? *Yes, now that you mention it. Recently I've been waking up some nights about midnight, which is unusual for me.*

TELL ME MORE ABOUT YOUR WAKING UP.

CASE 2.6
PATIENT SCRIPT TO PRACTICE CHRONIC VISIT HISTORY-TAKING

WHAT CAN I HELP YOU WITH TODAY?
I'm here for my scheduled follow up appointment for my diabetes.

HOW HAVE THINGS BEEN GOING WITH YOUR BLOOD GLUCOSE SINCE YOUR LAST VISIT?
Not as well as I would have hoped. My morning results have been right around 200 and my bedtime results are even higher(230-250).

HOW HAVE THINGS BEEN GOING WITH YOUR DIET AND EXERCISE?
The exercise is going pretty well. I take my dog for an hour almost on weekends and Tuesday and Thursday evenings. The diet is another thing entirely! It is really hard to remember all the things I'm supposed to do especially with trying to cook for the family. If asked your family's big meal is in the evening usually including some type of dessert which you try and avoid but you can't resist your favorites.

WHAT KIND OF PROBLEMS HAVE YOU HAD REMEMBERING TO TAKE YOUR MEDICATION?
None really. I have a good routine. I keep my metformin in the kitchen so I remember to take them with breakfast and dinner.

WHAT KIND OF CHANGES HAVE YOU NOTICED SINCE YOUR LAST VISIT?
None really.

I WANT TO DOUBLE-CHECK AND MAKE SURE YOU ARE NOT HAVING ANY OF THE FOLLOWING PROBLEMS?

(control)   **HOW MANY TIMES DO YOU GET UP TO URINATE DURING THE NIGHT?** *Two to three times*

                        GENITAL ITCHING/RASHES? *No*

                        PAIN ON URINATION OR INFECTED CUTS/SORES? *No*

                        DROWSINESS, DIZZINESS, PALPITATIONS, SWEATING? *No*

(complications)   **CHEST PAIN?** *No*

                        DIFFICULTY BREATHING? *No*

                        DIFFICULTY SLEEPING? *No*

                        CHANGES IN VISION/SPEAKING/CHEWING/MEMORY? *No*

                        PROBLEMS MOVING ANY LIMBS? *No*

                        HEADACHES? *No*

                        BURNING/TINGLING IN FEET? *No*

                        LEG PAIN/CRAMPS? *No*

                        NAUSEA/ GI UPSET? *No*

                        DIARRHEA? *No*

                        CHANGE IN TASTE? *No*

CASE 2.7
PATIENT SCRIPT TO PRACTICE CHRONIC VISIT HISTORY TAKING

SO HOW HAVE THINGS BEEN GOING WITH YOUR ASTHMA SINCE YOUR LAST VISIT?

- Better I think. My albuterol use was about the same, but no ER visits this month. Only used it about four times/week, once a week at night.

- I turned off the swamp cooler function and have thoroughly cleaned up the bedroom and am remembering to close the bedroom door when we leave.

- The albuterol seems to be working better now that I know how to use it. On a couple of occasions one puff has been enough.

WHAT KIND OF PROBLEMS HAVE YOU HAD REMEMBERING TO TAKE YOUR MEDICATION?
I did really well the first few weeks with the beclomethasone evening dose, then things heated up at work and I have been working late and just forget when I get home some evenings. The morning dose hasn't been a problem.

WHAT KIND OF CHANGES HAVE YOU NOTICED SINCE YOUR LAST VISIT?
Other than the things I mentioned, none.

BEFORE YOU GO I WANT TO DOUBLE-CHECK AND MAKE SURE THAT YOU ARE NOT HAVING ANY OF THE FOLLOWING PROBLEMS:

HEARTBURN?   No

CHEST TIGHTNESS?   No

SHORTNESS OF BREATH?   Yes, about four times a week

COUGHING?   Yes, about once a week

WHEEZING?   No

TREMBLING/PALPITATIONS?   No

EXPOSURE TO DUST/ANIMALS/POLLEN?   No

RUNNY NOSE?   No

ITCHING SKIN/RASH?   No

DIFFICULTY SLEEPING?   Yes, one night a week

SORES OR PAINS IN MOUTH?   No

CHAPTER

THREE

Documentation

1. Describe the need and benefits of pharmacist documentation of patient encounters in all settings.

2. Create a problem list from a patient database.

3. Document a simulated patient encounter using a subjective, objective, assessment, and plan (SOAP) format.

• INTRODUCTION

Pharmacist documentation of patient encounters is an essential element of providing pharmaceutical care. There are several ways to document patient care activities in the patient medical record. Prior to 1970, free-flowing narrative was the predominant method of documentation. Its primary disadvantage was that it did not provide a mechanism for which multiple providers, who were involved in the care of a single patient, to effectively communicate with each other. The notes were organized differently by each provider and one had to read the entire note to get important information, and yet many times narrative notes would not contain critical information.

The second approach is the structured approach. In 1968, Lawrence Weed, the director of the family practice residency program at Western Reserve University, became frustrated with the difficulty and variety of ways residents approached the diagnosis and treatment of patients, many of whom had multiple health problems. Initially, he devised a logical, rational, problem-based method of thinking about a patient, which he called **SOAP**. S stands for Subjective or patient history. O stands for Objective, which includes diagnostic tests and physical examination. A stands for Assessment or diagnosis, and P stands for Plan, which includes treatment, education, and other logistical elements of the care plan. It provided a structure to the diagnostic process. As he implemented this logical approach with his residents, it grew into the problem-oriented medical record (POMR), using the SOAP format to document patient encounters by the patient's health problems. The advantage of the POMR and SOAP approach is that they improve the quality of patient care through better communication between members of the health care team. In addition, use of the SOAP format guides the provider in a logical stepwise fashion to collect data, evaluate the patient's problem, and develop a treatment plan. It also allows providers to more effectively follow patients' progress and evaluate the efficacy of any interventions. In contrast to the narrative style, finding and reviewing patient notes with POMR are very rapid due to the organization of the note. Finally, in addition to improving quality and efficiency it serves a valuable purpose from a medicolegal standpoint. Organized, concise SOAP notes reduce the chances of misinterpretation and have been shown to have a positive impact on malpractice outcomes. Some variations of the POMR and SOAP are the predominant methods of documentation today, even in electronic health records, many of which have a SOAP template that drives writing a visit note. While this chapter teaches the process according to Weed's original process, the reader should be aware that there are many variations in use today. DAP is data, assessment, and plan. HOAP is history, observation, assessment, and plan. SOAPIER adds intervention, evaluation, and revision. The exact format differs by institution and facility. Academic medical centers tend to use a more elaborate and comprehensive version due to its use in teaching health care providers, while private practitioners tend to use more concise notes.

• PROBLEM-ORIENTED MEDICAL RECORD SYSTEM

The POMR has two main components: the problem list and individual visit notes done using the SOAP format. The problem list serves as a dynamic table of contents with numbered problems and contains all of the patient's *significant* active and inactive (past) health problems.

When reviewing a medical record to create a problem list, review each visit and record each new diagnosis for which the patient has been seen, along with the date of initial diagnosis. The next step is to distinguish between permanent problems that need to be put on the problem list and temporary problems that should not be placed on the problem list. Examples of permanent problems include chronic or recurring diseases such as diabetes or hypertension, past surgeries, adverse drug reactions, and vaccination status. The permanent problems are those that may impact current assessments. For example, a history of several C-sections 50 years ago (that caused scar tissue formation) may have an important influence when looking for causes in an 80-year-old woman presenting today with signs and symptoms consistent with intestinal obstruction.

Temporary problems are minor or self-limiting diseases, e.g., single episodes of acute otitis media, upper respiratory tract infection, sprained ankle, which will not have any impact on long-term health status. Temporary problems are *not* placed on the problem list. The problem list is a dynamic index to the medical record and changes as new information is added or evolves. For example, a single case of otitis media is a temporary problem. Six cases of AOM over 6 months become a *permanent problem* because now *recurrent AOM* may lead to serous otitis media, fluid buildup, and hearing loss or chronic suppurative otitis media due to the presence of a large central perforation. In those cases, we are going to consider many interventions to prevent hearing loss and slowed development of language skills such as prophylactic antibiotics, PE tubes, and tympanoplasty. This is now a permanent problem and it is a lifelong concern.

Once you have determined all the permanent problems, arrange them by date of initial diagnosis, oldest to newest, with the oldest permanent problem becoming problem number one. The remaining permanent problems are numbered in chronological order with the most recent diagnosis having the largest number. Some organizations will start with problem 00 and label it health maintenance, and use that to identify well-child visits, vaccinations, athletic physical examinations, and periodic preventive examinations as indicated by national standards, such as colonoscopies.

Finally, permanent problems must be separated into active and inactive. Active problems are those that the patient is currently being seen for or those that may have potential importance in the future. For example, if problem #1 was sulfa allergy, which represents the patient developing erythema multiforme to trimethoprim/sulfamethoxazole 20 years ago, that is an active problem because providers will want to avoid using that antibiotic again and possibly other sulfa drugs such as thiazide diuretics or sulfonylureas. Resolved problems such as surgeries or completion of 9 months of isoniazid prophylaxis for a positive tuberculin skin test are not current worries. However, in the case involving multiple C-sections, that information may aid in a more rapid diagnosis of intestinal obstruction. Similarly in the patient who has completed INH prophylaxis, closer monitoring for reactivation of tuberculosis in patients undergoing cancer chemotherapy or initiating use of immune suppressants such as ustekinumab would be warranted. Some institutions put the active and inactive problems in numerical sequence in separate columns, while others will make up two separate lists. The two-column approach can be seen in case 3.1 and is used in the exercises at the end of this chapter.

• SOAP NOTES

Labeling SOAP Notes

SOAP notes are always titled when documenting. This is to enable rapid perusal of the paper or electronic health record (EHR). Newer EHRs allow for search by diagnosis and problem number. For permanent problems, the title should include the problem

Pure Weed	Modified POMR SOAP note
<u>1/1/12 #2 DM</u>	<u>1/11/12 #2, 4, 6 DM, BP, CHOL</u>
S-	S-
O-	O-
A-	A-
P-	P-
	Pharmacist's Signature
<u>#4 BP</u>	
S-	
O-	
A-	
P-	
<u>#6 CHOL</u>	
S-	
O-	
A-	
P-	
Pharmacist's signature	

FIGURE 3.1 Titling entries for permanent problems.

number(s) and an abbreviation of the diagnosis. In a pure Weed system, each problem would have its own SOAP note, but over time physicians began to combine related disorders. So rather than having a SOAP note each for type 2 diabetes, hypertension, and dyslipidemia, many institutions allow physicians to combine related disorders. Temporary problems are titled as TP with the chief complaint serving as the title. If there are two chief complaints they are numbered consecutively. See Figures 3.1 and 3.2 for examples.

Signing the SOAP

Because encounter notes are medicolegal and quality assurance documents, they require the pharmacist's signature. In a manual health record, the pharmacist will sign only once at the bottom of the note(s) for that day and include their degree so other providers can readily identify who saw the patient. Some states may also require

<u>1/2/12 TP #1 Flu</u>
S-
O-
A-
P-

<u>TP #2 Laceration of L Knee</u>
S-
O-
A-
P-
Pharmacist's signature

FIGURE 3.2 Titling entries for temporary problems.

pharmacist's license numbers. In EHRs, entry into the record may automatically record the name, degree, and other requirements, others use a variety of checkboxes and codes, and others still require you to type in the appropriate information or will insert an electronic signature upon command. Regardless of the record format, all medical record entries require a provider's signature.

SOAP

Subjective data S stands for subjective information, which is information obtained during their interview. It also includes information given to you verbally by family, friends, or other health care providers and staff. Subjective information is the patient's and others' perceptions of the illness. When answers to closed-ended questions rule out (r/o) complications due to chronic diseases, such as diabetes, all negative answers can be lumped under the term "denies," e.g., "patient denies, visual disturbances, chest pain, shortness of breath (SOB), hypoglycemic symptoms, numbness and tingling in extremities, vaginal discharge, or dysuria." Any positive responses are further investigated using LOQQSAM and added to the note. "She states she has periodic headaches that are mild, of short duration and are, relieved by acetaminophen and are not associated with low blood glucose or neurological symptoms."

Objective Data O stands for objective data, which include laboratory or diagnostic test results, findings on physical examination, vital signs, and what you observe, e.g., labored breathing, splinting, or coughing, in addition to whatever is documented previously or found in the medical record by either yourself or other providers, including subjective information from previous visits, the problem list, etc.

Assessment A stands for assessment. Assessment includes the suspected diagnosis, level of control of chronic diseases, or provisional diagnosis while waiting for final confirmation of the diagnosis. For example, the 80-year-old lady with multiple C-sections might have her assessment read "Severe abdominal pain, nausea, and vomiting r/o intestinal obstruction." Later once the diagnosis is confirmed, it would change to intestinal obstruction. The degree of certainty in the diagnosis will be reflected in the problem list. In the case of a patient seen for a routine follow-up visit for diabetes, the entry might be "Type 2 diabetes nearly at target A1C, without complications."

Plan P stands for plan, which includes a variety of topics. Referrals, follow-up appointments ("Return to clinic in 3 months."), and further diagnostic tests are all included in the plan. In addition, the plan includes patient education performed and the treatment plan, which includes both drug and nondrug therapies. Students frequently ask where the pharmaceutical care plans go. The elements of pharmaceutical care plans, include most of the above things, and therefore, incorporating other elements of the care plan under P is appropriate.

• SUMMARY

Pharmacist documentation of clinical patient encounters is a required professional function. Structured documentation systems such as the POMR, along with its problem list and SOAP notes, are the most widely used of these structured approaches. Pharmacists should be able to develop a problem list by medical record review and to use SOAP notes to document each encounter.

CASE 3.1
DEVELOPING A PROBLEM LIST

Patient's Name:	Barnaby Jones	DOB 6/18/49

DIAGNOSES ABSTRACTED FROM B JONES MEDICAL RECORD

Appendectomy	1967
Hypertension	1993
Sore throat	4/4/94
Obesity	1990
Positive PPD	1981 (INH prophylaxis completed 2/82)
Ankle sprain	2/10/99
Open reduction	L Humerus FX 7/79
Cellulitis L hand	9/89
Congestive heart failure—mild	6/99
Constipation	5/55
Diaper rash (monilial)	7/50
Childhood immunizations completed	7/54
Penicillin allergy (hives)	10/60
Elevated liver function tests	5/91
Headache, vascular	1990
Diabetes mellitus	1999
Proteinuria	7/2003

Using Case 3.1

1. From this list, decide whether problems are permanent and go on the problem list, or temporary that do not go on the problem list.
2. Categorize the permanent problems into Active (A) and Inactive problems.
3. Arrange the Active and Inactive problems by date. The oldest will be problem 1 and the latest will be the last problem.
4. Now place the problems on the problem list in time sequence starting with 00 Health Maintenance and the oldest problem as #1. Active problems go in the left column and inactive in the right column.

PROBLEM LIST

Date of Onset/Number.		Active Problems	Inactive/Resolved Problems	Date Resolved
NAME	Barnaby Jones			
DOB	6/18/49			
SS/REG#				

PROBLEM LIST

Date of Onset/Number.		Active Problems	Inactive/Resolved Problems	Date Resolved
NAME	Barnaby Jones			
DOB	6/18/49			
SS/REG#				

CASE 3.2
WRITING A SOAP NOTE FOR A TEMPORARY PROBLEM

Directions

1. For each statement, place an SOA or P next to it.

2. Then combine all like data into a narrative or bulleted note.

CHIEF COMPLAINT   Runny nose with HA

• Trial of diphenhydramine LA 1 bid × 3 days

• Patient has marked allergic shiners bilaterally

• Patient presents with a 7- to 10-day history of a dull headache

• If no relief, see physician

• Patient sounds congested

• Headache only partially relieved by Ibuprofen 400 mg

• Also complains of blood shot eyes and increased sneezing

• Patient's eyes appear injected without discharge

• Denies physician visit for this problem previously, other health problems (thyroid, diabetes, heart, BP, or glaucoma) or diseases, other medications, breathing problems

• Warned about drowsiness, dry mouth

• Pain is located in front of head over maxillary sinuses

• Probable allergic rhinitis/conjunctivitis

• Pain now bad enough that it makes teeth hurt

• Has had it in the past, usually occurs in spring and fall

• Denies fever or purulent nasal discharge

• Patient has several crumpled Kleenex in R hand

• ENT negative transillumination, percussion/palpation of maxillary sinuses but has pale boggy turbinates

• If symptoms worsen, become febrile, or develop colored nasal discharge, go to physician ASAP

• Temperature/pulse/respirations (TPR)   99°F /84/15 BP 124/78

• Last Ibuprofen 8 hours ago

CASE 3.3
WRITING A SOAP NOTE FOR A PERMANENT PROBLEM (HYPERTENSION PROBLEM #3)

Directions

1. For each statement, place an SOA or P next to it.

2. Then combine all like data into a narrative or bulleted note.

- Continue chlorthalidone 25 mg 1 qAM and clonidine 2 mg 1 bid
- Patient here for routine visit
- Weight down 6 lb in the past 2 months
- No problems since last visit except for a dry mouth
- Reinforce great job on weight and sodium
- BP
  - 148/88 L arm sitting
  - 140/86 R arm sitting
- Dry mouth started about 2 days after starting clonidine
- Weight 162 lb
- Continue home BP twice daily
- BP at home range from 160-130/95-88
- Better control since starting clonidine
- Dry mouth has gotten slowly better since onset
- 7/10/95 SMAC-12 wnl
- RTC 2 months
- Denies dizziness or other problems
- No edema
- Working real hard to lose weight and reduce Na$^+$ intake
- Monitor dry mouth
- Will be going on vacation for 5 weeks and requests extra medication to last until next visit

FOUR

Dealing With Patients and Health Care Professionals

LEARNING OBJECTIVES

1. Describe potentially new attitudes, roles, and skills needed to effectively develop pharmacist-patient relationships that facilitate optimal care.

2. Describe important factors and variables that impact the effectiveness of the pharmacist as a primary patient educator.

3. Describe effective techniques for communicating about patients with other members of the health care team.

• INTRODUCTION

As the profession of pharmacy moves toward more active involvement in direct patient care, pharmacists will face new practice environments such as health care teams, which will require learning new methods to communicate with other health professionals. Pharmacists will also enter new roles as a provider with primary responsibility to help patients manage their chronic diseases. In those roles, developing effective pharmacist-patient relationships is essential to be successful in helping patients optimize their health. Finally, pharmacists in new roles will now be a primary educator of patients about their chronic disease and the medications to treat them, rather than just verifying that patients understand how to properly use their prescription medication.

• DEVELOPING EFFECTIVE PATIENT RELATIONSHIPS

Changing Patient Attitudes

In previous decades, health care providers were the sole owners of the knowledge regarding health, diagnosis, and medicines. They were perceived as an "all-knowing" authority figure whose recommendations were to be followed. Today, that model of patient-provider relationship has all but disappeared. Patients currently have a wide variety and depth of information regarding health issues available at their fingertips through the Internet. Scandals involving politicians, businessmen, and other traditional authority figures have eroded patient trust and respect of authority figures. Research has shown that patients rely more on peers and the Internet than health professionals for information about diseases and medication. Finally, most patients want a more active role in decisions about their health care.

Changing Provider Roles and Patient-Provider Relationships

Inter- and intraprofessional language still reflects those golden decades, where providers were the knowledgeable authority figures. Comments such as "That diabetic patient in bed 3B" or "I manage Mrs. Jones diabetes" are still heard today in hallway conversations. In reality, the only time a provider manages a patient's chronic disease is during the 20-minute office visit, two to four times a year. For the remainder of the time, the patient manages their chronic disease. The patient follows the diet, exercises regularly, and remembers to take medications in a timely fashion. Today's patients want to be considered by health care providers as a person, not as a disease, and tend to view approaches of past decades as noncaring attitudes. Patients want to be active participants in their care and view the preferred patient-provider relationship as a *partnership*. In this partnership, the provider's role is to facilitate optimal patient self-care of both acute and chronic illnesses and serve as the patient's advocate. Also, remember that the patient's desire for participation is dynamic. During times of severe illness, patients, not feeling well, may prefer to temporarily defer to the provider's judgment.

Changing Pharmacist Skill Requirements

To operate effectively in these new partnership roles, the pharmacist will likely need to augment his/her current skill set. Newer skills include enhanced communication skills, including reflecting responses, motivational interviewing, "I" messages, opened-ended questions; patient assessment skills including history taking; limited physical examination skills; primary patient education skills, e.g., teach-back methods; improved cultural sensitivity; and adherence support skills, which include enhanced knowledge of human behavior, effective communication skills, and interventions to improve adherence with prescribed therapy. The content of the textbook attempts to provide many of the important new skills and knowledge pharmacists require to effectively perform in newer patient-centered roles.

• PRIMARY PATIENT EDUCATION

Primary patient education, i.e., understanding pertinent facts about their disease, diet, exercise, home testing, etc, is the foundation of a patient's ability to adhere to prescribed therapy for their chronic disease. Primary patient education is that given to patients initially by the provider and their staff. Pharmacists traditionally have been providers of secondary education, primarily regarding medication, verifying that patients understand how to take their medication properly. In new patient-centered roles, the pharmacist will more frequently function as the primary educator and need to familiarize themselves with key factors that impact patient understanding of key elements of knowledge.

Adult Learners

Most primary education will be delivered to adults as either patients or caregivers. Adult learners have several unique characteristics that require different teaching approaches. First, adult learners are already very knowledgeable, given their considerable life experiences and the ready availability of technical material on the Internet. Therefore, standard comprehensive lecture formats have low utility, since significant amounts of the material may already be known by the participants. Needs-based, individualized, highly interactive techniques, with or without initial needs assessment, are the preferred learning style in patients. The goal of primary education is not to provide information, but to verify patient understanding of important information and skills. The verification of understanding requires the use of *teach-back*. For example, after being shown how to test blood glucose, the patient is then asked to verify their understanding by demonstrating proper technique. Many pharmacists are familiar with this education approach. The Indian Health Service counseling technique for prescription medication is a needs-based, interactive technique that uses teach-back methodology. The three open-ended questions assess patient knowledge, allowing the pharmacist to fill in the knowledge gaps. The consultation ends using a teach-back process, by asking the patient to go over how they are going to take the medicine this allows the pharmacist to verify patient understanding of proper medication use. One of the reasons teach-back methods are so effective is that by verbalizing or demonstrating understanding the patient remembers more information for longer periods of time.

Self-Efficacy

The principle of self-efficacy discloses that patients will only attempt an activity or learn material that they think they can accomplish. If overwhelmed with multiple activities to initiate or large volumes of material to learn, they give up and do not try. Therefore, 8-hour marathon comprehensive diabetes education classes are not nearly as effective as smaller more focused sessions that build upon each other, allowing a slower accumulation of knowledge. The principle of self-efficacy also applies to adherence to therapeutic regimens. If a patient with diabetes is simultaneously asked to start diet and exercise programs, begin to take medicine, and start home blood glucose testing all at the same time, many patients will be overwhelmed and just give up. So in both adherence and primary patient education, small focused steps, done sequentially that build upon previous sessions, are much better than large one-time comprehensive approaches.

Other Confounding Patient Variables

There are multiple factors that can impact the efficacy of educational efforts or necessitate changes in educational technique. Using teach-back techniques and open-ended questions for needs assessment or interactive teaching techniques helps the pharmacist quickly identify these potential problems. *Health literacy* is an important factor. Try to avoid using potentially confusing medical jargon or be sure to explain medical terms that need to be used in more lay language. *Age* can be a factor. Geriatric patients may have impaired hearing or vision, or lack of dexterity needed to administer medications. *Culture, language, and health beliefs* can also impact education a approaches. Pharmacists need to be alert to their presence and can use teach-back and open-ended questions to detect potential issues. Even the *disease* can impact receptivity to educational efforts. Asymptomatic diseases are the most difficult to educate about since patients feel well. However, some symptoms may help provide an effective approach. In a patient with diabetes whose primary compliant is fatigue and excessive urination at night, starting medication to lower the blood sugar first might be the right approach, since fatigue limits patient focus during educational sessions. Drastically reducing fatigue and nocturia may facilitate making the patient more receptive to educational efforts.

Individualize Education Approaches

The older approach to patient education was to give everyone the same material in the same way. This approach has been shown to produce suboptimal results. Today, with the availability of information, patients come into educational sessions with a wide range of knowledge levels, requiring assessment of each individual's knowledge, preferred learning styles, attitude toward their disease, and availability. To emphasize the need for individualized primary patient education, one diabetes educator applies an adage from a famous public speaker to patient education. In designing education approaches remember that each patient has three personal questions that the educator must answer in order to be effective: So what? Who cares? and What's in it for me? Good advice for all patient educators!

• EFFECTIVE COMMUNICATION WITH HEALTH CARE PROFESSIONALS

As pharmacists begin to practice in health care teams, they will notice that each health profession has unique appropriate communication protocols within the profession. Many times use of your profession's unique communication style interferes with the accuracy of critical communication about patients with other health care providers. In effect, each profession has its own language and protocols. When you are speaking to a member of another profession in your profession's language, you are immediately recognized as a "foreigner" and different from them. Dialogues between different professionals can be confusing and fraught with misunderstanding. One solution is to become multilingual and fluent in each profession's language. An alternative solution is for everyone to use a common language when discussing patients. With the advent of nurse practitioners and physicians' assistants, who also diagnose and prescribe, the most widely used communication protocol in health care is that used by physicians to communicate to each other about patients. While this protocol may have variations depending on locations, it generally has four major steps. First, a brief description of the patient, including name, age, gender, and relevant prior medical history is presented. Next, the reason for the call and the

TABLE 4.1	Medical Communication Protocol Based on Chief Complaint History

LOQQSAM

LOCATION
- **Where is the symptom located?**
- **Where does it move to?**

ONSET
- **When did it start?**
- **How long have you had it?**

QUALITY
- **What does it feel like?**
- **Describe the feeling in your own words.**
- f/u if not specific answer, e.g., pain. Is it dull, sharp, crushing, aching, or burning?

QUANTITY
- **How frequently does it happen?**
- **How bad is it? Pain rated on 1-10 scale**
- **How much does it interfere with your usual daily activities?**

SETTING
- **How did it happen?**
- **When do you notice it?**
- **In what circumstances does/did it occur?**
- **What happened just before it started?**

ASSOCIATED SYMPTOMS
- **What other symptoms do you have?**
- **What else happens?**
- **How else do you feel bad or different around the time it happened?**

MODIFYING FACTORS
- **What makes it better?**
- **What makes it worse?**
- **What have you tried for this? How did it work?**

IMPORTANT ANCILLARY QUESTIONS
- **What do you think caused this problem?**
- **What medications are you currently taking?**

current situation are discussed using a chief complaint medical history protocol, such as LOQQSAM, one of several similar methods of efficiently structuring the process (Table 4.1). Objective data such as physical examination and laboratory results can be added if available. After completing the description of the patient's problem in the chief complaint history format, pause to allow the physician to assimilate and analyze the information presented. Usually, the physician will quickly arrive at the correct assessment. If that does not happen, the presenter can put forward his/her assessment or recommendation using "I" messages. See Table 4.2 for a sample conversation by a pharmacist using this process when notifying the patient's primary care provider of a patient symptom. One similar process used for nurse-physician communication in many hospitals is the SBAR technique. SBAR stands for Situation, Background, Assessment, and Recommendation (Table 4.3). Under Situation one describes pertinent patient demographic data and the reason for the call. Background describes detailed medical information about the patient that is relevant to the situation. Next, the callers Assessment is presented. Finally, they provide a Recommendation or tell the physician what action the caller is requesting. While the first two parts are similar to the medical communication protocol, the lack of a pause, plus making an assessment and a recommendation before the physician can analyze the information presented are major differences.

TABLE 4.2	Sample Dialogue Using Medical Model
Pharmacist:	Dr. Brown, this is Rick Herrier at Jones Pharmacy. Your patient Doris Smith came in today to pick up her second refill for lisinopril 5 mg for her hypertension. While I was talking with her about medication I noticed that she coughed several times. She told me that she has had this dry hacking cough **(Quality)** for a little over a month **(Onset)**. She coughs 10 to 20 times an hour, but while it is annoying it doesn't interfere with her normal activities. **(Quantity)** She denies any previous respiratory illness or any symptoms other than the cough. **(Setting/Associated Symptoms)** She has tried throat lozenges and cough syrup without success. **(Modifying Factors)**
Pharmacist pauses	
Physician:	Given the timing, it sounds like it may be an ACE inhibitor cough. Why don't we switch her to amlodipine 5 mg qAM #30 with one refill and have her call for an appointment in a month.
Pharmacist:	Fine
	OR
Physician:	Why don't we give her 180cc Phenergan Expectorant with Codeine 1-2 teaspoonfuls every 6 hours and see how that works. Have her give it a week and if it persists come see me.
Pharmacist:	After talking with her, I became concerned that the cough might be due to lisinopril that she started 2 months ago and that's why I called.
Physician:	I hadn't thought of that. Sounds like a good pick up! What would you suggest?
Pharmacist:	If you want to stay in the same therapeutic target, then losartan 25 mg would be an option, or I know you use amlodipine quite a bit.
Physician:	Why don't we switch her to amlodipine 5 mg qAM #30 with one refill and have her call for an appointment in a month.

TABLE 4.3	SBAR Technique
SITUATION	*State what is happening to warrant the communication.*
	Identify self, patient, room number.
	Briefly identify the problem including when it started and how severe/urgent it is.
BACKGROUND	*Present pertinent background information related to the patient.*
	Symptoms, vital signs, history, lab results, current medications, IV fluids.
ASSESSMENT	*What is the caller's assessment?*
	In addition to assessment, a brief rationale behind it.
RECOMMENDATION	*What is the caller's recommendation or what does he/she want?*
	Order change.
	Patient needs to be seen now.

• KEY REFERENCES

1. Herrier RN, Boyce RW. Establishing an active patient partnership. *Am Pharm.* 1995;NS35:48-57.
2. Thistlethwaite J. Patient-doctor interactions: emotional cues and discussing prognosis. *InnovAiT.* 2009;2:598-604.
3. Martin LL, Barkan H. Clinical communication strategies of nurse practitioners with patients. *J Am Acad Nurse Pract.* 1989;1:77-83.
4. Brown JB, Lewis L, Ellis K, Freeman TR, Kaperski MJ. Mechanisms for communicating within primary care teams. *Can Fam Physician.* 2009;55:1216-1222.
5. Herrier RN, Boyce RW. Why won't physicians accept my advice? *J Am Pharm Assoc.* 1996;NS36:224-225.
6. Herrier RN, Boyce RW. Communicating more effectively with physicians. *J Am Pharm Assoc.* 1996;NS36:573-574.
7. Haig KM, Sutton S, Whittington J. SBAR: a shared mental model for improving communication between clinicians. *Jt Comm J Qual Patient Saf.* 2006;32:165-175.

Dealing With Patient Adherence Issues

1. Describe the relationship between terms used to define medication adherence including persistence, compliance, adherence, and concordance.

2. List appropriate responses in dealing with potential adherence problems.

3. Discuss the methods to measure adherence including limitations.

4. Describe common misconceptions about medication adherence.

5. List eight common adherence risk factors.

6. Describe behavioral interventions to improve adherence.

• INTRODUCTION

Medication nonadherence is a major public health problem. Nearly half of the 187 million people who take medications in the U.S. do not take them as prescribed. Poor medication adherence costs over $100 million annually. Patients with poor adherence to diabetes medication cost the health care system twice as much as patients with high adherence. While adherence to medication is a problem, adherence to diet and exercise, and other therapeutic modalities is even less than for medications. There is great confusion about what medication nonadherence is. Are you nonadherent if you miss or are late for any dose? Or are you considered adherent if you take 80% or more of your medication? Every study or review article uses different definitions. There is also confusing terminology. *Compliance* was the original term, but was considered to be politically incorrect by some because it implied following the providers' orders. *Adherence* came next because it is more politically correct than compliance and is the current "in" term in the United States. *Persistence* refers to how many pills are picked up from the pharmacy and is more of an economically focused term. Finally, experts in the United Kingdom thought that adherence was as bad as compliance and used *concordance* to better represent that the patient was in partnership with their provider and worked closely together to optimize patient outcomes. Finally, we have classified medication adherence into two categories: intentional and nonintentional (Table 5.1). This classification has some utility because it does generally relate to potential interventions to improve medication adherence.

• PROVIDER MISCONCEPTIONS ABOUT MEDICATION ADHERENCE

There are numerous misconceptions about medication adherence among health care providers. The major misconception is that they "manage" a patient's chronic disease. In reality, the only time a health care provider manages a chronic disease is the 15 to 30 minutes during periodic follow-up visits. The remainder of the time the patient manages their chronic disease. One expert said that providers need to recognize "whose disease is it anyway?" A corollary problem with providers is the

TABLE 5.1	Types of Nonadherence

INTENTIONAL NONADHERENCE

Capricious nonadherence—Solely for oppositional reasons (resistance)
Intelligent nonadherence—Does not meet one of the three reasons patients take medication
Lack of perceived efficacy
Perceived adverse effects
Do not care to take medicine
Altering dose schedule for convenience
Stop to see if still needed
Excess cost

UNINTENTIONAL NONADHERENCE

Forgetfulness
Confusion
Trouble swallowing
Trouble with device, eg, inhaler
Lack of understanding of necessity
Trouble reading labels
Lack of a routine

common belief that they can motivate patients to adhere with their therapeutic regimen. Unfortunately, behavioral sciences have shown that all motivation is self-motivation and that cheerleading style approaches have limited utility and may lead to decreasing rates of adherence. Similarly, some feel that if they clearly explain the risk of suboptimal adherence, patients will automatically be motivated to take their medication as prescribed. Some providers tell patients that if they do not take *all* their medications they *will have* a stroke or heart attack in hopes of motivating them toward better adherence. This threatening, chastising approach, like the cheerleader approach, has limited utility and may lead to results that are opposite of what they are trying to accomplish. Because of this class of misconceptions, some providers perceive patient's suboptimal adherence as a personal rejection of their advice and become angry with patients who do not perfectly control their chronic disease.

Many providers are also unaware of how much medication adherence is required to cure acute illness or gain benefit from chronic disease therapy. For years, pharmacists counseled patients that they had to take all 10 days of their antibiotic or the infection would come back. We now know that is not true. For a variety of common bacterial infections, we now successfully use single dose, 3-day regimens, 5-day regimens, and 7-day regimens to treat bacterial infections that were previously thought to require 10 to 14 days of antibiotic therapy. For chronic disease therapy, an 80% adherence rate has been hailed, albeit without any evidence, as the amount needed to get benefit. However, the original Veterans Administration study that initially demonstrated the efficacy of antihypertensive therapy in preventing complications, such as congestive heart failure, did not measure adherence and used a three times a day medication regimen, which carries an adherence rate of only 60% to 65%. Yet the study still managed to show considerable benefit. Similarly, providers insist that reaching target goals is necessary to get benefits such as preventing diabetic retinopathy, yet studies show that at A1C levels of less than 8.0%, the incidence of retinopathy drops drastically. The ACCORD studies showed that lower targets of glucose and blood pressure related to current guidelines did not have a positive effect on complication rates and even increased the risk of mortality in the lower target groups. Another common provider misconception is that elderly patients have lower medication adherence rates than younger populations. In reality, studies show that while the elderly generally take more medications and have more barriers to adherence, their actual adherence rates are better than younger populations. Finally, many providers feel that educating the patient should be enough to ensure optimal adherence. However, studies repeatedly show that traditional educational programs have little or no effect on medication adherence in *asymptomatic chronic diseases.*

• REQUIREMENTS FOR MEDICATION ADHERENCE

There are three things required for patients to adhere to medication regimens: sufficient understanding of the chronic disease and the medications being used to treat it, motivation to take the medication, and implementation of necessary behavior changes. The impact on adherence to medications for each of these three requirements differs between acute and chronic medications (Figure 5.1). In patients taking acute medication, patient understanding plays a major role, since most patients with acute diseases have symptoms and it is easy to be motivated to take medications that will end the symptoms. Similarly, the behavioral changes (taking medication) are short lived, lasting for only a few days. Therefore, it is not surprising that

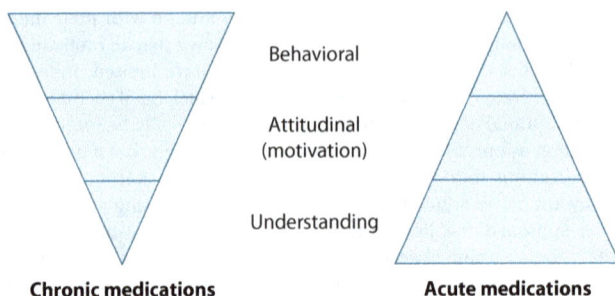

FIGURE 5.1 Requirements for medication adherence.

education and verification of patient understanding have been shown to have a significant impact on subsequent medication adherence in patients with acute symptomatic diseases. In patients with asymptomatic chronic diseases, such as hypertension,
and hypercholesterolemia, understanding about their disease and medications is still
the foundation for ultimate patient adherence, but has far less impact on subsequent
adherence because motivation and behavioral changes are the major forces in determining subsequent medication adherence. Since there are no obvious symptoms of
these chronic diseases such as diabetes, it is more difficult for patients to motivate
themselves to take medication to prevent some vague future complications. To be motivated to take medication and adhere to medication for prolonged periods, patients
must feel and accept that something is wrong with them, feel motivated to prevent
future problems by using medication, and believe that the pros of taking medicine will
in the long run outweigh the cons. The behavioral aspects are even more daunting,
since patients with chronic diseases are required to make lifelong changes in diet and
exercise, plus take medications for the rest of their lives. Therefore, it is not surprising
that studies show the lack of impact of education alone on medication adherence in
patients with chronic asymptomatic diseases. Finally, for adherence to both acute and
chronic medications, the traditional "telling people" educational approaches are not
effective. The educator must use "teach-back" techniques to verify that patients understand the instructional material by either demonstration or verbalization of their
understanding.

• ASSESSMENT OF RISK FACTORS FOR SUBOPTIMAL ADHERENCE

There are multiple theoretical and actual factors that can negatively impact medication adherence issues. Two theoretical tenets have been shown to have impacts on
rates of medication adherence (Table 5.2). Locus of control is a concept that deals
with patient confidence. Patients with an external locus of control feel that events are
either in the hands of a deity or are determined by fate and that they as an individual
have little control over what happens. Patients with an internal locus of control feel
that they have great influence over what happens to them. Studies have shown that
generally patients with an internal locus of control have significantly higher medication adherence rates than patients with an external locus of control. Therefore, an
external locus of control is a risk factor. The transtheoretical model describes five
stages of readiness for change. Patients in the bottom two stages, precontemplation
and contemplation, have not even considered making any changes in behavior and

TABLE 5.2	Risk Factors for Suboptimal Medication Adherence

Mental status
   Dementia
   Depression
Difficult living conditions
   Homeless
   Family stress
   Job stress
Substance abuse
Language/culture/health beliefs
Ability to pay
Complex treatment
Lack of transportation
Physical handicaps
Previous compliance history
Disease state
Locus of control
Transtheoretical model stage

are unlikely to start taking medication. For readers interested in these two theoretical concepts, there are several articles in the Key References section with a more detailed description of both topics.

The remaining risk factors are real world issues that in most cases are fairly obvious to most health care providers (Table 5.2). Patients with mental illness traditionally have had problems with medication adherence. Studies document that the presence of dementia, schizophrenia, or depression markedly increases the risk for suboptimal adherence. Studies in patients with substance abuse issues also show significant problems adhering to therapeutic regimens. Difficult living conditions also negatively impact medication adherence. Homeless patients many times have nowhere to store medications, low income, and nominal daily routine. In addition, a significant percentage of the homeless have been diagnosed with some type of mental illness, plus their medications are constantly at risk for theft. Similarly, job or family stress makes it difficult to remember to take medications in a timely fashion. Patients with language barriers, cultural factors, and different health beliefs are also at greater risk for adherence problems. The cost of medication is one of the most significant risk factors for poor adherence. Every pharmacist has had patients ask for advice about which of their several chronic medications they could go without due to excessive cost. Prescribers many times use expensive branded medications when older, but therapeutically equivalent generic medications would be just as effective. Therefore, due to similar efficacy and lower cost, cheaper generic medications should always be initially prescribed, unless *no other effective or safer alternatives* are available. When it becomes necessary to use more expensive medications, many manufacturers have programs to provide branded medication at little or no expense. Complex treatment regimens, with complicated administration technique or which require three or more doses/day for efficacy, should be avoided. However, due to the minimal difference in adherence rates between drugs taken once daily compared to those taken twice daily, there are very few patients who require branded extended release products to optimize adherence rates instead of generic medications that require twice daily dosing. Patients who are on six or more medications are also at risk for adherence issues. A careful review of a patient's previous compliance with a chronic medication regimen can also reveal issues that may impair adherence. Patients who previously had poor or suboptimal adherence with chronic medications usually will have a similar pattern of medication adherence in attempting to control both old and new chronic diseases. The disease state also impacts adherence. Adherence rates to medications used to control asymptomatic diseases such as hypertension, and hyperlipidemia are generally much less than with a symptomatic disease like rheumatoid arthritis. Finally, providers must be alert for more subtle risk factors that can negatively impact medication adherence. Difficulties in picking up medications in a timely fashion due to lack of transportation to get to provider visits and picking up medications from the pharmacy are an all-too-common problem that patients often are embarrassed to mention. Similarly, physical handicaps that interfere with proper administration of eye drops, inhalers, nasal sprays, as well as limited ability to open child-resistant prescription bottles often results in less than optimal outcomes from those medications.

• ASSESSING MEDICATION ADHERENCE PROBLEMS

Medication adherence can be assessed by both subjective and objective means. The principle subjective method is interviewing the patient about adherence problems during their routine primary care visit. A question such as: "Since your last visit, what kind of problems have you been having remembering to take your medications?" initiates the discussion about adherence. If the patient shares the fact that they are having problems, the provider needs to probe for more details with questions such as "How many times has it happened since the last visit? Why do you think it happened? Tell me about the circumstances the last time it happened." Historically, experts cite the lack of accuracy of the interview and in effect feel that patients routinely lie about their medication adherence. If patients do "lie" about their adherence, it is due to atrocious provider-patient communication techniques on the part of the provider! When patients fail to truthfully answer about adherence, it is because they are trying to avoid the embarrassment of the provider chastising them about adherence issues. From experience with previous providers or with the current provider, they have learned to avoid the punishment by telling the provider what he wants to hear. The impact of a threatening approach is discussed in more detail under the Provider Misconceptions About Medication Adherence section of this chapter. The way to prevent patients from altering their responses to prevent chastisement is to avoid the threatening approach and instead "set the stage" at the initial visit by confirming it is the patient's disease and their accurate input is important. You realize that there will be some difficulties in working medication taking into their daily routine and you are going to work with the patient to get the best possible results. Table 5.3 contains specific dialogue for setting the stage. By removing the punishment and recognizing

TABLE 5.3	Setting the Stage at the Initial Visit

a. Introduce your perspective on taking medication.

"Together, we want to find a medicine that you are genuinely interested in taking because it controls your disease without side effects. You are the one who is putting the medication into your body, so it's your opinion that is most important, not mine. So please always let me know exactly what you think about the medicines we are trying. I'm counting on your input. In addition, most people have problems figuring out how to fit taking medication and other changes into their existing life."

b. Tell them at each visit you are going to ask about each of those three issues.

"Therefore, because I need your honest input to make this medicine work best for you, at each visit I'm going to ask you how it's working, what kind of problems you think the medication might be causing, plus ask about problems you may be having in remembering to take your medicines. We can then work together to resolve any issues that may arise."

that it is their disease that you are helping them manage, it removes any need to embellish the truth about their medication adherence.

Objective measures include the refill record, pill counts, control of the chronic disease, and serum medication levels. The refill record can be used in several ways to measure persistence, an approximation of actual adherences rates. In using the pharmacy profile, there are two issues that need to be addressed. The first is the fact that physicians and providers operating outside organized health care delivery systems such as the Veterans Administration, Group Health, and Kaiser do not have access to patient refill records. Second, patients may occasionally use another pharmacy to get their medications, so a single missing refill may only indicate that they got it filled elsewhere, not unequivocal evidence of poor adherence.

The first and easiest method to analyze refill records is the "eyeball" method, which entails taking one prescription and tracking the dates of refills longitudinally to make sure they are getting it filled roughly every 30 days or whatever the third-party payer allows. Next is the medication possession ratio (MPR), a more formal approach than the "eyeball" method. The time period specified in days, e.g., 6 months = 180 days, is the denominator and the number of *days supply of medication filled* during the 6 months is the numerator. For example, a patient on enalapril 20 mg bid has received 300 tablets over a 180-day period; 300/2 = 150 days supply filled. The 150 days supply filled divided by the 180 days in the 6-month time period equals an MPR of 0.83 or 83%. Patients with near perfect adherence will have MPRs ranging between 0.9 and 1.1, depending on the refill dates within the period. Variable medication possession ratios (VMPR) and proportion of days covered (PDC) make adjustments for refill dates and are more accurate, so perfect adherence should be 100% with those two measurements. Unless this is calculated for the provider, generally, it is too time consuming to be practical. These measures are primarily used to analyze adherence in large claims databases. Some providers have the patients bring their prescription bottles or pill organizers, e.g., Medi-Set, to each visit and then count the number of pills remaining to measure adherence. This can be time consuming and impractical. Also, if patients discover that they are being chastised because of pill counts, they will learn to make sure that the number of pills left agrees with what the provider expects. Logically, the degree of control of the disease can indicate the level of medication adherence. If the chronic disease is not adequately controlled, then investigating adherence issues through subjective and objective means as a cause of poor disease control is required. Good control of the disease is not necessarily indicative of good adherence. Some patients who are intentionally nonadherent can mask their poor medication adherence by taking it for just the week before their primary care provider visit to avoid the chastising that comes with less than optimal control. This "white coat compliance" can be very effective in hypertension and was effective in diabetes mellitus until the A1C, which measures long-term blood glucose, became the laboratory test of choice for diabetes control. However, poor disease control may not be due to poor adherence. The medication regimes may be inadequate for control. For those drugs with readily available therapeutic serum level determinations, serum drug levels can be used to assess medication adherence. However, like all measurements of adherence, there are potential pitfalls. Low serum drug levels can also be indicative of genetic polymorphisms, individual variations in absorption and excretion or nonbioequivalent products. Adherence aids are thought to be the ultimate answer to measuring adherence. While they are of great help to some patients, unfortunately, most are easily defeated. For example, use of a computerized prescription lid to measure adherence through the number of times the lid was removed was thought to be the answer. However, once patients discovered what the lids did (by being chastised by the provider), they easily defeated them by leaving the lid off, or substituting an old lid. Even observed oral administration can be defeated by cheeking the medication until they leave the facility, then spitting it out. Therefore, the moral of this story is that there is no absolutely foolproof method to determine medication adherence. So the most accurate approach is to set the stage and use patient interview, plus one or more objective measures of adherence.

How do you approach the patient when the objective measures of adherence are inconsistent with the subjective measures? A lot depends on the situation. As the provider, one approach is the *supportive adherence probe.*

"I noticed there were some missing refills of beclomethasone inhaler and I'm concerned that there might be a problem." This use of an "I" message makes your concern the main issue and not their behavior and encourages them to talk about issues (cost, side effects, etc) that caused them not to refill the medication. Alternatively, "What's been your experience with the new medication?" can initiate dialogue regarding adherence problems. If this is a first visit, when asking how they take their current medication, look for pink flags during the interview that may indicate adherence issues. Answers such as "The doctor *wants me* to take it...." or "I'm *supposed* to take it...." are clear indicators that they are not taking it the way it is prescribed. These should be answered with a reflective response to encourage further discussion. "Sounds like you're not sure about how to take your medicine." If this is a new patient and you want to encourage an open discussion about adherence issues, a *universal statement* can be used in place of a more direct question: "Many of my patients have some difficulties remembering to take their medication. What kind of problems have you experienced?"

• TECHNIQUES TO HELP PATIENTS IMPROVE MEDICATION ADHERENCE

There are multiple techniques and approaches to assist patients in optimizing the benefits of their medication. Specific behavioral interventions that have been shown to be highly effective will be discussed. Also, some important issues mentioned previously will be discussed again along with comments regarding other popular approaches.

Behavioral Interventions

Develop a Routine Probably the most important thing to improve adherence is to help patients develop a routine for taking their medication. In an unpublished study, over 150 patients, taking four or more prescription medications every day, and who had an MPR of greater than 0.9, were asked what their "secret" was to their success in remembering to take their medications. Surprisingly, without prompting, 94% of patients immediately began to describe their routine, i.e., how they linked medication taking to their regular activities of daily living. While each had their individual unique approach, they all clearly had developed a routine. When asked how they developed their routine, their overwhelming responses were things such as common sense, by trial and error, over time, etc. Only a handful had help from others and none had help from a health care provider in establishing their routine.

Simplify the Treatment Regimen In general, the more doses one has to take and dosing regimens greater than twice daily, both negatively impact medication adherence. Therefore, reducing the number of medications and the frequency of dosing improves adherence. This is consistent with findings in adherence studies in transplant patients who take 10 or more medications and in patients undergoing antiretroviral therapy due to the required >90% adherence rates required to prevent the development of resistance. Once effective dosages of individual medications have been established, look for combination products in those strengths to reduce the number of pills that have to be taken every day.

Alter regimens so that no medication has to be taken more than twice daily. Simplifying the regimen helps patients more readily establish the routine needed to enhance adherence.

Minimize the Cost The importance of cost has already been discussed as a risk factor. Wherever possible use generic medications, reserving expensive extended release for those patients whose unusual routine absolutely requires them. If a combination product is far more expensive than both drugs alone, then talk with the patient and let them choose which one is more acceptable to them.

Tailor the Regimen Adapting the regimen to individual patient routines, schedules, and clinical findings can improve both medication adherence and disease control. Particularly difficult are people who work rotating shifts, or have other variable work schedules. Once again, working closely in partnership with the patient can usually resolve scheduling issues. Clinical situations can warrant regimen changes to maintain disease control without additional medications. For example, a patient on a branded statin and three once-daily antihypertensive medication. The patient's blood pressures upon awakening are in the 150/98 range, but are well below 140/90 the rest of the day. Rather than add a fourth antihypertensive medication, move one of the antihypertensive medications from the morning to evening and to help create a routine, switch the branded statin to a generic statin that has to be taken in the evening. This way they take two in the morning and in the evening, providing better control the morning blood pressure, and reducing the cost.

Confirm Appropriate Administration Technique Patients who use medication administration devices that require a specific technique for efficacy (i.e., inhalers, eye drops) and who are experiencing suboptimal disease control warrant a check for proper administration technique. For example, in a patient on several topical glaucoma preparations, have them demonstrate how they administer each one. The literature clearly shows that the majority of patients with glaucoma regularly make significant errors in administration technique, so suboptimal control may be solely due to poor technique, not poor adherence. When an additional glaucoma medication is added due to poor control, the pharmacist should require the patient to demonstrate appropriate techniques and verify understanding of appropriate waiting times between medication administrations.

Reward Patient Success Rewarding patient successes verbally or in more formal ways helps improve medication adherence. Verbal rewards even for partial success or substantial progression toward target values are highly effective. More concrete rewards (money, concert tickets) are also effective, provided the patient selects the nature of the reward themselves. Just offering a standard reward or cash reward is not effective in improving adherence.

Increase Attention Increasing the frequency of contact with the patient improves medication adherence. Even periodic telephone calls by the provider or his staff are effective. Using other health professionals such as pharmacists to see the patient monthly between less frequent physician visits has been shown to improve adherence and disease control. Normally, when starting medication after diagnosis of a chronic disease, provider visits are frequent (weekly, every 2 weeks) to allow time for patient education, monitoring the effect of the medication, and helping patients integrate medication taking into their daily routine. As the disease is better controlled, and the patient has developed an effective routine for taking medication, the intervals between visits can be increased. This also serves as a very powerful tangible reward for patient success. Should control of the disease and adherence regress to suboptimal levels, increasing the frequency of contact many times restores adherence and disease control to previous levels.

Enlist Support of Others Enlisting the support of others can be a critical factor in improving adherence to the treatment regimen. This is especially true in implementing dietary or exercise changes. Therefore, whoever does the cooking needs to be part of the patient education process. Enlisting spousal support to do exercise together, e.g., jointly walking the dog for 30 minutes every morning, is also effective. Many times patients have caregivers; they too need to be included in the therapeutic process. However, in those situations where the caregiver accompanies the patient, make sure that you focus your conversation on the patient, not on the caregiver.

Use Adherence Aids Many providers see compliance aids as a panacea, yet studies have shown that pill organizers have little or no impact *by themselves*. However, the literature has shown them to be effective as part of a comprehensive adherence support program. For patients who have trouble developing a routine, those devices can be effective. However, only a small part of the population falls into that category. That is why studies that force patients to use devices show limited efficacy. In addition, providers should never suggest adherence aids because the meta-message to the patient is "You are not competent to take care of yourself," which most elderly patients do not want to hear and may refuse to acknowledge because it is likely untrue in functioning seniors. The good thing is that many patients themselves select devices and use them effectively because it was their idea. Patients are much more likely to do something if it is their idea as opposed to the provider's. An alternative approach is to offer a device as part of a group of choices couched in terms of what other patients have found to be successful. "My other patients who have had the same trouble have found several things that seem to help. One leaves their evening medicine by her bedstand, another puts it next to her toothbrush, another uses a pill organizer for her warfarin, and another sets her alarm clock as a reminder. Do any of these ideas sound like they might work for you?"

Motivational Interviewing Motivational interviewing (MI), like adherence aids, is seen by some as a potential panacea to improving adherence. Unfortunately, like adherence aids, the use of motivational interviewing *by itself* has not been shown to have significant positive effects on medication adherence. However, in patients who are highly resistant to taking medications, portions of the MI portfolio can be useful. Ask, Listen, and Summarize is an excellent way to begin a dialogue about the reasons behind suboptimal adherence. Ask, Provide, Ask is an excellent way to provide necessary information in resistant patients. As with adherence aids, very few patients are candidates for formal motivational interviewing, since once the reason for nonadherence is discovered, other useful techniques can be used to help patients optimize the effectiveness of their medication.

Guiding Principles of Adherence Support

Whose Disease Is It Anyway? Always remember that the patient manages their own disease! Become a learned partner whose job is to help the patient decide which medications to try, help them develop routines, celebrate success, and help patients resolve problems integrating medication, diet and exercise into their daily routine. In effect, view yourself as a helpful coach. Remember that patients are more likely to carry out activities if it is their idea rather than something you suggest. Couch your suggestion as what you learned from your other patients' successes and give them several options to choose from.

All Motivation Is Self-Motivation The provider's job is to create an environment where patients can comfortably motivate themselves to adhere to the therapeutic regimen. Avoid the threatening/chastisement or cheerleading approaches as they are counterproductive to the development of self-motivation.

Making Long-Term Changes in Behavior Is Not Easy Remember that medication adherence in chronic diseases is a long-term behavior change that will take time and effort to accomplish. Be patient and supportive as patients learn to integrate this new behavior into other daily activities, usually by trial and error.

One Step at a Time Remember the principle of self-efficacy and initiate changes slowly, one step at a time, building self-confidence as you progress rather than have them try to make changes in diet, exercise, taking medication, and self-testing all at once, potentially overwhelming the patient.

Do Not Chase Numbers For the last three decades it has been all about the target objective measures. In addition, if you do not achieve exact target values, you are a poor provider. Recent iterations of national guidelines for diabetes mellitus, hyperlipidemia, and hypertension have all recognized the fallacy and futility of that approach, providing greater flexibility in establishing target lab values for each patient. If your patient started out with an A1C of 12% or a blood pressure of 190/110 and you help the patient get it down to 7.2% or 145/92 and the patient decides that they are unwilling to make more changes, accept it. It is their disease and their life. The marked reductions in glucose and blood pressure measurements have added decades to their life, and a reduction of 0.5% or a few more millimeters of mercury is unlikely to significantly decrease their potential for disease-related complications.

Help the Patient Establish a Routine Since good compliers all have developed a routine for remembering to take their medication, helping your patient develop a routine that integrates medication behavior into existing activities should be a primary focus of provider adherence support activities.

Regularly Assess Adherence Levels At your initial visit, set the stage (Table 5.3) to enhance the accuracy of the interview process and at every visit inquire about problems with adherence to dietary, exercise, and medication aspects of the therapeutic regimen. Look for "pink flags" during the interview and respond accordingly. In addition to the patient interview, use two objective measurements, such as disease control and refill records, to assess the presence of potential adherence issues.

• KEY REFERENCES

1. Herrier RN, Boyce RW. Establishing an active patient partnership. *Am Pharm.* 1995;NS35:48-57.
2. Herrier RN, Boyce RW. Myths about compliance. *Am Pharm.* 1995;NS35:12-13.
3. Krueger KP, Berger BA, Felky B. Medication adherence and persistence a comprehensive review. *Adv Ther.* 2005;22:313-356.
4. Herrier RN. Medication compliance in the elderly. *J Pharm Pract.* 1995;8:232-244.
5. Voils CI, Steffens DC, Flint EP, Bosworth HB. Social support and locus of control as predictors of adherence to antidepressant medication in an elderly population. *Am J Geriatr Psychiatry.* 2005;13:157-165.

6. Ahmedani BK, Peterson EL, Wells KE, et al. Asthma medication adherence: the role of God and other health locus of control factors. *Ann Allergy Immunol.* 2013;110:75-79.
7. Omeji O, Nebo C. The influence of locus of control on adherence to treat regimen among hypertensive patients. *Patient Prefer Adherence.* 2011;5:141-148.
8. Levinson W, Cohen MS, Brady D, Duffy FD. To change or not to change: "sounds like you have a dilemma." *Ann Intern Med.* 2001;135:386-391. (Transtheoretical Model)
9. Zimmerman GL, Olsen, CG, Bosworth ME. A "stages of change" approach to helping patients change behavior. *Am Fam Physician.* 2000;61:1409-1416. (Transtheoretical Model)
10. Benner JS, Glynn RJ, Mogun H, et al. Long term persistence in use of statin therapy in elderly patients. *JAMA.* 2002;288:455-61.
11. Kozma CM, Dickson M, Phillips AL, Meletiche DM. Medication possession ratio: implications of using fixed and variable observation periods in assessing adherence with disease-modifying drugs in patients with multiple sclerosis. *Patient Prefer Adherence.* 2013;7:509-516.
12. Rollnick S, Miller WR, Butler CC. *Motivational Interviewing in Health Care: Helping Patients Change Behavior.* New York: Guilford Press; 2008.
13. Shea SC. *Improving Medication Adherence: How to Talk With patients About Their Medication.* Philadelphia: Lippincott Williams & Wilkins; 2006.

Organizing Patient Visits

1. Describe the functions of a patient visit for a chronic disease.

2. Describe the typical structure of a patient visit for a chronic disease.

3. Describe the purpose and process for pre-visit planning and establishing visit agendas.

• INTRODUCTION

One of the topics infrequently taught in health profession schools is how to organize a patient visit. The primary exposure to the topic occurs informally during clerkship rotations and residencies. This informal approach tends to leave large gaps in provider knowledge, and may even teach inappropriate and/or inefficient practices. Because pharmacists are relatively new to providing primary care for patients with chronic diseases, it is an important topic as they increasingly enter roles in chronic disease management.

• PURPOSE OF PATIENT VISTIS FOR CHRONIC DISEASES

There are four broad functions of patient visits (Table 6.1). The first and most obvious is to collect data to assess disease control, patient adherence to all aspects of the therapeutic regimen (drugs, diet, exercise), and assess the presence of un-wanted complications due to the disease and the medication used to manage that disease. The second function is to develop and maintain rapport with the patient, which facilitates joint efforts to manage their disease. This includes dealing with patients' concerns, perspectives, and emotions regarding their chronic diseases. The third function involves assisting the patients in implementing jointly developed plans to optimize disease control and minimize complications. Subfunctions include patient education, assistance to optimize medication adherence, modification of therapeutic regimen, referral to specialists, etc. The last function is to ensure that patients receive appropriate levels of preventive care. Common to all practice areas is the tertiary preventive services whose aim is to prevent complications from the patient's chronic diseases. Some examples for patients with diabetes include routine diabetic foot examinations, annual dilated ophthalmoscopic examination, and annual microalbuminuria testing. Most of these tertiary prevention services can be found in national organization diagnosis and treatment guidelines. Secondary prevention includes screening for the development of comorbid diseases such as hypertension and hyperlipidemia in patients with diabetes mellitus or colonoscopy in older patients. Last are primary prevention services such as immunizations, weight control, and others recommended by the US Preventive

TABLE 6.1	Functions of a Patient Visit for Chronic Disease

1. Collect objective and subjective data for diagnostic and evaluation of disease status
    Disease control
    Regimen adherence
    Unwanted complications
2. Develop and maintain rapport with the patient
    Deal with patient concerns, perspectives, and emotions
3. Assist patients in implementing joint therapeutic plans
    Patient education
    Optimize adherence
    Modify therapeutic regimens
    Referrals to specialists
4. Preventive services
    Prevent complications (tertiary prevention)
    Identify comorbid diseases (secondary prevention)
    Immunizations, weight control (primary prevention)

Services Task Force. Depending on the practice site and extent of clinical privileges in preventive health, pharmacists' responsibilities range from recommendations to the primary care provider, to ordering the tests/procedures and making appointments for those tests and procedures. In the community pharmacy setting, pharmacists may be limited to "coaching" roles. In that situation, the pharmacist's role in preventive health would be limited to recommendations to the primary care provider and point-of-service laboratory testing. Pharmacists working in organized health care delivery systems, such as health maintenance organizations, the Veterans Administration, or the Indian Health Service, are expected to identify those preventive needs and order appropriate testing in a timely fashion.

• TYPICAL STRUCTURE OF A CHRONIC DISEASE VISIT

Initial Versus Follow-Up Visits

There are two basic types of visits. The initial visit is the first time you meet the patient. These visits take as much as 60 minutes since collection and verification of data are more comprehensive, plus time is needed to get to know them personally and to develop rapport. Follow-up visits usually require 20 to 30 minutes since you have established rapport and are working together toward a common goal. The amount of data collected is far less than an initial visit. Patients whose chronic disease is under good control and with few problems, less than 15 minutes may be sufficient. While those times are approximate, the duration of visits usually decreases over time and with improved control of the chronic disease. Remember, the time required to complete a visit needs to include time for any physical examination, time to document the visit in the patient record, and time to conduct any point-of-service testing. Some providers feel that patients' attention spans are limited and that a 60-minute appointment may be too long to maintain efficiency and effectiveness. They prefer to split the initial visit into two or three shorter visits a week apart. Similarly, some patients will require longer and more frequent follow-up visits during the first year because therapy adjustments and resolution of adherence issues are more significant and frequent. Finally, in organized health care systems there are usually standardized appointment systems and times that require adjustment to what might be optimal timing for the provider. Patients with multiple chronic diseases may require more time for both initial and follow-up visits. Fortunately, the exception to this rule is the most common encountered multiple disease situation: diabetes, hyperlipidemia, and hypertension. Since these all end up with the same complications if not controlled, you ask the same set of closed-ended questions for complications due to all three diseases, increasing efficiency.

Pre-Visit Planning

Pre-visit planning is one of the keys to improving efficiency and getting the most out of the time allotted for a patient visit, as well as potentially reducing the length of time required for the visit. Twenty-four to 48 hours before the upcoming visit, the patient's health record is reviewed to determine what needs to be done at that visit. Usually, preplanning for an initial visit takes far more time than follow-up visits, since there is a larger volume of patient data and potential barriers to optimal adherence to identify. While the pre-visit planning for an initial visit is usually done by the provider, some systems use experienced clinic nurses for follow-up visit pre-visit planning. The record review identifies the following: lab tests or diagnostic procedures due for this or future visits, preventive or health maintenance services such as

TABLE 6.2	Components of Pre-Visit Planning

1. Review patient records to determine what needs to be done at this visit
    Laboratory tests to monitor for disease control or complications
    Preventive or health maintenance services
        Periodic lab tests
        Annual physical examination
        Immunizations
    Patient education needed
    Barriers/issues to regimen adherence
    Efficacy of previous interventions/changes
2. Develop preliminary visit agenda
3. Complete needed manual and/or electronic orders

vaccinations or complete physical examination, patient education needs, evaluation of changes in therapy or routines implemented at the previous visit to enhance adherence (Table 6.2). From the review, a preliminary agenda is developed to remind the provider of all the items that need to be covered during the visit. In addition, any paperwork for specialist appointments, lab tests, or other testing procedures is completed manually or electronically before the visit and placed in the patient's folder or health record. The record review, agenda, and much of the paperwork can also be done electronically. Many organized health care delivery systems with electronic health records deliver prompts regarding items that are due as the record is reviewed. Similarly, providers can insert other prompts for the next visit, so much of the record review and preliminary visit agenda are completed electronically. Table 6.3 shows a sample agenda developed from pre-visit planning for a follow-up visit.

TABLE 6.3	Sample Visit Agenda

NEEDS BMP, LIPID PROFILE, MICROALBUMINURIA FOR NEXT VISIT
REVIEW REASONS FOR MISSED REFILLS ON METFORMIN
APPOINTMENT WITH OPHTHALMOLOGIST FOR ANNUAL DILATED EYE EXAMINATION
REVIEW SICK DAY PROTOCOL
CHECK ON UNDERSTANDING/EXPERIENCE WITH NEW STATIN PRESCRIPTION
INFLUENZA VACCINATION THIS VISIT OR NEXT

Introduction

One of the more frustrating things to happen is to arrive at the end of the visit when you have used almost all the allotted time, and the patient says "By the way, I have this _____ I want to ask you about" that is unrelated to the purpose of the visit. If you deal with the new issue, then you are late for your next appointment. If this happens several times a day, you get further behind schedule. If you do not address the new problem immediately, that patient is frustrated with you. Regardless of how you handle these situations, you end up with multiple unhappy patients. Fortunately, there is a simple solution. During the introduction and before you get to the patient history just ask: "In addition to your regular visit for diabetes, what other issues do we need to deal with today?" This gets the patient's agenda into the discussion at the start of the visit and you can jointly negotiate priorities for the visit before proceeding. The provider can go through his/her agenda more quickly, or postpone items, such as planned patient education, making time for the patient's new issues.

Organizing the Flow of the Patient Visit

Universally, there are only three sets of information required to evaluate every chronic disease: control of the disease, compliance with the therapeutic regimen, and complications due to the disease and the drug therapy used to manage it. This schema provides a simple structure to conduct a comprehensive visit effectively (Table 6.4). Some organized health care delivery systems use flow sheets to guide the visit and partially document patient responses and findings. Others use disease-specific structured checklists as a guide or disease-specific structured progress notes in the electronic medical record to guide the visit and/or document findings (Table 6.5).

TABLE 6.4	Three Cs for Organizing Chronic Disease Visit For Diabetes

1. CONTROL (level of disease control)
    Subjective—nocturia
    Objective—A1C

2. COMPLIANCE
    Subjective
        What kind of problems are you having remembering to take your medication, follow your diet, exercise regularly?
    Objective
        Review pharmacy records for refill history
        Weight
        Vital signs

3. COMPLICATIONS due to
    DISEASE
        Subjective
            Numbness, tingling, or pain in feet
        Objective
            Diabetic foot examination
    DRUGS
        Subjective
            Diarrhea, GI upset, change in taste
        Objective (assess renal function for risk of lactic acidosis)
            Serum creatinine
            Urine microalbuminuria

TABLE 6.5	Sample Disease-Specific Structured Provider Checklist

CONTROL

Subjective

"How have things been going with your diabetes since your last visit?
What have your home blood glucose readings been? How many times a day do you test?
How many times do you get up to go to the bathroom each night? **(nocturia)**
Skin rash, vaginal rash, or discharge? **(decreased immunological competence due to hyperglycemia)**
How about dizziness, palpitations, mental changes, sweating, hunger? **(hypoglycemia)**

Objective

Hemoglobin A1C *(HA$_{1c}$, glycosylated hemoglobin)* <7% **(measures long-term [last 3 months] blood glucose)**
Weight

COMPLIANCE

Subjective (Medication)

What do you take for your diabetes?
"What kind of problems have you been having remembering to take your medications?
How frequently does it happen? When was the last time it happened?
When did you take your last dose? How much?

Subjective (Exercise)

"How are you doing with your exercise?
What kind of exercise do you do? How frequently do you exercise?
What kind of problems have you been having getting your regular exercise done?

Subjective (Diet)

How's your diet going?
"What kind of problems have you been having following your diet?
What did you have for dinner last night?

Objective

Have patients draw up insulin dose if applicable
Check refill records/do pill count

COMPLICATIONS

Subjective Disease

"What changes have you noticed since your last visit?
How have your foot checks been going? How frequently do you check?

CLOSED-ENDED QUESTIONS

Numbness/tingling/ pain in your feet? **(neuropathy)**
Chest pain, SOB, DOE, PND? **(angina, CHF)**
Dizziness, memory loss, headache? **(CVA,TIA)**
Visual changes (especially color vision)? **(retinopathy)**
Pedal edema, weight gain, fatigue, nausea, decreased appetite? **(nephropathy)**
Dysuria, frequency ? **(UTI)**
Any sores, cuts, rashes? **(vasculopathy)**

Objective Disease

BP
Screening diabetic foot examination including sensory examination with monofilament

ANNUALLY OR AS INDICATED

Diabetic foot examination **(checks for macrovascular, microvascular, and neuropathic changes/complications)**
Microalbuminuria (sensitive for greater than 30 mg/L but less than 300 mg/L) (annually if no previous problem).
    Reported as mg/L or albumin to creatinine ratio (ACR) as mg/gm
BUN/serum creatinine
Dilated ophthalmoscopic examination including visual field
Complete Lipid Panel

TABLE 6.5	**Sample Disease-Specific Structured Provider Checklist (*Continued*)**

Subjective Medication
   Hypoglycemia **(sulfonylureas, insulin)**
   Nausea, vomiting, diarrhea, heartburn **(metformin, exenatide, gliptins)**
   Abdominal pain **(exenatide, gliptins)**
   Abnormal taste **(metformin)**
Objective Medication
   Edema **(glitazones)**
   Weight gain **(sulfonylureas, insulin, glitazones)**
   Serum amylase/lipase **(exenatide, gliptins)**
   Tachypnea **(glitazones, metformin)**

*Initial broad open-ended questions to begin discussion of control, compliance, and complications.

• KEY REFERENCES

1. Marvel MK, Epstein RM, Flowers K, Beckman HB. Soliciting the patient's agenda: have we improved? JAMA. 1999;83:283-287.
2. Yawn B, Goodwin MA, Zyzanski SJ, Stange KC. Time use during acute and chronic illness visits to a family physician. *Fam Pract*. 2003;20:474-477.
3. Hampson SE, McKay HG, Glasgow RE. Patient-physician interactions in diabetes management: consistencies and variations in structure and content of two consultations. *Patient Educ Couns*. 1996;29:49-58.
4. Haas LJ, Glazer K, Houchins J, Terry S. Improving the effectiveness of a medical visit: a brief visit structuring workshop changes patient perceptions of primary care visits. *Patient Educ Couns*. 2006;62:374-378.

TWO

Assessment
of Symptoms

Symptoms Related to the Ears, Nose, and Throat

1. Accurately identify the most likely etiology when patients present with a runny nose, sore throat, or earache, through history, diagnostic tests, and patient findings on examination, to enable the pharmacist to recommend effective treatment or refer the patient to an appropriate provider.

2. Use the knowledge of the pathophysiology, etiology, and common presentation of upper respiratory tract diseases to review prescription orders for appropriateness and to accurately educate patients about their disease and its treatment.

3. Use the knowledge of the pathophysiology, etiology, and common presentation of upper respiratory diseases to accurately interpret the diagnostic process to enable the pharmacist to advise providers regarding the most appropriate prescription therapy.

Common disorders of the upper respiratory tract are among the most frequent disorders dealt with by all health professionals. The runny or stuffy noses, earaches, and sore throats are universal afflictions dealt with by everyone. They may also be associated with a cough that is not the predominant symptom. Differential diagnosis of cough as the most significant symptom will be covered in more detail in the Chapter 8. These symptoms can occur alone or in combination, and carefully identifying the cause can allow prompt and effective treatment or referral to definitive care.

• RUNNY/STUFFY NOSE

Two common viral infections, allergic rhinitis, vasomotor rhinitis, and bacterial sinusitis make up the most common among the vast number of diseases that present with the chief complaint of a runny or stuffy nose. Table 7.1 provides the diagnostic schemata and comparative presentations.

Common Cold (Upper Respiratory Infection)

Caused by rhinoviruses or coronaviruses, the common cold represents over 60% of all disorders with nasal stuffiness or discharge as the primary complaint. Generally, the onset is slow with symptoms progressing over 12 to 36 hours and lasting 5 to 9 days. Nasal discharge is initially clear but progresses to mucoid and the amount varies over the course of the disease. Most patients will notice a green tinge to the mucous after 3 to 5 days, which is indicative of a viral not bacterial infection as previously thought. Sneezing is generally not a prominent feature. Patients may complain of a dry cough that is worse at night. There may also be a mild sore throat upon wakening in the morning. Both symptoms may be attributable to post-nasal drip. The sore throat often resolves after eating. Examination of the nose reveals pink to red (normal color), but swollen turbinates with a mucoid discharge. Most patients present with either no fever or only a low-grade fever.

Many patients will present incorrectly saying they have "*the flu*". They probably do not have true influenza, but a more symptomatic form of the common cold or upper respiratory infection (URI). True influenza is a much more severe seasonal respiratory disorder in which runny nose, sore throat, and earache are *not* the predominant symptoms. (See Table 7.2 for differences between URI and influenza.) This "*super virus*" is caused by respiratory syncytial virus, adenovirus, or coronaviruses and tends to present with a more acute and rapid onset, often with fever, myalgias, and arthralgias. Patients with these super virus infections tend to *look sick*. The cough may be productive and the sore throat may be more bothersome. Physical findings other than fever are similar to those of rhinovirus infections. This form of URI generally lasts several days longer than the common cold. The mucoid discharge also develops a green tinge over time. It is still a viral infection, and antibiotics have no effect on duration or severity of the illness. Like the common cold, it occurs predominantly in the late fall and winter months.

Allergic Rhinitis

The signs and symptoms of allergic rhinitis (AR) are significantly different than with viral URIs. The nasal discharge is copious, clear, and watery. Sneezing is a prominent feature. Its onset is usually sudden, and it can wax and wane, depending on the exposure to the airborne allergen. Nasal congestion can be the most troublesome symptom. The nose and the palate of the throat may itch. Many patients will have red, itchy, and watery eyes (allergic conjunctivitis). Because the cause is often outdoor airborne allergens such as pollen, it occurs in most parts of the country beginning in spring and lasting until fall. Some patients have allergy symptoms year round, due to moderate winters, or they may have an allergy to one or more indoor allergens, such as house dust mites, cockroaches, or indoor molds. Many people are

TABLE 7.1	Stuffy/Runny Nose				

A. DIAGNOSTIC SCHEMATA FOR RUNNY/STUFFY NOSE

Allergic Rhinitis   Upper Respiratory Tract Infection (Common Cold)   Bacterial Sinusitis

Vasomotor Rhinitis   Upper Respiratory Tract Infection (Flu or Super Virus)

B. DIFFERENTIAL DIAGNOSIS OF STUFFY/RUNNY NOSE

SUBJECTIVE	Cold	Allergic Rhinitis	Vasomotor Rhinitis	"Flu"/Super Virus	Bacterial Sinusitis
Location	N/A	N/A	N/A	N/A	N/A
Onset	"Feel cold coming on" slow onset (12 to 48 hours) symptoms that progressively worsen	Relatively sudden onset. May be off and on	Similar to allergic rhinitis	Acute onset—quicker onset/progression than cold	Cold lasts >7 days. Starts to get better or plateau, then gets worse or allergic rhinitis active in spite of antihistamines/intranasal corticosteroids
Quantity	Varies	Usually copious	Usually copious	Varies	Varies
Quality	Nasal discharge that is initially clear and thin but progresses to mucoid, then to green tinged after 3 to 5 days	Nasal discharge that is clear and watery	Nasal discharge that is clear and watery	Nasal discharge like cold	Nasal discharge is purulent, opaque, foul tasting/smelling, and/or blood tinged, brown to dark yellow *throughout the day*
Setting	September–March "others have it"	March–September (may be year round) If seasonal, exposure to allergen History of allergy	During dry, windy, dusty conditions	September–March "others have it"	After a cold or allergic rhinitis
Associated symptoms	Minimal sneezing, feverish, cough usually worse at night, dry mild sore throat esp in AM	Sneezing, itchiness Itchy, watery red eyes	Sneezing and itching are much less common than in AR, dry red eyes	Fever, myalgia, arthralgia, *looks sick*, cough more than cold, may be productive	High fever, unilateral facial pain, *looks sick*, maxillary toothache
Modifying factors	None	Antihistamines or removal of allergen makes it better. Further exposure to allergen makes it worse	None	None	Bending over makes facial pain worse Failure on decongestants

(Continued)

TABLE 7.1	Stuffy/Runny Nose (Continued)				
OBJECTIVE	Cold	Allergic Rhinitis	Vasomotor Rhinitis	"Flu"/Super Virus	Bacterial Sinusitis
Fever	Usually mild to no fever	No fever	No fever	High fever	Fever
Nasal examination	Inflamed, red swollen nasal mucosa with mucoid discharge

May be green tinged after 3 to 5 days | Swollen, pale, boggy nasal mucosa with clear watery discharge | Dry irritated but otherwise normal appearing nasal mucosa with clear watery discharge | Same as cold | Purulent, dark yellow-brown or blood tinged nasal discharge

Unequal decreased or absent maxillary sinus transillumination |
| Lung A&P | Clear | Normally clear

May have expiratory wheeze if asthma | Clear | Usually clear, may have occasional scattered rhonchi that clear with coughing | clear |
| Other | None | Allergic shiners, nasal crease, Dennie's lines, elevated levels of serum IgE | None | None | Pain on palpation/percussion of frontal/maxillary sinuses

Upper tooth pain if maxillary |
| Usual causative agents | Rhinovirus, coronavirus | Indoor and outdoor allergens | None | Respiratory syncytial virus (RSV), some coronavirus, adenovirus, parainfluenza | Streptococcus pneumoniae

Haemophilus influenzae

Moraxella catarrhalis |

TABLE 7.2	Cold Versus Flu Symptoms	
Signs and Symptoms	**Influenza**	**Common Cold**
Symptom onset	Abrupt	Gradual
Fever	Abrupt onset; commonly 100 to 102°F lasting 3-4 days *Not everyone will have fever, especially elderly	Rare
Muscle Aches	Common often severe	Rare
Chills	Common	Slight
Fatigue/weakness	:Common; may last 2 to 3 weeks, especially in elderly	Sometimes; usually mild
Extreme exhaustion	Common	Never
Sneezing	Sometimes	Common
Stuffy Nose	Sometimes	Common
Sore throat	Sometimes	Common
Chest discomfort or cough	Common; may be severe	Common; mild to moderate hacking cough
Headache	Common	Rare
Complications	Pneumonia; worsening of chronic underlying conditions, secondary bacterial infection, encephalopathy, myocarditis, myositis; can be rapidly progressive and life-threatening	Sinus congestion, earache

Source: Cold vs. Flu Symptom Chart. From http://www.jointcommission.org/assets/1/6/Cold_vs_Flu_Chart_2013.pdf. Accessed June 12, 2014 © The Joint Commission, 2014. Reprinted with permission.

aware they have allergies or may have a history or a family of allergic rhinitis, atopic dermatitis, and/or asthma. Avoiding exposure to the allergen, if known, as well as taking an antihistamine will decrease the frequency and severity of the symptoms. Patients are afebrile, and on examination they generally have pale, boggy, swollen nasal turbinates with a clear watery discharge. In addition, if the allergic rhinitis is chronic or perennial they may have allergic shiners, dark areas on their face below the eyes, near the nose due to the vasodilation associated with the chronic nasal congestion, a nasal crease, and Dennie's lines. In patients with allergic rhinitis, a careful history regarding asthma and its symptoms, including early morning cough or a family history of asthma, should be elicited since a significant percentage of patients have concurrent asthma. Auscultation of the lungs should be performed to determine whether or not the expiratory wheezing typical of asthma is present.

Vasomotor Rhinitis

In parts of the country where it can be dry and windy, patients appearing to have allergic rhinitis symptoms may have vasomotor rhinitis. Symptoms are similar to allergic rhinitis in terms of the nasal discharge, and can present with red irritated eyes without the discharge. Vasomotor rhinitis is an irritant rhinitis, not an immune-mediated disease such as allergic rhinitis. The primary way to distinguish it is by examining the nasal mucosa. In vasomotor rhinitis, the nasal mucosa is dry but the normal pink-red color, not pale. Also, patients will fail to respond to antihistamines and do not have allergic shiners, and other physical findings of AR.

Acute Bacterial Sinusitis

Bacterial sinusitis is uncommon. In patients with nasal symptoms for 14 or more days, only 0.2% to 2% of patients have bacterial sinusitis. Bacterial sinusitis is not directly communicable: that is, one does not catch it as one does the common cold. Rather, it is usually caused by bacteria that colonize the upper respiratory tract, most commonly *Streptococcus pneumoniae, Haemophilus influenzae,* and *Moraxella catarrhalis.* The bacterial infectious disease is a secondary event, which invariably follows an inciting event, usually either a viral URI or active allergic rhinitis. The typical clinical course is that the patient has a viral URI or an exacerbation of allergic rhinitis. The manifestations of this primary event start to get better after a week, but then symptoms suddenly worsen. Patients may complain of a headache centered near one eye. The pain is often worsened by bending over, and there is a purulent (opaque, dark yellow, or brown) nasal discharge throughout the day. Patients should be asked about the color of the discharge during the afternoon or after they have been awake and ambulatory for at least 6 hours. This is because most patients have opaque, yellowish brown discharge in the morning due to evaporation of moisture during the night. However, if this persists throughout the day, it is more consistent with true bacterial sinusitis. In addition, the nasal discharge may be described as bad smelling or foul tasting. The presence of a toothache may be a manifestation of a maxillary sinus infection. Some patients notice impaired smell and taste. Infrequently, cough, usually nonproductive and which worsens at night, occurs with acute bacterial sinusitis. Another factor that favors bacterial infection is the failure of a decongestant. However, this must be interpreted with caution since most patients who use decongestants continually will quickly notice that they do not work as well as they did initially. This is due to the development of tachyphylaxis due to downregulation of adrenergic receptors with continuous exposure. This necessitates larger dosage and/or more frequent use to get the efficacy similar to the initial dose. Objectively, patients may present with pain on palpation or percussion of the maxillary and frontal sinuses. Remember to palpate gently first, and percuss only if there is no pain on palpation. Patients may also have unequal, decreased, or absent transillumination of the maxillary sinus. Patients usually are febrile, but in the absence of fever, check to see what the patient has taken in the last 4 to 6 hours. Analgesics such as acetaminophen and NSAIDs, given for pain, are also antipyretics and may mask the fever.

Summary
The key in diagnosis of causes of a runny, stuffy nose is to distinguish allergic rhinitis and bacterial sinusitis from viral URIs because the former two are the maladies for which there are effective treatments.

• EAR PAIN/DISCHARGE

There are multiple causes for ear pain or discomfort, purulent discharge from an ear, and even associated acute hearing loss including acute otitis media, serous otitis media (aka otitis media with effusion), otitis externa, chronic suppurative otitis media, and cerumen impaction. There are also some causes of ear pain that are not caused by ear problems. Examples of these include temporomandibular joint (TMJ) disorders (also called TMJ pain dysfunction syndrome and TMJ syndrome), dental disorders, and streptococcal pharyngitis. Table 7.3 provides the diagnostic schemata and the comparative presentations for the most common disorders related to the ear.

Acute Otitis Media
The development of middle ear infections requires the transit of colonizing bacteria or viruses from the nasopharynx or oropharynx, up into the eustachian tube followed by lack of normal patency or drainage from the tube. Several things are common causes of abnormal closure or dysfunction of the eustachian tube. These include any of the causes of swelling

TABLE 7.3	Ear Pain/Discharge

A. DIAGNOSTIC SCHEMATA FOR EAR PAIN/DISCHARGE

Acute Otitis Media

Otitis Media With Effusion (Serous Otitis Media)

Chronic Suppurative Otitis Media

Otitis Externa (Swimmer's Ear)

TMJ Pain Dysfunction Syndrome

B. DIFFERENTIAL DIAGNOSIS OF EAR PAIN/DISCHARGE

SUBJECTIVE	*Acute Otitis Media*	*Otitis Media With Effusion (Serous Otitis Media)*	*Chronic Suppurative Otitis Media*	*Otitis Externa (Swimmer's ear)*	*TMJ Pain Dysfunction Syndrome*
Location	N/A	N/A	N/A	N/A	N/A
Onset	Typically get URI for 2 to 3 days, then notice ear symptoms or allergic rhinitis symptoms for several days	Usually occurs post-AOM or when allergic rhinitis symptoms prominent	None	Occurs after periods of excessive moisture and/or trauma to the external canals	Variable with severity of TMJ disorder and presence of modifying factors
Quantity	Severe discomfort, although infants may just be fussy or irritable and toddlers, young children may just pull at ear Pain disappears if TM ruptures	Painless unless changes in atmospheric pressure	Severity varies from significant to none	Pain varies but can be severe	Severity of discomfort varies depending on severity of TMJ disorder and other modifying factors
Quality	Varies	Fullness in ear	Varies	Varies	Ache to muscle spasm
Setting	Requires eustachian tube dysfunction and the passage of viruses or bacteria from the nasopharynx	Requires eustachian tube dysfunction	None	Lots of moisture in the ear due to head sets, earphones, swimming Picks at ear with foreign object, e.g., Q-tip, bobby pin	None

(Continued)

TABLE 7.3	Ear Pain/Discharge (Continued)				
Associated symptoms	Purulent discharge on the pillow if TM ruptures; Decreased hearing	Ear popping when yawns; Decreased hearing; May have perennial allergic rhinitis and its symptoms	Purulent discharge on the pillow; Decreased hearing	Purulent discharge on the pillow; Potentially decreased hearing if canal mostly occluded	Headache, grinding or popping noise when open mouth. Jaw may temporarily lock when opening mouth wide
Modifying factors	None	None	None	Yawning, laying on the ear may worsen pain	Grinding teeth at night, chewing gum makes it worse
OBJECTIVE	*Acute Otitis Media*	*Otitis Media With Effusion (Serous Otitis Media)*	*Chronic Suppurative Otitis Media*	*Otitis Externa (Swimmer's ear)*	*TMJ Pain Dysfunction Syndrome*
Fever	Mild to moderate (38°C to 40°C)	None	Usually none	Usually none	None
Ear examination	Ear canal normal, may have purulent discharge if TM ruptures; Red, bulging TM with loss of landmarks (light reflex, malleus, short process); TM-reduced mobility	Ear canal normal. TM normal to retracted with prominent short process and malleus; Fluid-air levels or air bubbles behind TM; TM-reduced mobility	Ear canal normal unless discharge; Large central TM perforation with pus, red middle ear tissue, or cholesteatoma; TM normal if visualized	Pain on pinna traction or tragus pressure; External canal red swollen, with purulent discharge, picturesque growths; TM normal if visualized	Normal
Other					Palpation of TMJ reveals crepitus when opening mouth and/or muscle spasm; Underbite or other malocclusion; Mouth does not open straight vertically
Usual causative agents	Viral, Streptococcus pneumoniae, H. influenzae, Moraxella catarrhalis	None usually	Staphylococcus sp. Pseudomonas, fungi	Staphylococcus sp, Pseudomonas, fungi	None

or enlargement of posterior pharyngeal lymphoid tissue, like a cold (viral URI) or upper respiratory manifestations of allergies. Roughly half are caused by respiratory viruses; the remaining are caused by the respiratory tract bacteria, *Streptococcus pneumoniae, Haemophilus influenzae,* and *Moraxella catarrhalis.* Acute otitis media (AOM) occurs mostly in children under 6 years of age who have relatively short straight eustachian tubes. By 6 years of age, the eustachian tube is considerably longer and is curved, making the retrograde transit of microorganisms more difficult. Bottle propping in infants and toddlers who are lying on their back promotes passage of the ingested fluid with bacteria into the middle ear. In most cases, the onset of AOM symptoms is preceded by a 2- to 3-day history of viral URI or allergic rhinitis. In children who have not yet developed significant verbal skills, the ear pain is manifested by pulling at the affected ear or generalized fussiness or irritability. AOM is usually accompanied by a fever and decreased hearing in the affected ear. The natural course of AOM leads to increasing pain and pressure, finally resulting in a pinpoint perforation in the tympanic membrane (TM) with immediate cessation of severe pain due to the release of pressure. Over two-thirds of the cases resolve spontaneously without sequelae. This is true of virtually all viral causes and many cases caused by *Haemophilus* and *Moraxella.* While the cases caused by *Streptococcus pneumoniae* are less likely to resolve spontaneously, many still do. In less than 1% of the cases due to more virulent organisms such as *S. pneumoniae,* the mastoid bone is invaded, causing mastoiditis.

Objectively, most patients have a fever. On otoscopic examination, the TM is usually red. If tympanometry or pneumatic otoscopy is done, the TM is nonmobile. It may be bulging, and a pinpoint perforation may be visible. Normal landmarks are not visible. There may be a purulent discharge coming from the pinpoint perforation, and/or it may be noticed on the floor of the external canal. If the TM ruptures during sleep, the discharge can stain the pillow and the patient awakens to find the ear pain much better or gone. Current guidelines recommend that for most children 2 or over, only analgesic/antipyretics be given for 48 hours. Almost 75% will resolve without antibiotic therapy. Even for those patients referred to a primary care provider for severe symptoms for antibiotic therapy (whether <2 years old or not), OTC analgesics/antipyretic products are appropriate. However, follow-up visits are required to check for the potential development of otitis media with effusion.

Otitis Media With Effusion/Serous Otitis Media

The term otitis media with effusion (OME) more accurately reflects our knowledge of the inflammatory nature of the disease. Serous otitis media (SOM), an older but still frequently used term, reflected the belief (at the time) that there was only fluid behind the ear not caused by inflammation. It is now thought that there are two causes of OME: allergic rhinitis and post-AOM. In children who have had AOM, more than 60% will have some effusion remaining up to 8 weeks later. Like AOM, eustachian tube blockage/dysfunction is required for the development of OME. Usually OME resolves spontaneously without sequelae, but in some cases the inflammation creates bubbles of CO_2 in the fluid, which diffuse out into the blood stream, creating a vacuum that pulls the TM back against the middle ear bones, causing them to touch each other. Untreated, this can eventually cause permanent hearing loss when the bones fuse. Generally, OME is painless unless there are changes in atmospheric pressure as occurs during takeoff and landing of an aircraft. Patients may notice a sensation of fullness, decreased hearing, and ear popping when yawning. Otoscopic examination reveals a nonmobile TM, possibly with the presence of an air fluid level or air bubbles behind the TM. The landmarks, particularly the malleus and its short process, become very prominent because the TM is retracted against the middle ear bones in more severe cases. The TM may be somewhat bluish in appearance. Treatment of severe OME with a retracted TM requires the placement of pressure equalization tubes (PE tubes) through the TM. The tubes function to equalize the pressure, relieving the retraction induced contact with the bones of the middle ear, while allowing the inflammation to run its course. OME does not require antibiotic therapy. The efficacy of decongestants or corticosteroids is controversial.

Chronic Suppurative Otitis Media

Chronic suppurative otitis media (CSOM) differs considerably from AOM. First, it requires the presence of a large central perforation in the TM. The cause of this central perforation is unclear. Trauma, placement of PE tubes, high fever, and repeated episodes of AOM with perforation have all been identified as causes. Rather than respiratory tract bacteria, the pathogens come from the flora of the external canal with *Staphylococcus* species and *Pseudomonas aeruginosa* predominating as causative agents. Other gram-negative bacteria can also be involved. Bacteria migrate through the central perforation, often facilitated by water from swimming or showering. Once inside the middle ear, they infect tissue and with accompanying inflammation, cause a purulent discharge. If untreated, this process can destroy important middle ear tissue, and invade the mastoid and other bony structures of the cranium. In chronic cases, a whitish cyst made up of epithelial tissue called a cholesteatoma may form. This tissue can enlarge, become infected, and eventually destroy middle ear bones. The two major symptoms of CSOM are decreased hearing and a purulent discharge for >14 days. Pain is generally not a prominent feature except in more widespread disease. On otoscopic examination, there is a large central TM perforation with a purulent discharge. In long-standing disease, there may be a cholesteatoma seen as a whitish cyst in the middle ear. Patients with suspected CSOM should be referred to an otorhinolaryngologist, as soon as possible, for definitive treatment.

Otitis Externa (Swimmer's Ear)

Otitis externa (OE) is an infection of the external ear canal. Trauma from cleaning ears with foreign objects, wearing earpieces chronically, and constant moisture from sweat (especially while wearing earphones), or frequent immersion of the head in water (swimming) are all predisposing factors. Common pathogens include normal external ear canal flora including *Staphylococcus* sp, *Pseudomonas aeruginosa,* and multiple fungi. Patients generally have one or more predisposing factors and present with pain/discomfort and a purulent discharge. Hearing may or may not be affected depending on the amount of swelling and debris. Complete otoscopic examination may not be possible. However, to the extent that it is possible, usual findings include a red, swollen external canal with purulent material. With fungal infections, picturesque growths with colorful spores or hyphae may be seen. The TM is mobile on pneumatic ostoscopy, but swelling, debris, and especially pain in the external canal may prevent complete visualization of the TM. Since the canal is swollen and painful, the cardinal diagnostic finding is pain with a firm pull on the earlobe (pinna) or pressure on the tragus. Eliciting pain on pinna pull is generally diagnostic since patients with other ear disease will not experience any pain with this maneuver. In addition, there may be peri- or post-auricular lymphadenopathy. Finally, if you suspect OE, be careful during the otoscopic examination. That is gently pull the pinna and possibly use a small diameter disposable otoscope speculum.

Ear Pain With a Normal Otoscopic Examination

Occasionally, a patient complaining of ear pain will have a normal otoscopic examination. When that occurs, think of referred pain from a dental problem, pharyngitis, or TMJ pain dysfunction syndrome. Specific problems may include a tooth abscess or streptococcal pharyngitis. A normal otoscopic examination in this setting warrants a mouth and throat examination by applying pressure on each tooth with a tongue depressor to detect abscessed teeth. Also, palpation over the TMJ and observation of the mouth opening should be conducted.

TMJ Pain Dysfunction Syndrome

TMJ pain dysfunction syndrome can cause pain in the area of the ear due to muscle spasms caused by grinding the teeth (bruxism), or structural and/or functional abnormalities of the TMJ. Patients may complain of ear pain, headache, or tinnitus. These patients may admit to a grinding, clicking, popping, snapping sensation or noise when they open and close their mouth. Ask if they grind their teeth at night and how frequently they chew gum, as both are typical in TMJ pain dysfunction syndrome. A quick check for TMJ problems can be done when examining the peri- and post-auricular lymph nodes. Press gently against the TMJ (just in front of the ears) and have the patient open their mouth slowly. Any clicking, grinding, popping sensations palpated may indicate TMJ problems. Also, palpable muscle spasms may be felt over the joint, which is typical. Watch the opening of the mouth carefully. If it does not open smoothly straight up and down, there may be TMJ problems. Finally, check for dental malocclusions especially an underbite. Generally, patients with TMJ pain dysfunction syndrome will have multiple suspicious findings, e.g., an underbite, a history of chewing gum frequently, an irregular mouth opening, and the presence of grinding, clicking, popping over the TMJ on palpation. Patients suspected of TMJ problems should be initially referred to a dentist for further evaluation.

• SORE THROAT/HOARSENESS

There are multiple causes of sore throats, but most are due to either infections (bacterial or viral) or irritant/allergic disorders. The most common bacterial infectious cause of sore throat is *Streptococcus pyogenes* (Group A β-hemolytic strep or GABHS) also known as *strep throat*. Numerous other bacteria have been implicated as causes of sore throat, but are less common (including *Fusobacterium necrophorum, Arcanobacterium haemolyticum*, Group C and G streptococci, *Mycoplasma pneumoniae, Chlamydophila pneumoniae, N. gonorrhoeae,* and even *Corynebacterium diphtheriae*). There are many viral causes, but the most common are those associated with viral URIs, which create pharyngitis either directly or by post-nasal drip. Other viral causes of pharyngitis include influenza viruses, coxsackieviruses (including those that cause herpangina and hand, foot, and mouth disease), Epstein-Barr virus (EBV), which is the cause of mononucleosis, and cytomegalovirus (CMV). Since primary HIV infections often cause a syndrome like mononucleosis, with pharyngitis as a common component, depending on their individual risk factors, patients should have this diagnosis considered. Another common cause of sore throat, usually by a post-nasal drip mechanism, is allergic rhinitis. Distinguishing between causes of hoarseness is also important. Viral laryngitis is a minor self-limiting disorder, whereas acute epiglottitis and carcinoma of the larynx can both be fatal if not diagnosed early and accurately. Table 7.4 provides the diagnostic schemata and comparative presentations of sore throat.

Streptococcal Pharyngitis

Strep throat is caused by a Group A β-hemolytic strep (*Streptococcus pyogenes*). It represents between 10% and 30% of all patients reporting a sore throat as the primary or only symptom. It occurs most frequently in elementary school-age children (ages 5 to 11) and those in contact with them. Most cases occur during the school year, peaking during

TABLE 7.4	Sore Throat

A. DIAGNOSTIC SCHEMATA FOR SORE THROAT

Streptococcal Pharyngitis	Mononucleosis	Hand, Foot, and Mouth Disease (HFMD)
Viral Pharyngitis	Herpangina	Post-nasal Drip due to Allergic Rhinitis/URI (PND)

B. DIFFERENTIAL DIAGNOSIS OF SORE THROAT

SUBJECTIVE	Streptococcal Pharyngitis	Viral Pharyngitis	Mononucleosis	Herpangina	HFMD	PND
Location	May have referred ear pain					
Onset	Rapid onset of severe symptoms lasting 72 hours	Usually slower onset and last 5 to 10 days	Slow onset, lasting 5 to 7 days may be preceded by fatigue/malaise	Rapid onset lasts 7 to 10 days	12 to 36 hours onset, lasts 7 to 10 days	Slow onset, lasts as long as nasal symptoms
Quantity	Severe with difficulty swallowing all day	Wide range of symptoms from PND to strep, but usually milder	Mild to moderate lasting all day	Severe pain lasting all day difficulty swallowing	Severe pain lasting all day difficulty swallowing	Mildly painful upon awakening gets better during the day
Quality	N/A	N/A	N/A	N/A	N/A	N/A
Setting	Occurs in school-age children beginning in elementary school and those in contact with that age group / Occurs primarily during school year in fall/winter / Nausea vomiting in children	All ages	Adolescents/young adults (kissing disease)	Mostly children	All ages	All ages
Associated symptoms	Absence of cough or other nasal symptoms	Many also have cough and URI symptoms	Marked fatigue/malaise	Malaise	Malaise , skin manifestations	Symptoms of URI/allergic rhinitis
Modifying factors	Acidic or carbonated drinks make it worse	Certain forms can mimic strep	Acidic or carbonated drinks make it worse	Acidic or carbonated drinks make it worse	Acidic or carbonated drinks make it worse	Acidic or carbonated drinks make it worse

OBJECTIVE	Streptococcal Pharyngitis	Viral Pharyngitis	Mononucleosis	Herpangina	HFMD	PND
Fever	38.4°C to 40°C	Usually low grade	Low-grade fever	38.4°C to 40°C	Usually low grade	None
Throat examination	Beefy red posterior pharynx with swollen tonsils with exudate (pus) on tonsils or posterior pharynx	Variable from mild to severe inflammation	Mildly inflamed posterior pharynx, swollen tonsils. About half have pus. A few with sheets of pus. Frenulum of tongue may be jaundiced	Multiple vesicles and/or ulcerations with red border on posterior pharynx and tonsils	Similar lesions to herpangina only distributed all over oral cavity and throat	Mildly inflamed posterior pharynx with clear to mucoid nasal mucous drainage
Other	Painful anterior cervical lymphadenopathy. Fetid breath. Positive throat culture or rapid strep test	Many have viral URI findings	Elevated AST/ALT. Positive Monospot test. Painful anterior/posterior cervical lymphadenopathy. Lymphadenopathy may extend to arm pit	50% have truncal rash	67% have painful blisters on palms, soles, and buttocks	Findings of allergic rhinitis or viral URI
Usual causative agents	β-hemolytic *Streptococcus pyogenes*	Same as URI	Epstein-Barr virus	Coxsackievirus, enterovirus	Coxsackievirus, enterovirus	

the winter months. Circumstances associated with crowding of people, like a closed classroom, facilitate transmission of the organism. Recently, due to the large number of children in organized daycare or preschool, the age of suspicion for strep throat is considerably lower than previously seen. Concern for an accurate diagnosis is based on the possibility of nonsuppurative (autoimmune) inflammatory sequelae, acute rheumatic fever, in untreated patients. Acute rheumatic fever occurs between 2 and 5 weeks after the sore throat and presents with fever, carditis, migratory polyarthritis, and/or chorea. The carditis can result in permanent valvular damage and risk for developing bacterial endocarditis. Due to careful attention to its diagnosis and prompt treatment, the incidence has been drastically reduced since the late 1940s to just one per 1 million population.

Subjectively, patients present with sudden onset of fever and severe sore throat, difficulty swallowing with pain worsened when swallowing acid liquids such as citrus juices and carbonated beverages. The pain is severe and constant throughout the day. Cough and nasal symptoms are uncommon. Malaise is common, but arthralgias and myalgias are not. Gastrointestinal symptoms including nausea, vomiting, and abdominal pain may occur, but are more common in children. Generally, symptoms markedly improve by 72 hours after onset. Symptoms lasting longer than that should raise the suspicion of other causes such as viral pharyngitis and mononucleosis. A recent history of exposure to someone with a severe sore throat or diagnosed strep throat is common.

Objectively, examination of the throat and tonsils will reveal beefy red color, usually with purulent exudates and in many cases fetid (foul smelling) breath. Achieving complete visualization of the posterior pharynx and/or obtaining a culture or rapid strep test usually requires inducing the gag reflex with a tongue depressor. However, in a significant number of patients having them open their mouth wide, sticking their tongue out, and "panting like a dog" may preclude the need for a tongue depressor. Tonsillar tissue may be swollen. A marked fever (39°C to 40.5°C) is a significant feature. Painful anterior cervical adenopathy is typical. A small number of patients will have a skin rash comprised of fine red papules on the truck that spread to the extremities but not the palms and soles of the feet. Typically, it has a sandpaper-like feel and blanches upon pressure. This manifestation is called scarlet fever or scarlatina. The classic confirmation for diagnosis is considered to be the throat culture. However, due to the 48-hour delay in obtaining culture results and the need to start therapy as soon as possible, the Rapid Antigen Detection Test (RADT) for *S. pyogenes* is usually preferred. Results of these tests are available in minutes. Unfortunately, they have a relatively high rate of false-positive findings because as many as one-fourth of patients are carriers of β-hemolytic *Streptococcus*. There is also a significant number of false negatives, mostly a function of poor sampling technique. Therefore, practically speaking, the clinical diagnosis requires a combination of typical features plus bacteriologic confirmation to accurately make the diagnosis. More technically, to rule out the carrier state, a definitive diagnosis requires typical signs and symptoms, plus some confirmation of the presence of the organism in the pharynx by standard culture or an RADT, *and* a positive result of acute and convalescent serologic tests for GABHS (i.e., antistreptolysin O or ASO test). If one tonsillar pillar or the uvula is swollen and displaced and the patient has difficulty opening their mouth without pain, suspect the suppurative complication peritonsillar abscess, which requires immediate referral.

Viral Pharyngitis

Generally, viral pharyngitis presents with a wide range of symptoms and degrees of severity depending on the specific virus. Rhinovirus, adenovirus, coronavirus, herpes simplex, parainfluenza and RSV are common causes. Symptoms tend to have a slower onset, longer duration, and less pain than strep throat. Most patients with viral pharyngitis have additional symptoms such as nasal symptoms, cough, and conjunctivitis that are very uncommon in patients with strep throat. However, in some cases viral pharyngitis can mimic streptococcal pharyngitis in every aspect except the positive bacteriological findings.

Mononucleosis

Mononucleosis, caused by EBV, occurs most frequently in adolescents and young adults, hence its nickname the "kissing disease." The onset of the sore throat is slow and it lasts 5 to 7 days with mild to moderate pain. In addition, most patients experience significant fatigue and malaise that may last for 4 to 8 weeks. Sometimes it is the primary presenting symptom. Since the incubation period is 4 to 6 weeks, few patients remember any potential exposures. Objectively, examination of the throat reveals redness usually not as severe as in strep throat. About half the patients will have purulent exudates, with some having profuse exudates that is continuous over the posterior pharynx and tonsils. Painful anterior and posterior cervical lymphadenopathy is common, with some patients having swollen, painful lymph nodes as remote from the throat as the underarms. Patients have a low-grade fever and 90% have mildly elevated AST and ALT levels. Jaundice develops in less than 5% of patients. All patients develop some degree of splenomegaly that may not be evident upon physical examination. A CBC reveals lymphocytosis with the presence of >10% atypical lymphocytes. A positive Monospot test and elevated EBV antibody levels are diagnostic for the disease. Unfortunately, neither may be positive during the first 2 weeks of the disease and may need to be repeated to confirm the diagnosis.

Herpangina/Hand, Foot, and Mouth Disease

These two disorders are caused by viruses in the enterovirus group, which includes coxsackieviruses and others. Some sources actually consider them to be different manifestations along the same disease spectrum. Both diseases usually present with severe throat pain, malaise, and difficulty swallowing and symptoms last for 7 to 10 days. Herpangina has a rapid onset and occurs most frequently in children, whereas hand, foot, and mouth disease (HFMD) has a slightly slower onset of 12 to 36 hours and occurs in patients of all ages. Objectively, both have dermatological manifestations in more than 50% of patients. In herpangina, a maculopapular, vesicular rash appears on the trunk. In HFMD, the vesicular lesions with erythematous borders typically occur on the palms of the hands and soles of the feet, as well as the buttocks in some cases. In HFMD, the fever is generally low grade, where herpangina presents with temperatures of 38.4°C to 40°C. Examination of the throat reveals varying degrees of erythema with red vesicles that ulcerate and have a red border. In herpangina, lesions are limited to the posterior pharynx and tonsillar pillars, while in HFMD they occur all over the oral cavity including tongue and gingivae. Painful cervical lymphadenopathy is common in both disorders.

Pharyngitis Due to Post-Nasal Drip

Patients with both allergic rhinitis and viral URIs can have sore throats. However, they differ in several ways from other forms of pharyngitis. Rarely is sore throat the primary complaint. While the patient may awaken with the sore throat, it usually goes away after several hours. In contrast, with most other causes of pharyngitis the pain is constant throughout the day and night. Also, the sore throat when due to post nasal drip lasts only as long as the rhinitis does. Objectively, examination of the throat reveals drainage or discharge, often in two tracks, on the posterior pharynx. When present, this drainage is often of similar consistency and appearance as the nasal discharge. There may be some mild inflammation on the soft palate or posterior pharynx.

Loss of Voice/Hoarseness

Loss of voice or hoarseness at times accompanies sore throat or it can occur by itself. The most common cause of hoarseness is acute laryngitis. Respiratory viruses such as rhinovirus, adenovirus, and coronavirus are the most frequent cause. Allergies and voice strain due to overuse are other common causes. Smokers as well as patients with GERD may also experience the symptom. Onset of the hoarseness is slow and is accompanied by other symptoms of the causative disorder. Symptoms lasting longer than 2 weeks, especially in smokers, should be referred to an ENT specialist to look for more serious causes such as laryngeal carcinoma.

Croup, also known as viral laryngotracheobronchitis, is a disease of infants and young children in which the structures implicated in the name of the disorder become inflamed due to common respiratory viruses. Occurring mostly in the winter months, the hallmark signs are abrupt onset of a nocturnal cough that sounds like a seal barking along with inspiratory stridor and trouble breathing. Most cases are mild and require no treatment other than providing humidified air for the child to breath during attacks. This can be accomplished by taking the child into the bathroom, closing the door, and turning on the hot water in the shower to fill the room with steam. The warm moist air relieves the cough, stridor, and breathing difficulties. Severe difficulty breathing, continuous stridor at rest, retractions when breathing, early cyanosis, and lethargy are all signs of severe disease that may require immediate treatment and/or hospitalization. In short, if the steam does not work well, then the child needs to be taken to a facility for definitive care.

Finally, acute epiglottitis, while rare, deserves mention. The incidence has drastically decreased in countries where routine immunization of children against *Haemophilus influenzae* type b and *Streptococcus pneumoniae* has been implemented. These are/were the two most common causes of the disease, although many other bacterial (and even some viral and fungal) causes have been documented. However, the rate in adults has remained constant with the average occurrence at age 45 with a gender ratio of 3:1 for males to females. It is a life-threatening infectious disease, with a 7% mortality rate in adults. It typically presents with an acute onset of sore throat, and difficult or painful swallowing. The classic sign is the sudden loss of voice as opposed to the slow onset of hoarseness and laryngitis seen in viral conditions. Patients generally present with a high fever and in later stages may experience difficulty breathing and stridor. This is a medical emergency and may require tracheostomy to prevent asphyxia and death. Therefore, patients (especially older males) presenting with a severe sore throat and sudden loss of voice must be immediately referred.

• KEY REFERENCES

1. Slavin RG, Spector SL, Bernstein IL, et al. The diagnosis and treatment of sinusitis: a practice parameter. *J Allergy Clin Immunol*. 2005;116(6 suppl):S13-S47.
2. Anon JB. Upper respiratory infections. *Am J Med*. 2010;123(4 suppl):S16-S25.
3. Dykewicz MS, Hamilos DL. Rhinitis and sinusitis. *J Allergy Clin Immunol*. 2010;125(2 suppl):S103-115.
4. Neilan RE, Rolan PS. Otalgia. *Med Clin North Am*. 2010;94(5):961-971.
5. Ely JW, Hanson MR, Clark EC. Diagnosis of ear pain. *Am Fam Physician*. 2008;77(5):621-628.
6. Coker TR, Chan LS, Newberry SJ, et al. Diagnosis, microbial epidemiology and antibiotic treatment of otitis media in children: a systematic review. *JAMA*. 2010;304(19):2161-2169.
7. Schafer P, Baugh RF. Acute otitis externa: an update. *Am Fam Physician*. 2012;86:1055-61.
8. Wessels MR. Streptococcal pharyngitis. *N Engl J Med*. 2011;364(7):648-655.
9. Chan TV. The patient with sore throat. *Med Clin North Am*. 2010;94(5):923-943.

CASE 7.1

SM, a regular customer at your store, comes in to pick up her mother's prescription. As she pays for the prescription, she asks: "Is there anything better than Actifed for this cold I've got? I'm tired of being stuffed up. It's been six days!"

a. Based on the information above, what are three likely causes for SM's symptoms? Explain your rationale.

_____

_____

_____

_____

_____

b. List 10 questions you would ask, physical examinations you would conduct, or lab tests you would order to identify the etiology of SM's symptoms.

_____

_____

_____

_____

_____

CASE 7.2

Iloff Medkem, a first-year pharmacy student, has the " 2014 Crud," which began 8 days ago with fever, rhinorrhea, facial fullness, myalgias, and arthralgia. After 5 days he began to feel better. However, his rhinorrhea returned 2 days ago as a mucoid discharge. Today he presents with pain under both eyes and the discharge has markedly changed.

a. List three questions you would ask to clarify his problem.

_____

_____

_____

_____

_____

b. List three physical examinations you would perform to clarify the diagnosis.

_____

_____

_____

_____

_____

c. What is the most likely diagnosis if the questions and examinations you listed above are positive?

_____

_____

_____

_____

_____

![logo] **CASE 7.3**

Howican Paddle presents to the pharmacy with a 3-day history of right ear discomfort with decreased hearing. This morning he woke up with a small yellow stain on his pillow.

a. What are the two most likely causes of his symptoms? Explain your rationale.

_____
_____
_____
_____
_____

b. List two questions you would ask to help identify the cause. Explain your rationale.

_____
_____
_____
_____
_____

c. For each of the diagnoses listed in question a above, list expected findings on ear examination.

_____
_____
_____
_____
_____

CASE 7.4

FF, a 33-year-old fourth-grade teacher asks what would be good for this bad sore throat he has had for the last 48 hours.

List 10 questions/physical examinations/lab tests you would want to ask, conduct or order to confirm your assessment.

Cough

LEARNING OBJECTIVES

1. Accurately identify the most likely etiology of a cough, through history, diagnostic tests, and appropriate patient findings on physical examination to enable the appropriate recommendation of effective treatment or referral to an appropriate provider.

2. Use the knowledge of the pathophysiology, etiology, and usual presentation of common diseases with cough as a primary symptom to review prescription orders for appropriateness and to accurately educate patients about their disease and its treatment.

3. Use the knowledge of the pathophysiology, etiology, and usual presentation of diseases with cough as a primary symptom to accurately interpret the diagnostic process to advise regarding the most appropriate prescription therapy.

A cough is a natural protective process. Normal, healthy school-aged children experience 10 to 12 coughing episodes per day. Coughing has two main functions: (1) clearing the larynx, trachea, and bronchi of inhaled material, mucous, infectious agents, noxious substances, foreign particles, edema fluid, and pus and (2) increasing oxygenation in the blood via post-cough inspiration and breathing. These mechanisms are thought to partially contribute to the cough of exercise-induced asthma and the early morning cough typical of asthma.

Mechanical and chemical cough receptors are located primarily in the epithelium of the upper and lower respiratory tracts, but are also found in the esophagus, diaphragm, stomach, and pericardium. When irritated, they initiate a reflex arc via the vagus nerve to the cough center in the medulla, which then causes a reflex arc via the vagus, phrenic and spinal motor nerves to initiate a four-step process. First, there is an inspiratory phase, followed by a forced expiratory phase against a closed glottis to build up intrathoracic pressure. Second, the glottis opens with rapid expiration and causes the cough sound, followed by a deep inspiration. Prolonged or violent coughing can cause vomiting, fractured ribs, muscle spasm, urinary incontinence, and syncope.

• ETIOLOGY

The causes of a cough are numerous and can be due to disorders of the upper respiratory, lower respiratory, gastrointestinal, or cardiovascular systems. Viral upper respiratory infections, allergic rhinitis, and bacterial sinusitis all produce cough as an associated symptom, probably due to post-nasal drip of mucoid or purulent material. The lower respiratory tract is the primary source of cough as a symptom. Infections can be caused by viruses (acute bronchitis, viral pneumonia, and influenza), bacteria (pneumonia, tuberculosis, and whooping cough), or fungi (histoplasmosis, coccidioidomycosis, and candida). Inflammatory conditions of the lungs leading to cough include asthma, COPD, and smoking. Drug-induced pulmonary adverse effects also have cough as a major symptom complex. Gastroesophageal reflux disease (GERD) is an important gastrointestinal cause of cough. Various malignancies involving the respiratory tract may also present with a cough as the primary symptom. Finally, congestive heart failure is the most common cause of cough due to disorders of the cardiovascular system.

• DIAGNOSIS

The diagnosis of the cause of a cough is complex and requires a careful history, physical examination, and laboratory studies. The cough history and timing of the cough can provide important diagnostic clues. A good example of this is patients with a nighttime cough. Coughs due to GERD and upper airway cough syndrome (aka postnasal drip) usually occur shortly after lying down. Coughs caused by congestive heart failure typically occur 2 to 3 hours after lying down, whereas coughs due to asthma typically occur from 2 to 6 o'clock in the morning.

There are several ways of classifying coughs to facilitate diagnosis. Coughs are called acute if the duration is less than 3 weeks and chronic if the duration is greater than 3 weeks. They can also be classified based on amount of mucous brought up during coughing. Coughs that present with copious mucous are called productive or wet coughs and those with scant or no mucous production are called dry coughs. However, neither of these classification systems is absolute. Some have used the term subacute cough to describe a cough lasting 3 to 8 weeks, with chronic coughs defined as lasting more than 8 weeks. Similarly, there are some conditions that while usually presenting with a dry cough, but can generate a productive cough under specific circumstances such as time of day and severity of illness. These are called *mixed coughs.*

• ACUTE COUGH WITH PRODUCTIVE SPUTUM

The three main causes of an acute productive cough are bacterial pneumonia, acute bronchitis, and acute exacerbation of COPD (Table 8.1).

TABLE 8.1	Productive Cough		

A. DIAGNOSTIC SCHEMATA FOR PRODUCTIVE COUGH
  Bacterial Pneumonia
  Acute Bronchitis
  Chronic Obstructive Pulmonary Disease (COPD)

B. DIFFERENTIAL DIAGNOSIS OF PRODUCTIVE COUGH

SUBJECTIVE	Acute Bronchitis	Bacterial Pneumonia	COPD
Location	N/A	N/A	N/A
Onset	Gradual near the end of a URI	Gradual, 7 to 10 days after onset of viral URI or acute bronchitis	Very slowly after years and years of smoking, environmental or occupational hazard exposure
Quantity	Frequent coughing	Frequent coughing	Frequency varies because coughing is to clear excessive mucous from lungs
Quality	Mucoid sputum worse in the AM and night	Purulent (dark yellow/brown blood tinged) sputum throughout the day	Primarily mucoid sputum
Setting	Usually associated with the later stages of viral URI		Heavy chronic smoker
Associated symptoms	May have remnants of a viral URI	Elderly may present as primarily a behavior change, fatigue, malaise feverish, shortness of breath	Shortness of breath
Modifying factors	Nothing seems to help	Nothing seems to help	Nothing seems to help
OBJECTIVE			
Fever	Low-grade fever <100° F (37.8°C)	High-grade fever >100°F (37.8°C)	Afebrile
Chest x-ray	Normal	Consolidated infiltrates	Usually normal. May have markings indicating emphysema
Auscultation and percussion of lungs	Mostly clear, but may have rhonchi, which clear/change after coughing, rarely expiratory wheezes	Crackles around area of consolidated infiltrates. If large infiltrate may not hear breath sounds over central area. May have bronchophony, egophony	Usually rhonchi, which change/clear after coughing. Patients with emphysema may have faint breath sounds. Also in more advanced disease
Other findings	May have URI findings	Tachycardia, tachypnea, WBC >10,000/mL with >80% PMNs (mature plus immature)	Use of ancillary muscles in throat and neck to help breathing, well-developed sternocleidomastoid muscles. Cannot speak in complete sentences. May have tachypnea even on oxygen. Markedly reduced pulmonary function tests
Usual causative agents	90% viral, 10% pertussis	CAP: *Streptococcus pneumoniae, Haemophilus influenzae*, atypicals. Inpatient: gram-negative rods, e.g., *Klebsiella, Pseudomonas,* or MRSA	Smoking

Bacterial Pneumonia

Typically, community-acquired bacterial pneumonia (CAP) presents with a previous history of upper or lower respiratory infection that has transformed into a purulent productive cough *throughout the day* (mucous is opaque, dark yellow, brownish, or may be blood tinged). Typical objective findings include; fever >100°F (37.8°C), crackles upon auscultation of lung fields, tachypnea (normal is 12 to 20 breaths per minute), tachycardia (>100 beats/min), a chest x-ray with a consolidated infiltrate, and a white blood cell count greater than 10,000 cells per microliter, with >80% mature (polys, segs, PMNs), plus immature neutrophils (bands, stabs). Patients with more widespread disease may present with an inability or difficulty speaking in complete sentences or use ancillary muscles of the neck (sternocleidomastoids) to augment inspiration due to inadequate oxygen intake. For larger consolidated infiltrates, dullness on percussion, absent breath sounds, and the presence of bronchophony, egophony, or whispered pectoriloquy will correspond with the location of the infiltrate on the chest x-ray. Unfortunately, there is no individual or set of signs and symptoms that have a sensitivity and specificity greater than 65%, and because of the Medicare standard for starting antibiotics within 6 hours of admission for patients with potential CAP, the diagnosis ends up being primarily a clinical diagnosis. Therefore, in many cases empiric antibiotic therapy is started before the diagnosis is confirmed.

There are many confounding variables that interfere with quickly arriving at the diagnosis. In the elderly, they may not mount a vigorous febrile response or may be taking medications such as NSAIDs or acetaminophen for osteoarthritis that may mask a febrile response due to their antipyretic effects. Many times the elderly present without cough as a prominent symptom. Sudden changes in behavior, attention, or consciousness (obtundation) may be the primary symptom of bacterial pneumonia in the elderly. Also in patients with impaired swallowing or cough reflex, aspiration of gastric contents or food can occur, causing a bacterial pneumonia (aspiration pneumonia). All geriatric patients with a change in behavior or cough should be checked for pneumonia or other infectious processes such as urinary tract infections.

Common causative agents in CAP are *Streptococcus pneumoniae* and *Haemophilus influenzae*. Hospital-acquired bacterial pneumonia includes a wide range of bacterial pathogens typically gram-negative rods, such as *Klebsiella pneumoniae*, *Pseudomonas aeruginosa*, or penicillinase-producing gram-positive organisms such as *Staphylococcus aureus*. Other bacteria that cause about 25% of all community-acquired pneumonia are called atypical pneumonias or walking pneumonias. Their systemic symptoms tend to be milder; there is a lower incidence of productive cough and less of a febrile response compared to typical bacterial pneumonias. Similarly, patients with viral or atypical pneumonia do not mount as much of a neutrophilic response as seen with most bacterial pneumonias. Radiologically, viral and atypical infiltrates differ from bacterial findings because they tend to be interstitial rather than lobar in nature, yet can have great variability and overlap with bacterial pneumonia. While lung auscultation can reveal a range of findings from crackles to rhonchi, atypical and viral pneumonias have a much higher frequency of wheezing than bacterial infections. Also, viral and atypical pneumonias tend to have more extrapulmonary manifestations than bacterial infections. Recently, procalcitonin serum levels are being used to differentiate bacterial infections from atypical or viral infections. In bacterial pneumonias, serum procalcitonin levels are usually greater than 0.5 μg/L. Elevated procalcitonin levels usually are absent in viral and atypical infections. Because of the difficulty in many cases determining the etiology, standards for the treatment of CAP require coverage of common bacterial pathogens as well as common atypical pathogens.

Acute Bronchitis ("Chest Cold")

Over 90% of the cases of acute bronchitis in teens and adults are viral and antibiotics offer no benefit in terms of reducing symptoms or shortening the course of disease. Many times these are part of the latter stages of a viral URI. Symptoms include a productive cough with mucoid sputum, which may be green tinged, low-grade fever if any, and a normal chest x-ray. Auscultation of the lungs is normal most of the time with occasional rhonchi that clear with coughing. Tachypnea and tachycardia are uncommon and when they occur, pneumonia should be suspected. The pathogens are generally the same as those for the common cold with more severe presentations: rhinovirus, influenza, parainfluenza, respiratory syncytial virus, coronavirus, and adenovirus. Symptoms last from 1 to 3 weeks. Many patients with acute bronchitis develop bronchial hyperresponsiveness and may experience expiratory wheezes. For that reason, inhaled β-adrenergic bronchodilators such as albuterol are the treatment of choice.

• CHRONIC COUGH WITH SPUTUM PRODUCTION

Chronic Obstructive Pulmonary Disease

Chronic obstructive pulmonary disease (COPD) involves permanent changes to lung structure primarily due to long-term smoking. It is discussed in greater detail in Chapter 21. Patients generally present with a productive cough due to excess mucous production. In the early stages, smoker's cough, auscultation, and percussion of the lungs may be without findings. As the disease progresses auscultation reveals primarily rhonchi, but wheezing and occasional crackles may occur. In later stages known as emphysema, the alveoli lose their elasticity and air becomes trapped in peripheral lung fields. Auscultation of the lungs in patients with emphysema reveals faint or no breath sounds in certain areas due to decreased pulmonary function and the lack of air movement in areas of severe emphysema. Stable patients are usually afebrile, but due to poor pulmonary function have tachypnea and tachycardia. As pulmonary function deteriorates, patients are forced to use ancillary muscles in taking breaths. Many patients with COPD have enlarged sternocleidomastoid muscles that contract with each breath to try and force more air into their oxygen-starved lungs and body.

• SUBACUTE/CHRONIC COUGH WITH NO SPUTUM PRODUCTION

Asthma

Asthma is characterized by chronic inflammation of the small airways of the lungs, which leads to bronchospasm and the symptoms of asthma (see Table 8.2). Roughly 80% of asthmatics have involvement of IgE and up to 75% have a personal or family history of one or more of the atopic triad (allergic rhinitis, atopic dermatitis, or asthma). Asthma attacks typically include a decreased peak expiratory flow rate due to bronchoconstriction, cough, expiratory wheezing, and difficulty breathing (dyspnea) that may be manifested by *a tightness in the chest*. In severe attacks, which may be called status asthmaticus if they do not respond quickly to standard treatments, tachypnea and tachycardia can occur and patients may feel like they are suffocating. Asthma may present with an acute attack, but frequently presents in a more subtle form as a cough. Because the vital capacity of the lungs is lowest between 2 and 6 in the morning, patients with subclinical bronchospasm become hypoxic and begin a series of coughs. These coughs serve to increase oxygen intake. Therefore, repeated coughing episodes between 2 and 6 AM can be an indicator of mild asthma and should be investigated. Additionally, people may get coughing spells while running or during exercise, causing them to stop

TABLE 8.2	Subacute/Chronic Nonproductive (Dry) Cough

A. DIAGNOSTIC SCHEMATA

Asthma	Gastroesophageal Reflux Disease (GERD)
Tuberculosis (TB)	Medication (ACE Inhibitors)
Lung Cancer	Pertussis

B. DIFFERENTIAL DIAGNOSIS OF DRY HACKING SUBACUTE OR CHRONIC COUGH

SUBJECTIVE	Asthma	TB	Cancer	GERD	Drugs	Pertussis
Location	N/A	N/A	N/A	N/A	N/A	N/A
Onset	After running for a short while. Daily at 2 to 6 AM	Worse at night in some stages	N/A	Starts within 1 hour after lying down	Within days to years of starting on medication	Sudden and dramatic initially. May last for up to 8 weeks
Quantity	Between 2 and 6 AM coughs several times then stops	Varies	Varies	Varies	Varies	Worse at night
Quality	Dry, hacking	Usually dry, hacking	Dry, hacking	Dry, hacking	Dry, hacking, very mild, not forceful. Can be almost like clearing throat, irritation, urge to cough	Dry, hacking cough >90% have episodic coughing spasm
Setting	Same as onset	Living in close quarters with someone with a chronic cough. Travel to potential endemic TB area	Smoker, history of smoking	Same as onset	Same as onset	Same as onset
Associated symptoms	History or symptoms of allergic rhinitis and/or atopic dermatitis	Weight loss, night sweats, fatigue, malaise	Weight loss, night sweats, fatigue, malaise	History of GERD or frequent heartburn, that is worse at night	None	>15% have trouble breathing after coughing spasm. 30% to 40% of patients have at least one episode of vomiting due to violent coughing spasms

	Asthma	TB	Cancer	GERD	Drugs	Pertussis
Modifying factors	Cough preparations ineffective; Exercising may exacerbate cough; Cough stops shortly after ceasing to exercise	Cough preparations ineffective	Cough preparations ineffective	Cough preparations ineffective. Better with antacids, PPIs, H$_2$ blockers	Cough preparations ineffective	Cough preparations ineffective
OBJECTIVE						
Fever	None	Uncommon in early stages	None	None	None	None or low grade
Auscultation and percussion of lungs	Normally clear but can have expiratory wheezes	Normal breath sounds	Normal breath sounds	Normal breath sounds	Normal breath sounds	Mostly clear but can have inspiratory stridor or expiratory wheezes
Chest x-ray	Normal	Varies	Varies	Normal	Normal	Normal
Other	Evidence of active atopic dermatitis and or allergic rhinitis; Peak flow (PEFR) <80% of predicted value	Positive PPD; Positive acid fast stain of sputum sample; Positive interferon-γ release assay	None	None	Stops several weeks after drug discontinued	None
Usual causative agent	IgE-mediated allergic reaction	*Mycobacterium tuberculosis*	N/A	Acid reflux	ACE Inhibitor	*Bordetella pertussis*

exercising or playing due to the coughing. Sometimes the coughing is so subtle that patients may not associate it with breathing difficulties, so a careful history into the timing and setting of any dry cough is essential to ruling out asthma as a cause. Asthma and the pharmacist's use of assessment skills in the management of patients with asthma are found in Chapter 21.

Tuberculosis

Tuberculosis (TB) is an infectious disease caused by *Mycobacterium tuberculosis.* The infection most commonly develops in the lungs, but extrapulmonary TB is not uncommon and can be found in the pleura, lymphatic system, kidney, central nervous system, and bone or joints. It is commonly transmitted by aerosolized droplets released into the air by coughing. When enough TB bacilli pass through the body's protective barriers (respiratory tract mucosa, nasal hair, and cilia) and begin to grow in alveolar lung tissue, more than 90% of infected patient's immune systems begin working to isolate the infection. Macrophages wall off the small number of TB bacillus forming a granuloma, and no further growth or clinical disease occurs. In more than 90% of patients, this primary infection is asymptomatic or patients think it is a "mild chest cold" as the body walls off the invading bacillus. Patients whose immune systems are functioning have no symptoms and normal chest x-rays. Six to eight weeks later, the only evidence of infection is a positive TB skin test. These walled off infections are called latent TB infections (LTBI). Because of this pathophysiology, more than 90% of the patients who eventually develop active TB do so because of a reactivation of a latent primary infection when the immune system fails to continue to hold the infection in check. The risk for developing active TB is highest within 2 years of the initial infection. In patients with LTBI, the chance of developing active TB can be drastically reduced by using daily isoniazid prophylaxis for 6 to 9 months, which kills off the remaining bacilli within a granuloma. In patients with a compromised immune system (AIDS, organ transplant recipients, and those on $\geq$ 15 mg prednisolone/day or TNF-α inhibitors), an immediate infection ensues usually in the form of an acute pneumonia called a primary progressive TB infection.

While there are many myths and fears regarding the transmission of TB from patients, the body's mechanical defense systems remove most of the bacilli before they reach the alveoli. Generally, people who become infected have been exposed to large numbers of bacilli for a long period of time, meaning they have to live with someone with active TB in a poorly ventilated or closed environment. That is why TB is most common outside the United States and in indigent populations who live in closed cramped living conditions.

Active TB typically presents as a dry hacking cough. Patients have a history of travel to endemic areas, living with indigent families in foreign countries, or being around a person with a chronic cough for a prolonged period. Generally, auscultation and percussion of the lungs are normal and less than half the patients present with fever and/or night sweats. Fatigue, malaise, and weight loss can frequently accompany other symptoms. Patients with active TB generally have abnormal chest x-rays, and a positive TB skin test using PPD (tuberculin purified protein derivative), which is administered intradermally using the Mantoux technique. Generally, >15mm induration (the lump, not the redness) is called a positive test. Greater than 10mm or 5mm are used depending on patients' risk and immune status. Unfortunately, in many countries children are immunized with BCG vaccine (containing an attenuated form of bovine TB that is noninfectious), which confers partial immunity, but generally leaves patients with a lifelong positive PPD. For those patients, a new interferon-γ release assay such as QuantiFERON-TB Gold Test or T-Spot TB Test is much more specific for *Mycobacterium tuberculosis* and results are not altered by previous BCG vaccination as is the PPD.

Cancer

There are two main types of lung cancer. The first is small cell lung cancer (SCLC) previously called oat-cell lung cancer. The other main type is non-small cell lung cancer (NSCLC). More than 85% of all primary lung cancers are due to smoking. The risk of lung cancer increases directly with cumulative cigarette smoking exposure. Fortunately, even for long-term smokers, stopping smoking reduces the patient risk for subsequent lung cancer. Cancers that originate in other organ systems can metastasize to the lungs and cause symptoms mimicking primary lung cancer.

Patients with primary lung cancer present with a subacute or chronic dry hacking cough. Patients with COPD or a productive smoker's cough might note a change in cough frequency or severity or notice blood in their sputum. Patients generally have a significant history of smoking or exposure to secondhand smoke. Most patients without COPD present with normal findings on auscultation and percussion of the lungs. Fever is rare. Patients may present with fatigue, malaise, unexplained weight loss, or some change in their ability to breathe normally. Patients suspected of having lung cancer need a referral for a chest x-ray or computerized tomography of the lungs. Definitive diagnosis of cancer type requires invasive procedures such as lung biopsy to obtain a specimen from the tumor or lesion.

Gastroesophageal Reflux Disease

Reflux disease causes a dry hacking cough when stomach contents reflux into the distal esophagus via an esophageal-tracheobronchial reflex. Classically, associated with heartburn or sour taste in the mouth, more than 40% have no gastrointestinal symptoms. While proton pump inhibitor therapy can help in many patients, in others normalizing the pH has no impact on the cough. Generally, the cough occurs most frequently within an hour of lying down horizontally. Chest x-rays and auscultation of the lungs are normal.

Angiotensin-Converting Enzyme Inhibitors

Angiotensin-converting enzyme (ACE) inhibitors cause a dry hacking cough because they also interfere with the normal breakdown of bradykinins in the lungs. This leads to a stimulation of nitric oxide synthetase, which leads to a local accumulation of NO, an irritant to lung tissue, causing a characteristic cough. The cough is described as mild or hardly a cough at all. Some people feel a sensation in the throat and may seem to be clearing their throat. While incidences have been reported as high as 15%, many times subtle symptoms are overlooked and most literature lists an incidence between 3% and 10%. Like the GERD-induced cough, radiological and physical examination findings are negative. The cough usually occurs within a week to 6 months after initiating ACE inhibitors or increasing the dose. It typically stops within a week of discontinuation of ACE inhibitor therapy, but may take up to a month.

Pertussis (Whooping Cough)

Caused by the bacteria, *Bordetella pertussis*, whooping cough has recently increased in frequency in teenagers and adults because the vaccination only provides protection for about 10 years. Previously, pertussis vaccination was limited to infancy and a booster prior to elementary school because the antigen caused severe adverse effects in teens and adults. The availability of the new, less toxic to adults, acellular antigen in vaccines has enabled the current recommendation of vaccination for teens and adults to prevent the increasing incidence in these groups. While potentially fatal in unvaccinated infants, pertussis presents in a much milder form in adults and teens, without the classical "whoop" seen in infants. It typically presents as a dry hacking cough. Over 90% of adults have violent coughing spasms that can leave patients breathless after the coughing spasm. Over 80% cough during the night, and over one-third have at least one vomiting episode due to a coughing spasm. The cough can last up to 8 weeks. The chest x-ray is negative as is auscultation of the lungs in most patients. In some patients, inspiratory stridor or expiratory wheezes can be heard. Fever is either low grade or absent. Pertussis currently is the primary non-viral cause of acute bronchitis in adults and teenagers, representing less than 10% of all acute bronchitis infections.

• ACUTE/SUBACUTE/CHRONIC COUGH WITH MIXED OR VARIABLE PRODUCTIVITY

Upper Airway Cough Syndrome (Post-Nasal Drip)
Any disease that causes post-nasal drip can cause a cough (see Table 8.3). Usually dry and nonproductive during the day, accumulation of drying discharge overnight can produce some nominal mucous during the first few coughs in the morning. Most patients with upper airway cough syndrome (UACS) have a recent history or signs and symptoms of either allergic rhinitis or a viral URI. The cough is most notable in the first hour immediately after lying down for sleep due to drainage from the sinus cavities and into the throat. Physical examination of the lungs is negative.

Post-Infectious Cough Syndrome
Viral respiratory infections that involve the lower respiratory tract can result in a lingering cough lasting 2 to 8 weeks' with few physical findings consistent with infection. While the exact mechanism is unknown and probably multifactorial, the viral infection is thought to create enough irritation and inflammation to cause the cough to continue long past the presence of an infectious process. The continuing cough is the result of bronchial hypersensitivity and hyperresponsiveness manifested as a cough. In one study of 184 adults with subacute cough, 82% had either post-infectious cough syndrome (PICS) or UACS. Physical findings are minimal. If a cough lasts more than 8 weeks, then further diagnostic workup is warranted, looking for chronic causes including asthma, allergic rhinitis, TB, and cancer.

Influenza/Viral Pneumonia
Viral pneumonias represent about 20% of community-acquired pneumonias in adults and a much higher percentage in children. Influenza is the most common and best studied viral infection. Other common causes are respiratory syncytial virus, adenovirus, parainfluenza, and coronavirus. The presentation is quite variable, ranging from influenza with abrupt onset, severe systemic symptoms such as fever, malaise, aches pains, and chills. The development of a cough due to other viruses causes milder symptoms, and the illness evolves more slowly with many having symptoms of a viral URI as the initial presentation. Leukocytosis with a neutrophilic response and elevated serum procalcitonin levels are uncommon.

Congestive Heart Failure
In older patients with a long history of hypertension or coronary heart disease, congestive heart failure can be a cause of cough. Typically, fluid accumulates as edema in the lower extremeties during the daytime. Approximately 2 to 3 hours after laying

TABLE 8.3	Acute/Subacute Mixed/Variable Productivity Cough

A. DIAGNOSTIC SCHEMATA

Upper Airway Cough Syndrome (UACS)   Influenza/Viral Pneumonia   Atypical Pneumonia
Post-Infectious Cough Syndrome (PICS)   Congestive Heart Failure (CHF)

B. DIFFERENTIAL DIAGNOSIS OF ACUTE/SUBACUTE/CHRONIC COUGH OF MIXED OR VARIABLE PRODUCTIVITY

SUBJECTIVE	UACS	PICS	Influenza/Viral	CHF	Atypical Pneumonia
Location	N/A	N/A	N/A	N/A	N/A
Onset	During or after a viral URI or allergic rhinitis	After a viral respiratory infection	Sudden onset	Starts about 2 to 4 hours after lying down	Develops over several days/weeks
Quantity	Thought to be caused by post-nasal drip (PND) occurs frequently during the first hour after lying down to sleep	Lasts 2 to 8 weeks postinfection	Varies	Excess fluid pooled in lower extremities redistributes to vascular system	Mild symptoms that may worsen with time
Quality	Usually dry. Potentially, some productivity in the morning	Usually dry. Potentially some productivity in the morning	Initially dry, can change to mildly productive	Dry or unknown in early stages. Productive as pulmonary edema progresses	Initially dry but can progress to productive
Setting	Same as onset	Recent viral respiratory tract infection	Exposure to influenza	Same as onset	Same as onset
Associated symptoms	History or symptoms of allergic rhinitis and/or viral URI	Recent history of URI	High fever, malaise, myalgia, arthralgia, sore throat, runny nose (20%)	PND, orthopnea, pedal edema	Fever, malaise, myalgia, arthralgia, sore throat, possible GI symptoms
Modifying factors	Antihistamines and decongestants can help with cough	Cough preparations ineffective	Cough preparations effective in pneumonia phase	Goes away in minutes after patient sits or stands. Cough preparations ineffective. Sleeping propped up with extra pillows prevents awakening	Cough preparations effective

(continued)

TABLE 8.3 Acute/Subacute Mixed/Variable Productivity Cough (*Continued*)

OBJECTIVE	UACS	PICS	Influenza/Viral	CHF	Atypical Pneumonia
Fever	None or low grade	None	High fever	None	Yes, but severity varies, generally low grade
Auscultation and percussion of lungs	Normal breath sounds	Normal breath sounds, occasionally expiratory wheezes	Clear to rhonchi, crackles, and expiratory wheezes	Crackles in both lung bases. May have dullness over crackles	Crackles, rhonchi with occasional expiratory wheezes
Chest x-ray	Normal	Normal	Normal to feathery interstitial infiltrates	Enlarged heart, fluid in base of both lungs	Various infiltrates (feathery, consolidated, interstitial)
Other	Signs of allergic rhinitis or viral URI	None	Positive POS tests for influenza A or B	Edema, tachypnea, tachycardia	Elevated cold agglutinin titers in *Mycoplasma* (50% to 75%)
Usual causative agent	Post-nasal drip	Hyperresponsive/hypersensitive airways	Type A and B influenza viruses, RSV	Fluid in alveolae	Atypical bacteria (*Chlamydiophila, Mycoplasma, Legionella*)

down, the edematous fluid redistributes itself in the vascular compartment, overcoming the failing heart's pumping capability and causing fluid to leak into the lungs. Patients wake up coughing, and/or short of breath several hours after retiring. Sitting up or standing up causes the excess fluid to repool in the periphery, reducing cardiac workload and causing the symptoms to go away. This is called paroxysmal nocturnal dyspnea or PND. Patients realize over time that sleeping propped up with several pillows or sleeping in a recliner prevents those nocturnal events. That is called orthopnea and is typically described in terms of the number of pillows required to sleep (e.g., three pillow orthopnea). The cough can range from dry to productive depending on the severity of the heart failure with frank pulmonary edema presenting with a productive cough. Physical examination of the lungs in the early stages is generally normal except for cardiac enlargement upon percussion and peripheral edema due to excess fluid. Once pulmonary edema occurs at any posture, crackles in both lungs or absent breath sounds predominate physical findings along with a productive cough.

Atypical Pneumonia

Atypical pneumonia was coined to describe pneumonias that presented differently from typical bacterial pneumonia. While *Mycoplasma, Chlamydia*, and *Legionella* species are usually included in the definition of *atypical*. Also many experts include viral and other bacterial or rickettsial pathogens. All three primary agents are bacterial but do not cause the classical symptoms or responses of bacterial pneumonia. Because of its relative lack of acuity, atypical pneumonia has been referred to as "walking pneumonia." Atypical pathogens represent almost 25% of the causes of community-acquired pneumonia in adults.

Mycoplasma pneumoniae is most common in school-aged children and young adults. The onset of illness is gradual and initial symptoms may include headache, malaise, and low-grade fever. Patients generally feel worse than physical findings would indicate. The cough is usually nonproductive to mildly productive and symptoms involving the upper respiratory tract while not typical are not uncommon. The white blood count is normal in the vast majority of patients, but in severe disease the body does mount a neutrophilic response typical of bacterial pneumonias. Chest x-ray abnormalities are typically feathery rather than consolidated infiltrates.

Chlamydophila pneumoniae is a less frequent cause of atypical pneumonia, but parallels *Mycoplasma* in terms of clinical presentation. *C. pneumoniae* differs from *Mycoplasma* in its 21-day incubation period and the presence of laryngitis in most patients as a typical symptom.

Legionella infections are the least common atypical pathogen. Clinical presentation most closely resembles that of classical bacterial pneumonia with the exception of minimal to mild sputum production. *Legionella* infection should be suspected in patients with pneumonia accompanied by a high fever (>39°C), gastrointestinal symptoms, especially diarrhea, a Gram stain of sputum that reveals lots of neutrophils but no bacteria. Smokers, patients with chronic lung disease, or immunosuppressed patients are at higher risk. Elevated liver function tests are also a common finding. Radiologically, *Legionella* infections tend to be more like bacterial pneumonia. Urinary antigens can be diagnostic for the main serotype but vary with severity of disease.

• KEY REFERENCES

1. Gonzales R, Sande MA. Uncomplicated acute bronchitis. *Ann Intern Med*. 2000;133:981-991.
2. Horsburgh CR, Rubin EJ. Latent tuberculosis infection in the united states. *N Engl J Med*. 2011; 364: 1441-1448.

3. Pai M, Zwerling A, Menzies D. Systematic review: T-cell based assays for the diagnosis of latent tuberculosis infection: an update. *Ann Intern Med.* 2008;149:177-184.
4. McCool FD. Global physiology and pathophysiology of cough. *Chest.* 2006;129:48S-53S.
5. Pratter MR. Overview of common causes of cough. *Chest.* 2006;129:59S-62S.
6. Kwon NH, Oh MJ, Min TH, Lee BJ, Choi DC. Causes and clinical features of subacute cough. *Chest.* 2006;129:1142-1147.
7. Goldsobel AB, Chipps BE. Cough in the pediatric population. *J Pediatr.* 2010;156:352-358.
8. Chung KF, Pavord ID. Chronic cough 1: prevalence, pathogenesis and causes of chronic cough. *Lancet.* 2008;371:1364-1374.
9. Eversten J, Baumgardner DJ, Regenry A, Banerjee I. Diagnosis and management of pneumonia and bronchitis in outpatient primary care practices. *Prim Care Resp J.* 2010;19:237-241.

CASE 8.1

Roby Tussin, a 68-year-old male, presents to the pharmacy 4 months after a bout of viral pneumonia. When you ask how he is feeling, he tells you that while he occasionally still gets tired, he has not been able to get rid of his cough, which is dry and hacking and worse at night.

List three possible causes for his cough. Explain your rationale.

_____

_____

_____

_____

_____

List three questions you would ask Roby. Explain your rationale.

_____

_____

_____

_____

_____

List four diagnostic tests or physical examinations you would order or perform to help make the diagnosis. Explain your rationale.

_____

_____

_____

_____

_____

CASE 8.2

You are introduced to TW, a famous 82-year-old golfer at a Tucson AZ golf function. He has been visiting here for the last 3 months overseeing the construction of a golf course he designed. When he finds out you are a pharmacist, he asks if there is anything stronger than promethazine with codeine for coughing spells that have been bothering him for the last 4 weeks. It seems to be worse at night. He finished a 10-day course of amoxicillin 2 weeks ago for a cough "that went to his chest." He also complains about his recent 10-lb weight gain and the shot of him on TV last night made him look "fat as a hog." "Even my feet are getting fat! Why even my favorite slippers are getting tight." An excellent historian, TW tells you about his long-standing hypertension, which is treated with carvedilol and doxazosin (also for his prostate), and coronary artery disease that resulted in a tiny heart attack that led to a four-vessel CABG 15 years ago. He also takes aspirin, tiotropium inhaler for his smoking-induced COPD, and atorvastatin. You notice that his breathing appears to somewhat rapid.

Given TW's history and his current complaints, list three possible causes for his coughing attacks. Explain your rationale.

_____

_____

_____

_____

_____

List six questions, examinations, or tests you would ask/order/perform to help clarify his diagnosis. Explain your rationale.

_____

_____

_____

_____

_____

Chest Pain

1. Accurately identify the most likely etiology when patients present with chest pain, through history, diagnostic tests, and patient findings on examination to enable the appropriate recommendation of effective treatment or referral to an appropriate provider.

2. Use the knowledge of the pathophysiology, etiology, and common presentations of chest pain as a primary symptom to review prescription orders for appropriateness and to accurately educate patients about their disease and its treatment.

In 2006, chest pain and symptoms related to myocardial ischemia were responsible for almost 10% of the 120 million visits to emergency rooms. In the U.S. chest pain and the diseases associated with chest pain are commonly dealt with by pharmacists in almost all practice settings. Approximately, 15 million prescriptions for statins are filled by pharmacists every month, not to mention the larger number of prescriptions for other drugs used to treat angina and causative diseases. National guidelines recommend that most patients discharged after myocardial infarction be placed on as many as four to five medications in addition to their pre-hospital medication regimen. At every visit, pharmacists involved in the management of patients with diabetes, dyslipidemia, and essential hypertension screen patients for symptoms of angina pectoris as a complication of those diseases. Similarly, pharmacists involved in anticoagulation clinics screen for symptoms of pulmonary embolism, a complication of deep vein thrombosis. Therefore, it is important for the pharmacist to understand the various causes of chest pain.

• ETIOLOGY

Not all chest pain is cardiac in nature. In addition to angina, pulmonary embolism, pleurisy, pericarditis, esophagitis, various musculoskeletal causes, and hyperventilation may present with symptoms of chest pain. The most common serious cause of chest pain is atherosclerotic heart disease or coronary artery disease. The specific pathological process of how cholesterol-laden plaques build up in the coronary arteries and eventually cause a myocardial infarction is discussed in more detail in the Chapter 19 on dyslipidemia. Atherosclerotic strokes are discussed in the Chapter 13 on headaches. The most common initial symptom of coronary artery disease is angina pectoris. However, the disease can also present either as a ventricular dysrhythmia that causes sudden death or as a myocardial infarction. Plaque buildup begins as young adults slowly increase the occlusion of the coronary arteries. Once a coronary artery reaches 75% occlusion, patients may begin to have symptoms of angina at times of increased myocardial oxygen demand due to exercise, strong emotions, and cold temperatures. Local tissue hypoxia in cardiac muscle creates the classical cardiac pain seen in angina. Occlusions above 90% may lead to chronic hypoxia and symptoms even at rest. Patients with significant plaque deposition are at risk for a myocardial infarction. As part of the process of plaque deposition and eventual occlusion of the artery lumen, an inflammatory process is created between the plaques and the intima of the artery. For unclear reasons, that inflammation eventually causes the plaque to rupture, exposing the intimal wall to platelets, which begin adhering to the rupture area and quickly aggregating to form a clot. Clot formation may result in 100% occlusion. This lack of oxygen causes the cardiac muscle distal to the clot to die, leading to a myocardial infarction and its complications.

• DIAGNOSIS

Diagnosis of the exact cause of chest pain requires a careful history of the nature of the pain, circumstances surrounding its onset, physical examination, as well as multiple diagnostic examinations, such as electrocardiogram (ECG) or spiral computerized tomography (Table 9.1). In addition, a variety of blood tests, such as troponin I and D-dimer, may be used to discover the likely cause.

• CORONARY ARTERY DISEASE

Coronary artery disease (CAD) consists of a sequence of symptoms usually indicating progressively worsening atherosclerosis and narrowing of the coronary artery. Angina pectoris (the chest pain of CAD) has the smallest amount of obstruction

TABLE 9.1 Chest Pain

A. DIAGNOSTIC SCHEMATA FOR CHEST PAIN

Angina Pectoris

Unstable Angina

Non–ST-Segment-Elevation Myocardial Infarction (NSTEMI)

ST-Segment-Elevation Myocardial Infarction (STEMI)

Hyperventilation Syndrome

Pulmonary Embolism

B. DIFFERENTIAL DIAGNOSIS OF CHEST PAIN

SUBJECTIVE	Angina Pectoris	Unstable Angina	NSTEMI	STEMI	Hyperventilation Syndrome	Pulmonary Embolism
Location	Substernal with radiation down left arm	Substernal with radiation down left arm	Substernal with radiation down left arm	Substernal with radiation down left arm	Substernal with radiation down left arm	Peripheral, anywhere in lung field
Onset	Sudden	Sudden	Sudden	Sudden	Slow onset	Sudden
Quality	Episodic crushing, squeezing, tightness	Prolonged crushing squeezing, tightness	Prolonged crushing, squeezing, tightness	Prolonged crushing, squeezing, tightness	Crushing, squeezing, tightness	Varies. Usually sharp and pleuritic
Quantity	Severe pain, forcing patient to stop activity	Severe pain, forcing patient to stop activity	Severe pain, forcing patient to stop activity	Severe pain, forcing patient to stop activity	Severe pain, forcing patient to stop activity	Varies
Setting	Brought on by specific activity such as exercise, emotion	Hx of previous angina	Hx of previous angina	Hx of previous angina	Hyperventilation brought on by severe anxiety, fear, or panic attack	Post-op, hx of DVT, bedridden
Associated symptoms	SOB	SOB	Diaphoresis, nausea, SOB, vomiting, syncope	Diaphoresis, nausea, SOB, vomiting, syncope	Circumoral paresthesia	SOB, dyspnea, calf pain
Modifying factors	Made worse in cold weather, during exercise or periods of high emotion	None, unremitting pain unaffected by sublingual NTG	None, unremitting pain unaffected by sublingual NTG	None, unremitting pain unaffected by sublingual NTG	Anxiety, fear, panic bring it on	Shallow breaths
	Pain relieved by Nitroglycerin (NTG)				Breathing into a paper bag makes it better	

OBJECTIVE						
	ST segment depression	ST segment depression	ST segment depression	ST segment elevation	Tachypnea, tachycardia	No breath sounds over infarct area. Elevated D-dimer levels. Lesions or deficits on spiral CT or V/Q scan. Ultrasound of calf shows clot
	No change in cardiac enzymes	No change in cardiac enzymes	Elevated troponin levels	Elevated troponin, CK^{MB}, AST, S&S CHF		

(Continued)

TABLE 9.1	Chest Pain (Continued)

A. DIAGNOSTIC SCHEMATA FOR CHEST PAIN (continued)

Pericarditis
Pleurisy
Esophagitis
Costochondritis
Chest Wall Twinge Syndrome
Mitral Valve Prolapse

B. DIFFERENTIAL DIAGNOSIS OF CHEST PAIN (continued)

SUBJECTIVE	Pericarditis	Pleurisy	Esophagitis	Costochondritis	Chest Wall Twinge Syndrome	Mitral Valve Prolapse
Location	Substernal with radiation to left trapezius	Peripheral lung fields	Epigastric	Cartilage between rib and sternum	Left anterior chest	Over the apex of the heart
Onset	Sudden	Sudden	Slow onset	Slow onset	Slow onset	Sudden
Quality	Sharp	Sharp	Burning, gnawing sensation	Dull ache	Sharp	Sharp, sticking
Quantity	Severe continuous pain	Severe pain worse when breathing	Varies	Mild to moderate pain only when breathing	Moderate to severe pain only when breathing	Episodic lasts seconds to hours
Setting	May coincide with heartbeat	Lung infection or malignancy	Worse when lying down, hx of large meals or ethanol ingestion	None	N/A	None
Associated symptoms	SOB	SOB	N/A	N/A	N/A	Fatigue, palpitations
Modifying factors	Lying down, swallowing, deep breath, movement make it worse; Leaning forward, breathing shallowly make it better	Deep breaths make it worse; Shallow breaths make it better	Worse when lying down, hx of large meals or ethanol ingestion	Breathing or movement can make it worse; Shallow breathing and NSAIDs make it better	Bending over and taking deep breaths make it worse; Shallow breathing makes it better	None
OBJECTIVE	ECG changes; Friction rub during systole; Splinting	Friction rub on auscultation; Splinting	None for acute. For GERD then endoscopy is performed	Pain on palpation of the painful area (point tenderness)	Splinting with pain	Upon auscultation of the heart, a systolic click followed by a late systolic murmur. Timing and loudness of sound changes with standing and squatting

of the coronary lumen. The presence of angina means that the patient is at serious risk of atherosclerotic plaque rupturing and causing a clot and more complete lumen occlusion as occurs in a myocardial infarction. Myocardial infarction, which can lead to fatal complications, such as dysrhythmias, congestive heart failure (CHF), and cardiogenic shock, is one of the leading causes of death worldwide. Chest pain of CAD is classically described as a crushing, squeezing, or tightness, "like there is an elephant on my chest," and is usually located beneath the sternum (substernal). Pain may radiate to the left arm, jaw, shoulder, and back. Angina may be confused with indigestion, or other causes such as panic disorders especially in women, who are more likely than men to have other sensations/symptoms, e.g., burning or stinging sensations. Also, women may perceive other symptoms, e.g., heart flutter, SOB, and lightheadedness as anxiety, whereas men usually perceive them as chest pain.

Angina Pectoris (Ischemic Heart Disease)

Pain occurs when cardiac muscle oxygen demand exceeds its supply. The fixed decrease in the lumen of the coronary arteries prevents on-demand increases in the supply of oxygen. This is the definition of *ischemia*. There are three primary causes of angina. First, myocardial oxygen demand increases with increased cardiac workload. Things that increase workload and cause the pain of angina include hypertension (pumping against high peripheral resistance), physical activity or exercise, which increases the heart rate, increased intravascular volume (heart is forced to work harder), and CHF. Second, because epinephrine and norepinephrine increase the force and rate of contraction, anything that causes the release or mimics catecholamines will increase myocardial oxygen demand. So emotions such as anger or fear, cold temperatures, hypoglycemic episodes, CHF, and drugs that stimulate the adrenergic branch of the autonomic nervous system such as cocaine, nicotine, decongestants, and sympathomimetic bronchodilators such as albuterol will cause angina. Finally, diseases that create overall hypoxemia such as cigarette smoking, asthma, and COPD can make the patient more susceptible to angina pain.

Angina pain goes away when the cause for increased myocardial oxygen demand is removed or corrected, e.g., stopping physical activity, calming down, or using nitroglycerin to decrease cardiac workload by decreasing venous return to the heart by dilation of peripheral veins in the legs.

In addition to the history suggestive of angina, stress ECGs will show classical ST-segment depression as the affected area of the heart muscle becomes ischemic with increased cardiac workload. Also, CT coronary artery angiography can pinpoint the specific location of the lesion(s). Myocardial perfusion imaging at rest, with technetium or thallium, can also be used to identify ischemic areas.

Acute Coronary Syndrome

Acute coronary syndrome (ACS) is one of three conditions: unstable angina (UA), an immediate harbinger of one of two types of myocardial infarctions; non–ST-segment-elevation myocardial infarction (NSTEMI); and ST-segment-elevation myocardial infarction (STEMI). In all three syndromes, thrombosis of a coronary artery has begun and chest pain continues at rest or lasts 20 to 30 minutes and does not stop when the inciting cause is discontinued or does not stop with the use of sublingual nitroglycerin (NTG). ACS is a medical emergency and if the diagnosis is confirmed for any of the three syndromes, then immediate and intensive interventions are required to prevent serious myocardial damage and death. Diagnosis of ACS depends on clinical presentation, the presence or absence of serum biomarkers, and an abnormal ECG.

While most patients present with classical angina-like chest pain, as many as 20% to 30% of patients present with atypical symptoms and may complain of different kinds of chest pain or no chest pain at all. Women, the elderly, and patients with diabetes more commonly present with atypical symptoms. In patients with risk factors (smoking, hypertension, dyslipidemia, males >55 years of age, family history of CAD, and diabetes), care must be taken not to assume that absence of classical angina like pain eliminates the potential for ACS or angina pectoris.

The three cardiac biomarkers currently used to evaluate ACS are substances that are released into the blood stream when cardiac muscle is damaged. Troponin I and T are regulatory proteins associated with cardiac muscle contraction. Currently, high-sensitivity serum troponin I and T are the most specific and accurate in diagnosis of myocardial infarction. Levels begin to rise 3 to 12 hours after infarction, peaking at 24 hours. Any other type of damage to cardiac muscles, e.g., contusion, myocarditis, or catheter ablation, as well as impaired renal function may also lead to troponin elevations. Myoglobin is a low molecular weight muscle protein found in cardiac and skeletal muscle. Serum levels are detected from 1 to 4 hours after cardiac muscle damage and peak 6 to 7 hours later, making it the earliest marker to be affected. Any kind of muscle injury, trauma, and renal impairment can also elevate myoglobin levels. Finally, the MB fraction of creatine kinase (CK^{MB}), an enzyme involved in the transfer of high-energy phosphate groups is specific for cardiac muscle. The pattern of release is similar to troponin. Because of the kinetics of their release, CK^{MB} and troponin I and T should be reevaluated 6 to 12 hours after the original levels were drawn.

ECG changes are important in distinguishing between the three entities that comprise ACS. In UA and NSTEMI, the findings are typical of ischemic ST depression or T-wave inversion. Because there is little or no scarring, Q waves are formed so the ECG returns to normal within weeks after the insult. STEMI on the other hand shows acute ST-segment elevation, usually followed by a depressed Q wave, which develops hours later and remains as evidence of a past myocardial infarction. Old terminology used to refer to NSTEMI as non–Q-wave myocardial infarction and STEMI as a Q-wave myocardial infarction.

Unstable Angina
Patients with UA usually have a history of stable angina pectoris with a recent history of acceleration in frequency, or persistence of angina, or angina that is induced by less activity than usual. The pain of UA is similar to angina, but it persists or is unresponsive to usual sublingual NTG. ECG findings range from normal to either ST-segment depression or T-wave inversion. Serum troponin I and T, creatine kinase, MB fragment (CK^{MB}), and serum myoglobin levels are normal.

NSTEMI
NSTEMI is a form of heart attack. Patients who tell you they had a "mild" heart attack probably are referring to NSTEMI. Patients with NSTEMI have enough occlusion to cause heart muscle damage, which releases cardiac biomarkers (serum troponin I/T, CK^{MB}, and myoglobin), but not enough damage to permanently alter ECG findings.

STEMI
STEMI is the classical form of myocardial infarction with increased levels of cardiac biomarkers and marked changes in the ECG, primarily ST-segment elevation. Previously known as Q-wave myocardial infarction because the amount of muscle mass

damaged by the infarction is enough to create significant scar tissue that causes a negative deflection of the Q wave. They may take several days to develop and are an indicator of a previous myocardial infarction. STEMIs can be regularly accompanied by other symptoms such as nausea, vomiting, diaphoresis, and SOB.

• OTHER CARDIAC CAUSES OF CHEST PAIN

The heart can be the origin of other causes of chest pain.

Pericarditis

Pericarditis is an inflammation of the lining or sac surrounding the heart. It can be caused by a variety of infectious agents, e.g., bacteria, fungi, and viruses, autoimmune disorders, renal failure, and trauma. The pain is generally described as sharp with radiation to the left trapezius area. Swallowing, lying down, and deep breathing make it worse, while shallow breathing and leaning forward make it better. Uremic pericarditis typically presents with little or no pain. Objective findings may include fever if infectious, or evidence of trauma to the chest. Auscultation of the heart may reveal a pericardial friction rub in 60% to 85% of patients, usually associated with systole and the movement of the heart against the inflamed pericardium. Echocardiogram can be used to detect pericardial effusion.

Mitral Valve Prolapse

Seen in 5% of the population with women having twice the incidence of men, mitral valve prolapse (MVP) is asymptomatic in most patients. Abnormal growth of valve tissue causes a portion of the valve to "flop back" into the atrium. Pain associated with MVP is generally described as sharp and sticking, lasting from seconds to hours and located at the apex of the heart. Auscultation of the heart reveals a midsystolic click, followed by a late systolic murmur. Timing of the click, length of murmur, and occasional loudness change from supine to standing or squatting or during a valsalva maneuver, can be diagnostic.

• RESPIRATORY CAUSES OF CHEST PAIN

Pulmonary Embolism

A pulmonary embolism (PE) is an infarct of the lung due to the release of a venous blood clot from the periphery that makes its way into the pulmonary arteriolar system, usually due to a deep vein thrombosis (DVT) in the calf or leg. Infarct size is determined by the size of the pulmonary vessel occluded by the clot. Large infarcts can be fatal. The onset of chest pain is sudden and is described as a sharp pleuritic type pain associated with dyspnea. Patients may also have calf pain and/or swelling.

Objectively, the patient may have both tachypnea and tachycardia depending on the size of the infarct. Palpation of the calf may be painful and a Homan sign is positive in about 25% of patients with thrombophlebitis, an inflammation of the veins that leads to clot formation. Stasis and trauma are the two leading causes of DVT. DVT development is so common that hospitalized patients, patients going to surgery, and those with cancer are either fitted with mechanical devices that increase venous return from the lower extremities or are placed on injectable anticoagulants such as enoxaparin to prevent them.

There are several diagnostic tests that are used for PE and DVT. To detect the presence of a DVT, an ultrasound of the calf is used. Spiral CT scans of the lungs is the test of choice for PE. Also, occasionally, a V/Q scan (lung scan) that identifies perfusion defects through scintilography. Finally, D-dimer levels, a fibrin fragment that stays in the blood stream for several days after a thrombotic event, are elevated. Levels < 500 µg/L can help rule out PE as a cause of chest pain.

Pleurisy

Pleurisy is chest pain associated with inflammation of the pleural lining of the lungs. Bacterial pneumonia, TB, PE, and malignancy are possible causes. Chest pain is described as sharp and is made worse when taking a deep breath (pleuritic pain) and is usually located laterally at the periphery of the lung fields. Sometimes pleurisy with pneumonia may be described as a right upper quadrant abdominal pain. Objective findings on auscultation may include a friction rub over the inflamed area and findings typical of pneumonia (crackles, absence of breath sounds over consolidated areas).

Hyperventilation Syndrome

Patients present with a crushing, squeezing substernal chest pain that may radiate down the left arm. It is caused by fear or panic induced hyperventilation, which blows off too much carbon dioxide, leading to chest tightness or pain. Many patients also present with circumoral paresthesias (numbness and tingling). Breathing into a paper bag relieves the chest pain by increasing carbon dioxide blood levels.

• MUSCULOSKELETAL CAUSES OF CHEST PAIN

Chest pain due to musculoskeletal causes is very common. Any chest pain that can be reproduced by palpation of the location of the pain or by movement of the upper extremities is likely musculoskeletal in origin. So both history and physical examination are important in establishing a musculoskeletal cause.

Trauma/Rib Fracture

Trauma to the chest and ribs is a common cause of chest pain. A careful history for even minor trauma or muscle overuse is important. Do not overlook hard coughing due to a respiratory infection, which can occasionally induce a rib fracture. Physical examination can help rule out trauma-related chest pain. First, observe the thorax for trauma (hematomas, bruises, lacerations, etc.). Next, have the patient point to the location. Palpate that area for tenderness, as well as other areas of the chest. Next, flex each arm horizontally by lifting the elbow and pulling it across the chest. Next, have the patient look up at the ceiling while you pull both arms backward. If a rib fracture is suspected, do the compression test by pushing the sternum toward the spine, while supporting the patients back with the other hand. Replication of the pain by these maneuvers confirms traumatic causes. Thoracic x-ray can demonstrate fractures.

Chest Wall Twinge Syndrome (Precordial Catch)

Patients complain of a sharp pain or "catch" lasting 30 seconds to 3 minutes usually located on the left anterior chest, which is worse with deep breathing and better with shallow breathing. It can be located elsewhere on the chest and some report onset while bending over at the waist. The cause is unknown but is thought to be due to intercostal muscle spasm.

Costochondritis

Costochondritis, an inflammation of the cartilage between the rib end and the sternum, is another common cause of chest pain. Costochondritis presents with a dull pain near the sternum, which can be made worse by respiratory motion and shoulder or arm movement. Palpation over rib cartilage near the sternum, where the patient has indicated the pain's location replicates the pain.

• GASTROINTESTINAL CAUSES OF CHEST PAIN

Esophagitis, Acute or Chronic (GERD)

Esophagitis is the most common cause of chest pain seen in the emergency room. Patients present with a history of recent overindulgence of food and ethanol or intermittent pain when lying down. While the pain is usually described as "heartburn" (a gnawing, burning-like pain), it can present in other forms. A "GI cocktail" may be given to confirm esophagitis as a cause after ECG and biomarker tests are negative. GI cocktails are usually a combination of liquid antacid and viscous lidocaine occasionally with a liquid anticholinergic. However, the literature indicates the combination is no better than liquid antacid alone.

• KEY REFERENCES

1. Kontos MC, Diercks DB, Kirk JD. Emergency department and office-based evaluation of patients with chest pain. *Mayo Clin Proc.* 2010;85:284-299.
2. Steurer J, Held, U, Schmid D, et al. Clinical value of diagnostic instruments for ruling out acute coronary syndrome in patients with chest pain: a systematic review. *Emerg Med J.* 2010;27:896-902.
3. Kosowsky JM. Approach to the ED patient with "low risk" chest pain. *Emerg Med Clin North Am.* 2011;29: 721-727.
4. Fichet DH, Theroux P, Brophy JM, et al. Assessment and management of acute coronary syndromes: a Canadian perspective on current guideline-recommended treatment—Part 1: non-ST-segment elevation ACS. *Can J Cardiol.* 2011;27:S387-S402.
5. Fichet DH, Theroux P, Brophy JM, et al. Assessment and management of acute coronary syndromes: a Canadian perspective on current guideline-recommended treatment—Part 2: ST-segment elevation myocardial infarction. *Can J Cardiol.* 2011;27:S402-S412.
6. Amsterdam EA, Kirk JD, Bluemke DA, et al. Testing of low risk patients presenting to the emergency department with chest pain: a scientific statement from the American Heart Association. *Circulation.* 2010;122:1756-1776.
7. Yiadom MY. Acute coronary syndrome clinical presentations and diagnostic approaches in the emergency department. *Emerg Med Clin North Am.* 2011;29:689-697.
8. Arslanian-Engoren C, Engoen M. Physioligical and anatomical bases for sex differences in pain and nausea as presenting symptoms of acute coronary syndromes. *Heart Lung.* 2010;39:386-393.

CASE 9.1

Ferf Barfel, a 56-year-old overweight male, is playing golf when he has a sudden onset of severe chest pain. A 911 call brings him to the ER. The only other recent history is a visit 2 days ago for various aches and pains of 3 days' duration after falling off his golf cart when he forgot to set the brake and it rolled over his left lower leg. To stop it Ferf had to hang on for dear life, putting all his considerable weight behind it to keep it from rolling down the hill. He hurt his chest, back, and shoulder in the process. Examination and x-rays were negative at the time. Ferf's problem list is as follows.

1990	Obesity
2001	Hypertension
2001	Hypercholesterolemia
2008	Type 2 diabetes mellitus

List four likely causes of Ferf's chest pain. Explain your rationale.

_____

_____

_____

_____

_____

List 10 questions, diagnostic tests, or physical examinations you would ask, order, or perform to find the cause of his chest pain. Explain your rationale.

_____

_____

_____

_____

_____

Heartburn and Abdominal Pain

1. Accurately identify the most likely etiology when patients present with heartburn or abdominal pain, thorough history, diagnostic tests, and ppropriate patient findings on examination, to enable the appropriate recommendation of effective treatment or referral to an appropriate provider.

2. Use the knowledge of the pathophysiology, etiology, and common presentation of abdominal complaints as a primary symptom to review prescription orders for appropriateness and to accurately educate patients about their disease and its treatment.

3. Use the knowledge of the pathophysiology, etiology, and common presentation of diseases with heartburn or abdominal pain as a primary symptom to accurately interpret the diagnostic process to advise regarding the most appropriate prescription therapy.

• ETIOLOGY

Heartburn and abdominal pain plus associated symptoms are common presentations in ambulatory and urgent care. Gastroenteritis, appendicitis, and peptic ulcer disease are common causes of abdominal pain. Each accounts for 11% to 13% of patients seen with abdominal pain in the emergency room. Similarly, gynecological and urinary tract problems account for 9% and 7%, respectively. The most common cause (20%) is nonspecific. Patients who present with symptoms usually associated with the gastrointestinal tract (heartburn, indigestion, nausea, vomiting, diarrhea, bloating, or abdominal distention) may actually have diseases in the genitourinary tract, central nervous system, cardiovascular system, or endocrine system, or they may be due to medications or metabolic abnormalities. Therefore, the assessment of abdominal symptoms must include considerations of problems associated with multiple other organ systems or exogenous issues. Most of these disorders require referral to definitive care, so it is important for pharmacists to recognize common features when patients request help with self-care with nonprescription products.

• DIAGNOSIS

The diagnosis of the exact etiology of abdominal pain and heartburn can be difficult as evidenced by the high percentage of cases in which no specific cause can be found on the first encounter in the emergency room. Part of the problem is the lack of specific innervation of the visceral organs. Pain in one organ may be felt in any of several places. The literature is full of descriptions of "classical presentations" of diseases of the abdomen. However, atypical presentations are common especially in the elderly. For example, the classic pain of gallbladder disease is described as sharp, colicky right upper quadrant pain. Unfortunately, 25% of patients with biliary disease do not present with the "classical" symptoms. Figure 10.1 shows the location of "classical" pain by external anatomical location of the abdominal surface.

Diagnostic accuracy is dependent on a careful history and physical examination, since there are few laboratory tests that can specifically diagnose diseases that produce abdominal symptoms (Table 10.1). Location of the pain, the type of discomfort, and associated symptoms are usually required to narrow the list of possible diagnoses. Due to expense and exposure to radiation, imaging studies are reserved to diagnose more severe symptoms, or those which evade diagnosis on initial evaluation, especially if something potentially life threatening is suspected. Usually, abdominal x-ray, endoscopy, abdominal ultrasound, or CT scan are used to obtain a specific diagnosis.

• DISEASES THAT PRESENT WITH HEARTBURN OR INDIGESTION

These related disorders usually present with a burning, gnawing discomfort located in the epigastric area of the abdomen. Some describe it as heartburn or indigestion. Medically, it can be called dyspepsia. Peptic ulcer disease is either a duodenal or gastric ulcer. Ulcers occur when an imbalance occurs between acid production and mucosal defense mechanisms. Medications such as NSAIDs, corticosteroids, and *Helicobacter pylori* (*H. pylori*) facilitate the breakdown of mucosal barriers in both the stomach and the duodenum. Peptic ulcer disease, if untreated, may lead to upper gastrointestinal bleeding and/or perforation. Treatment of these disorders centers on

```
                    xiphoid process
                     (substernal)
                         |
                    /  epigastric  \
                   /  duodenal ulcer  \
                  /       PUD          \
                 /        GERD          \
  right         /    gastric ulcer       \     left
costal margin  /           |              \  costal margin
              /            |               \
- - - - - - -/             |                \- - - - - - -
  RUQ    hepatitis/hepatomegaly |   splenic abscess
         cholecystitis      |   splenomegaly         LUQ
         colon (hepatic flexure)|  colon(splenic flexure)
                            |
                            |
                  acute pancreatitis
                            |
                     umbilical
- - - - - - - - - - - - - - -|- - - - - - - - - - - - - - -
                  early appendicitis
                            |
                            |
                            |
  RLQ    appendicitis       |   colon(transverse)
         colon (cecum)      |   kidney stone        LLQ
         hernia             |   hernia
         kidney stone       |   diverticulitis
         gynecological (testicular)| irritable bowel syndrome
                            |   gynecological(testicular)
                            |
                           UTI
                            |
                       suprapubic
                            |
                     gynecological
```

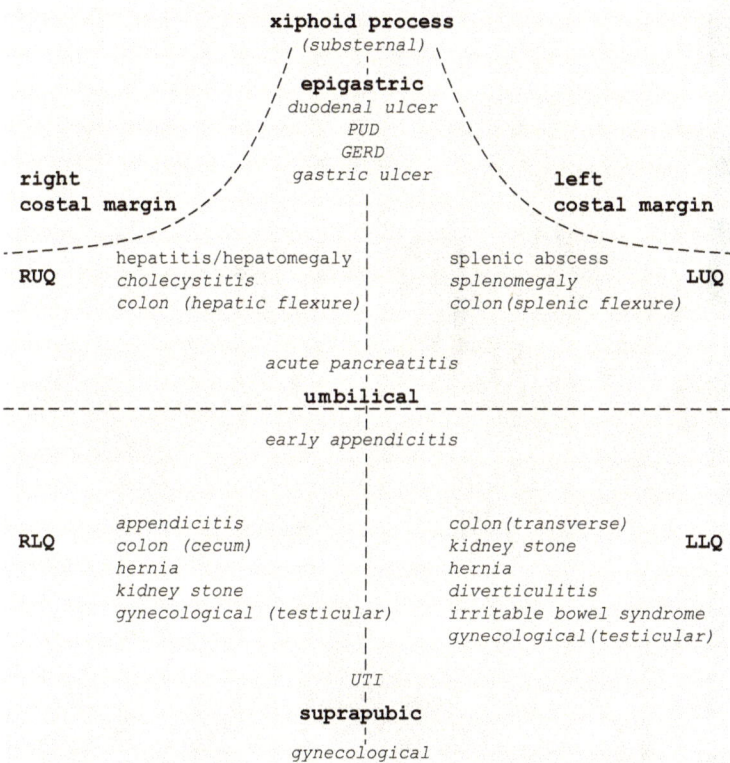

FIGURE 10.1 Abdominal architecture.
RUQ = Right upper quadrant, RLQ = Right lower quadrant, LUQ = Left upper quadrant, LLQ = Left lower quadrant.

decreasing acid production in the stomach and eradication of *H. pylori*. Diagnosis of more severe forms of heartburn may require esophagogastroduodenoscopy (EGD) to allow direct observation and biopsy of the lesion.

Duodenal Ulcers

Duodenal ulcers are thought to be due to a combination of excess acid production and a breakdown of the mucosal barrier by *H. pylori*, a gram-negative bacillus, which is able to live between the mucous layer and the surface epithelial cells of the stomach and duodenum. It attaches to the epithelial cells and by several mechanisms disrupts the mucosal barrier, leading to erosion and ulceration.

Classically, duodenal ulcers present with heartburn that is relieved by meals but returns 1 to 2 hours after eating. Food raises the pH of the stomach, temporarily buffering the acid and causing relief of symptoms. Once the food passes through the duodenum, the pain recurs. Neutralization of stomach acid with antacids or suppression of acid production with H_2 blockers or PPIs also relieves the pain. Ulcers will heal with acid directed treatment, but 80% will recur unless *H. pylori* is simultaneously eradicated.

TABLE 10.1 | **Heartburn/Abdominal Pain**

A. DIAGNOSTIC SCHEMATA FOR HEARTBURN/ABDOMINAL PAIN

Duodenal Ulcer

Gastritis/Gastric Ulcer

Esophagitis(Including GERD)

Gallbladder Disease

Gastroenteritis(GE)

Appendicitis

B. DIFFERENTIAL DIAGNOSIS OF HEARTBURN AND ABDOMINAL PAIN

SUBJECTIVE	*Duodenal Ulcer*	*Gastritis/Gastric Ulcer*	*Esophagitis/GERD*	*Gallbladder Disease*	*Gastroenteritis*	*Appendicitis*
Location	Epigastric	Epigastric	Epigastric	Right upper quadrant (RUQ) may radiate to back	Variable (epigastric/umbilical/RLQ/LLQ)	May begin epigastric or umbilical. Migrates to RLQ
Onset	1 to 2 hours after meals	Variable, may be brought on by spicy food/ETOH, NSAIDs	After laying flat	3 to 4 hours after fatty meal	Variable, usually sudden or rapid onset	Variable
Quality	Burning, gnawing	Burning, gnawing	Burning, gnawing	Sharp	Usually sharp and may be cramping in nature	May resemble heartburn initially but progresses to severe and sharp in nature
Quantity	Variable severity	Variable severity	Variable severity	Variable. May resemble heartburn in early stages but becomes severe	Severe pain, forcing patient to stop activity	May become severe
Setting	Usually 1 to 2 hours after meal	Variable	Variable	3 to 4 hours after fatty meal	History of ingestion of potentially contaminated food or in close contact with others who have similar symptoms

Lasts 24 to 72 hours | N/A |
| **Associated symptoms** | If bleeding, melena, hematemesis, coffee ground vomitus | If bleeding, melena, hematemesis, coffee ground vomitus | Belching regurgitation, bloating | Radiates to back, nausea | Nausea, vomiting, and diarrhea | Nausea, vomiting |

	Duodenal Ulcer	Gastritis/Gastric Ulcer	Esophagitis/GERD	Gallbladder Disease	Gastroenteritis	Appendicitis
Modifying factors	Food, antacids, H₂ blocker, PPI make it better	Antacids, H₂ blocker, PPI make it better. NSAIDs, EtOH spicy food may make it worse	Variable relief with antacids, H₂ blockers, PPI. Made worse by lying down	Fatty food makes it worse	None	None
OBJECTIVE	Esophagogastroduodenoscopy (EGD) with *H. pylori* culture	EGD with *H. pylori* culture	EGD to check for esophageal erosion	Gallbladder ultrasound	Hyperactive bowel sounds on abdominal auscultation	Abdominal ultrasound, X-Ray or CT scan
	Positive stool for occult blood if bleeding ulcer	Positive stool for occult blood if bleeding ulcer		Positive Murphy sign		RLQ pain with guarding or rigidity. Positive Blumberg, Markle, Rovsing, Psoas, Obturator signs
						WBC >10,000 with 80% PMNs

A. DIAGNOSTIC SCHEMATA FOR HEARTBURN/ABDOMINAL PAIN (continued)

Intestinal Obstruction	Gynecological	Kidney Stones
Pancreatitis	Urinary Tract Infection	MI/Angina

B. DIFFERENTIAL DIAGNOSIS OF HEARTBURN ABDOMINAL PAIN (continued)

SUBJECTIVE	Intestinal Obstruction	Pancreatitis	Gynecological	Urinary Tract Infection	Renal Calculus	MI/Angina
Location	Any area of the abdomen. RLQ, LLQ most common	Periumbilical, epigastric. May radiate to lower back	Suprapubic, LLQ, RLQ	Lower back, urethral, abdomen or suprapubic	Lower back, may be described as abdominal in initial attack or suprapubic	Substernal/epigastric may radiate down extremities
Onset	Sudden to slow onset	Sudden to slow onset	Variable	Variable	Sudden	Sudden/or upon exercise

(Continued)

TABLE 10.1	Heartburn/Abdominal Pain (Continued)					
SUBJECTIVE	*Intestinal Obstruction*	*Pancreatitis*	*Gynecological*	*Urinary Tract Infection*	*Renal Calculus*	*MI/Angina*
Quality	Sharp, colicky, cramping	Sharp	Variable	Stinging, burning dull flank pain	Sharp	Typically crushing and squeezing but can present as heartburn/abdominal pain especially in women
Quantity	Severe	Constant severe pain	Variable	Mild to moderate pain	Severe pain	Severe
Setting	Older patient with history of abdominal surgery, severe constipation	Heavy ETOH use, Hx of gall bladder disease	Female patient	Pain upon urination, urgency, frequency	N/A	Patient with hypertension/hyperlipidemia/diabetes
Associated symptoms	Nausea, vomiting, and paradoxical diarrhea early in the course	May have nausea and vomiting	Vaginal bleeding or discharge, bloating	Flank pain, nausea, and vomiting with acute pyelonephritis	N/A	Palpitations, nausea, vomiting, diaphoresis
Modifying factors	None	None	None	None	None	Rest relieves angina, not MI
OBJECTIVE						
	Mass on abdominal palpation, tympanic bowel sounds on percussion. Ultrasound, flat plate of the abdomen, CT scan	Elevated serum amylase, lipase; Abdominal ultrasound, CT with IV contrast; Abdominal tenderness/guarding on palpation, fever	Pregnancy test, pelvic examination, fever; WBC >10,000 with >80% PMNs in PID	MSCC urinalysis with culture and sensitivity; Flank pain on firm percussion	Hematuria upon urinalysis; Flank pain on firm percussion	Classical ECG finding, elevated cardiac enzymes (see Chapter 9)

Gastric Ulcers

Gastric ulcers or ulcers in the stomach also present with typical gnawing, burning epigastric pain, but with no pattern of relief by food. Ethanol can aggravate symptoms and ulcers caused by NSAIDs or corticosteroids are typically located in the stomach. Neutralizing stomach acid or suppressing its production relieves pain in most cases. Here too, treatment requires eradication of *H. pylori* to prevent recurrence.

Three other disorders have presentations similar to gastric ulcers but may not involve *H. pylori* in the pathology. First is *gastritis*, which is an acute event caused by excessive ethanol ingestion or temporary use of irritating medication such as NSAIDs alone or in combination with spicy food and/or ethanol. A short trial of acid suppression and avoidance of inciting issues usually causes the symptoms to disappear until the next inciting event. If symptoms recur without an inciting event, then further diagnostic workup is in order to rule out ulceration or malignancy. *Functional dyspepsia* is common and has symptoms similar to gastritis and gastric ulcer. The pathology is unclear but appears to be related to delayed gastric emptying time, and intestinal motility issues, but not *H. pylori* and acid. Not surprisingly, acid suppression has variable efficacy in relieving the symptoms. Finally, in patients over 55, dyspepsia of new onset or heartburn that fails to respond to a short course of acid suppression, *gastric carcinoma* must be considered. Generally, response of symptoms to acid suppression is variable. The primary reason for the 14-day restriction for the use of H_2 blockers and proton pump inhibitors is to prevent partial treatment of symptoms that may be a malignancy, an incompletely healed ulceration, or continued bleeding.

Testing for *H. pylori* is usually done via biopsy during EGD. The sample can be tested in several ways. The most common and inexpensive is the *rapid urease test* with >90% sensitivity and specificity. *Histological examination* is more accurate but is more expensive. Finally, *culture* of the biopsy specimen is 100% accurate, but is generally reserved for patients who fail initial antibiotic therapy. There are several noninvasive tests for the presence of *H. pylori*. The first is the *urea breath test,* which involves ingestion of radiolabeled urea. The urea is hydrolyzed by *H. pylori* into CO_2, which is measured as radiolabeled carbon in the breath. Its accuracy is as good as many of the tests of biopsy materials. Unfortunately, concurrent ulcer therapy interferes with the test, so it is only accurate before any therapy or after therapy is completed because both classes of therapeutic agents cause false-negative readings. Antibodies to *H, pylori* can be detected in office-based blood and urine tests. Usually they are not as accurate as other tests and cannot distinguish current from past infections. Finally, there is the fecal antigen test, which has accuracy similar to the urea breath test and may be less affected by therapeutic regimens.

Upper Gastrointestinal Bleeding

Both duodenal and gastric ulcers can bleed. Sometimes the bleeding is massive, causing the patient to vomit bright red blood (hematemesis). Smaller, but still significant amounts of blood, may make the vomitus appear as coffee grounds, which represents blood partially digested by stomach acid. Significant amounts of blood may not cause vomiting, but do cause the feces to have a black, tarry appearance and consistency (melena). A complete evaluation would consist of vital signs for tachycardia, tachypnea, and orthostatic changes in blood pressure; a BUN and serum creatinine to check for protein digestion from blood; a complete blood count, examination of nail beds conjunctiva or frenulum of the tongue for paleness indicative of anemia; and stool examination for melena or occult blood. See chapter 25 for more details.

GERD/Esophagitis

Gastroesophageal reflux disease or GERD represents a group of disorders that are caused by acid and bile reflux into the esophagus in patients whose lower esophageal sphincter (also called LES or cardiac sphincter of the stomach) does not function properly. In esophagitis, LES tone is either permanently or temporarily incompetent and fails to prevent acid and bile from refluxing from the stomach into the thinly lined esophagus. Decreased LES can be associated with ethanol ingestion, which relaxes the LES, anatomical variances, or a hiatal hernia. Acute esophagitis is caused by a temporary loss of LES tone. Typically, patients with acute esophagitis describe some combination of a large meal, spicy food, and ethanol followed by laying on their stomach as an inciting event. Chronic esophagitis is due to a permanent change in LES tone. There are two major forms of chronic esophagitis. Today, the term GERD refers to chronic *erosive* esophagitis, which if untreated can lead to Barrett's esophagitis, which is a precursor to esophageal carcinoma. *Nonerosive* chronic reflux disease is usually referred to as NERD. It *does not* carry the associated risk of esophageal carcinoma. All three forms of esophagitis present with typical heartburn symptoms, a gnawing, burning pain that is made worse when lying down, which splashes acid up past the incompetent LES, into the lower esophagus. Acid neutralization or suppression therapy usually relieves symptoms.

Hiatal Hernia

A hiatal hernia is a weakening, break or rupture in the diaphragm, where the opening that normally only allows the esophagus into the chest cavity, allows part of the stomach to slide up into the chest cavity during moments of increased abdominal pressure. While normally asymptomatic, it may cause symptomatic reflux disease. Suspected causes are obesity, poor posture, frequent bending over, or heavy lifting, as well as hereditary and congenital defects. It is common with up to 60% of patients over 60 having some degree of hiatal hernia. For patients with this condition, as well as GERD minimizing straining, heavy lifting, bending over, correcting slouched seating posture, and raising the head of the bed 4 to 6 inches on blocks all can decrease the frequency of esophageal symptoms. Similarly, no eating within 2 to 3 hours before bedtime, avoidance of alcohol intake, and eating smaller meals more frequently also can decrease the frequency of symptoms.

• OTHER CAUSES OF ABDOMINAL PAIN/DISCOMFORT

Cholecystitis (Gallbladder Disease)

Inflammation of the gallbladder is a common cause of abdominal pain. Classically, acute cholecystitis presents with severe, colicky (cramping) right upper quadrant (RUQ) pain, which may radiate to the right upper back and shoulder, which usually occurs 3 to 4 hours after a fatty meal. Many times it is associated with gallstones. About two-thirds of patients will stop inspiration due to pain when deeply palpating the right costal margin and deep breathing is attempted (positive Murphy's sign). Ultrasound may show thickened gallbladder walls, gallstones, or fluid around the gallbladder. Many patients will have a history of similar, but much milder symptoms in the past. While sharp colicky pain is common, 25% of patients present without it. Patients may complain of more vague symptoms such as heartburn, bloating, or discomfort, occurring 2 to 4 hours post-fatty meal intake. This is more common in ethnic groups such as Hispanics and Native Americans, where the incidence is significantly higher than the national average. In acute disease, patients may present with fever, and an elevated white blood cell count and elevated liver function tests.

Pancreatitis

The causes of pancreatitis range from gallbladder disease to medications. Acute biliary pancreatitis, the most common cause of pancreatitis, represents 35% to 60% of all causes. Gallstones lodge in the distal common bile duct, blocking off the ampulla of vater preventing drainage of digestive enzymes into the intestinal lumen. Heavy alcohol use is the second most common cause of pancreatitis and is called alcoholic pancreatitis. Other causes include medication, hypertriglyceridemia, trauma, and infections by a variety of microorganisms. In 30% of patients, no cause is immediately identified and is termed idiopathic pancreatitis. In patients initially diagnosed with idiopathic pancreatitis, further comprehensive diagnostic workups have identified a specific cause in almost 80% of cases.

Patients with acute pancreatitis present with sharp, constant, severe abdominal pain in the periumbilical, epigastric, or left upper quadrant areas and may radiate to the back. Nausea and vomiting may occur. Physical examination findings may include abdominal tenderness and guarding on palpation, as well as fever. Patients may prefer bringing their knees to their chest to help relieve the pain, instead of lying flat. Serum amylase and lipase if elevated more than three times the upper limit of normal are indicative of pancreatic damage. High sensitivity C-reactive protein may be significantly elevated when tested 48 to 72 hours after the onset of abdominal pain, indicating pancreatic necrosis. Abdominal ultrasound is the initial imaging study of choice for detecting gallstones. An abdominal CT scan with intravenous contrast is the imaging study of choice if gallstones are not detected on ultrasound.

Appendicitis

Classically, acute appendicitis presents as severe pain located in the right lower quadrant (RLQ). Accompanying peritoneal inflammation may induce the peritoneal reflex, which leads to constipation and urinary retention. In a significant number of cases, appendicitis begins as mild to moderate epigastric discomfort, which then migrates to the umbilical region before settling in the RLQ as more severe discomfort. A history of anorexia or nausea and vomiting are also common associated symptoms.

Examination of the abdomen can be helpful in diagnosing acute appendicitis. Gently palpating or percussing over the RLQ can confirm the location. Slow, light, steady pressure over the painful area followed by sudden release of pressure may increase the pain (Blumberg sign). Deep palpation and release, so-called rebound tenderness, adds nothing but unnecessary pain to the diagnostic process. More appropriate is the Rovsing sign where the *left* lower quadrant (LLQ) is slowly, but deeply palpated followed by a sudden release. A positive sign occurs when increased pain is elicited during the sudden release in the RLQ over the appendix. Having the patient walk, cough (cough test), and/or stand on their toes, then suddenly and firmly drop on their heels (Markle or heel drop test) may elicit localized RLQ pain by moving the peritoneum over the inflamed appendix. The Psoas and Obturator signs use muscle movement/irritation over the adjacent appendix to elicit increased localized RLQ pain. The Psoas sign is an increase in RLQ pain when the patient is asked to lift his straightened right leg up from the examination table against hand resistance on the thigh. The obturator sign is elicited when the provider, while supporting the right leg when lying on the examination table, bending both the hip and the knee at 90° elicits pain upon passive external or internal rotation. In addition, most patients present with fever and have a white blood cell count consistent with a bacterial infection (>10,000 white blood cells/mm³, with >80% mature plus immature neutrophils). Patients with several of these signs and symptoms will require ultrasound or CT scan if the ultrasound is inconclusive to confirm the diagnosis.

Intestinal Obstruction

Intestinal obstruction can be caused by multiple factors. Some common examples include; tumors or masses in the intestine, formation of scar tissue around the intestine adjacent to previous abdominal surgery sites, fecal impaction due to severe constipation, volvulus (twisting of the intestine), and intussusception (enfolding of the bowel lumen into itself). Pain is usually severe, cramping, or colicky. Locations varies and can be in any area of the abdomen but the lower quadrants are more common sites. Patients usually complain of constipation, but initially may have paradoxical diarrhea. It is more common in older patients. Nausea and vomiting are common and vomiting can bring temporary relief of the abdominal pain. Auscultation of the abdomen may reveal high-pitched tinkling bowel sounds or absence of bowel sounds. Palpation of the abdomen may reveal tenderness, guarding, as well as solid masses and percussion may reveal tympanic sounds. Abdominal ultrasound, x-ray, or CT scan is used to confirm the presence of intestinal obstruction.

Chronic/Recurrent Bowel Disorders (Ulcerative Colitis, Crohn Disease, Irritable Bowel Syndrome, Celiac Disease)

Recurrent episodes of cramping abdominal pain accompanied by *diarrhea* should lead to referral for definitive diagnosis, which usually requires colonoscopy and biopsy. The pain is usually sharp and cramping similar to intestinal obstruction.

Other Considerations

Abdominal pain, especially located in the lower quadrants in females, may represent gynecological or urinary tract problems so the history should include probing for dysuria, frequency, urgency, flank pain, and vaginal bleeding or discharge. Obviously any positive history will require referral.

Some gynecological causes include pelvic inflammatory disease (PID), ectopic pregnancies, and ruptured ovarian cysts. In PID, pain is usually mild to moderate located in lower quadrants and is associated with fever and vaginal discharge/bleeding. *Ectopic pregnancy* pain is usually severe, with a sudden onset (at the time of rupture), but can be located anywhere in the abdomen. Similarly patterned, but less severe pain is associated with a ruptured ovarian cyst. A pelvic examination followed by ultrasound or CT scan is required for definitive diagnosis.

While problems with the kidneys can be associated with abdominal pain, they generally present as suprapubic, flank or back pain. The pain associated with renal calculi (kidney stones) is usually described as extremely severe, sharp back pain or suprapubic pain as the stone moves down the ureter. However, the pain may be described as abdominal by patients during an initial episode. Pain in urinary tract infections (UTI) is generally described as occurring in the suprapubic, LLQ, RLQ, low back area or flank area in patients with upper tract UTIs (acute pyelonephritis). Pain and discomfort in UTIs are usually associated with dysuria, urgency and frequency. For acute pyelonephritis, fever, flank pain, and nausea or vomiting can be associated with dysuria and frequency. A midstream clean-catch urinalysis with culture and susceptibility is used to confirm the diagnosis. See Chapter 16 for more details.

Finally, pain due to myocardial infarction or angina can sometimes be perceived as heartburn or abdominal pain. See Chapter 9 for more details.

• KEY REFERENCES

1. Ragsdale L, Sutherland L. Acute abdominal pain in the older adult. *Emerg Med Clin North Am.* 2011;29: 429-448.
2. Petroianu A. Diagnosis of acute appendicitis. *Int J Surg.* 2012;10:115-119.
3. Kumar R, Mills AM. Gastrointestinal bleeding. *Emerg Med Clin North Am.* 2011;29:239-252.
4. McNamara R, Dean AJ. Approach to acute abdominal pain. *Emerg Clin North Am.* 2011;29:159-173.
5. Muniraj T, Gajendran M, Thiruvengadam S, et al. Acute pancreatitis. *Dis Mon.* 2012;58:98-144.
6. Cartwright SL, Knudson MP. Evaluation of acute abdominal pain in adults. *Am Fam Physician.* 2008;77:971-978.
7. Panebianco NL, Jahnes K, Mills AM. Imaging and laboratory testing in acute abdominal pain. *Emerg Clin North Am.* 2011;29:179-193.
8. Hayden GE, Sprouse KL. Bowel obstruction and hernia. *Emerg Med Clin North Am.* 2011;29:319-345.

CASE 10.1

Eddie Jones, a 78-year-old veteran, presents to clinic requesting something stronger for heartburn. A quick review of his health record reveals a history of recurrent bleeding duodenal ulcers starting 20 years ago. However, since treatment for *Helicobacter pylori* in 1989 he has been without problems. He says he first noticed this new problem about 6 weeks ago and OTC H$_2$ blockers have not helped very much. He has been taking ibuprofen 400 mg three to four times a day for the last year for "old age" aches and pains.

a. List three likely causes for Eddie's problem. Explain your rationale.

    _____

    _____

    _____

    _____

    _____

b. List four examinations, questions, or laboratory tests you would perform to differentiate between the probable causes listed above. Explain your rationale.

    _____

    _____

    _____

    _____

    _____

c. Just as you complete your interview, Eddie mentions that he has noticed his stools are much darker than usual and is concerned about a recurrence of his bleeding ulcers. List four questions, examinations, or laboratory tests that would help determine if Eddie is bleeding from his upper gastrointestinal tract.

    _____

    _____

    _____

    _____

    _____

ELEVEN

Nausea and Vomiting

LEARNING OBJECTIVES

1. Accurately identify the most likely etiology when patients present with nausea and vomiting, through history, diagnostic tests, and appropriate patient findings on examination to enable the appropriate recommendation of effective treatment or referral to an appropriate provider.

2. Use the knowledge of the pathophysiology, etiology, and common presentations of diseases with nausea and vomiting as a primary symptom to review prescription orders for appropriateness and to accurately educate patients about their disease and its treatment.

3. Use the knowledge of the pathophysiology, etiology, and common presentation of diseases with nausea and vomiting as a primary symptom to accurately interpret the diagnostic process to advise regarding the most appropriate prescription therapy.

• ETIOLOGY

Nausea and/or vomiting is a common presentation in ambulatory and urgent care centers, serving as the chief complaint in 3.7% of emergency room visits. While most causes are self-limiting, it can be a symptom of a variety of diseases throughout the body, many of which are serious or life threatening, affecting the central nervous system, genitourinary tract, gastrointestinal and surrounding organ systems. In addition, nausea and vomiting can be caused by medications, toxins, cardiovascular disease, and metabolic diseases. Causes can be iatrogenic, infectious, inflammatory, and mechanical in nature. Given the broad variety of causes and the potential for involvement of multiple organ systems, a very careful and comprehensive history and physical examination are essential.

• DIAGNOSIS

Because of the broad range of diagnostic possibilities, the key to identifying the cause of nausea and/or vomiting lies with the associated symptoms (Table 11.1). For example, gastroenteritis typically presents with a sudden onset, a history of exposure to potentially tainted foods, or others with similar symptoms. Most patients concurrently complain of abdominal discomfort, fever and diarrhea. Diagnostic accuracy is dependent on a careful history and physical examination, since there are few laboratory tests involving the gastrointestinal tract that can specifically diagnose the cause of nausea and vomiting. Laboratory tests and imaging studies are used primarily in diagnosing those causes not related to the stomach or intestines.

• COMMON CAUSES OF NAUSEA AND/OR VOMITING

Gastroenteritis

Gastroenteritis can be caused by both viral and bacterial pathogens (Table 11.2). Common viral gastroenteritis pathogens include rotavirus, norovirus, and adenovirus. Bacterial gastroenteritis pathogens include *Staphylococci, Campylobacter, E. coli, Shigella* and *Salmonella* species. Onset can occur hours to days after ingestion and the nausea and vomiting usually subsides within 24 to 48 hours. Patients with nausea and vomiting lasting more than 48 hours should be referred. The nausea and vomiting may occur alone but is usually accompanied by diarrhea, fever, cramping abdominal pain, and malaise. Usually patients have a history of recent travel, a sick family member, or recent attendance at a potluck, picnic, or other potential source of spoiled food. Physical examination is negative for abdominal tenderness and bowel sounds are hyperactive on auscultation.

TABLE 11.1	Associated Symptoms–Based Differential Diagnosis of Nausea and Vomiting
Nausea/Vomiting Plus	*Diagnosis*
Hematemesis, coffee ground vomitus	Upper gastrointestinal tract bleeding
Fever	Gastroenteritis, appendicitis, PID, UTI, meningitis
Constipation	Appendicitis, intestinal obstruction
Diarrhea	Gastroenteritis
Dysuria/vaginal discharge	UTI, PID
Amenorrhea	Pregnancy
Headache	Migraine, meningitis, stroke, head trauma
Abdominal pain	Cholecystitis, PID, gastroenteritis, appendicitis, pancreatitis, intestinal obstruction
Chest pain	MI

TABLE 11.2	Common Causes of Nausea and Vomiting

A. DIAGNOSTIC SCHEMATA FOR COMMON CAUSES OF NAUSEA AND VOMITING

Gastroenteritis	Motion sickness
Medication	Nausea and vomiting of pregnancy

B. DIFFERENTIAL DIAGNOSIS OF COMMON CAUSES OF NAUSEA AND VOMITING

SUBJECTIVE	*Gastroenteritis*	*Medication*	*Motion Sickness*	*Pregnancy*
Location	N/A	N/A	N/A	N/A
Onset	6 to 48 hours after ingestion	Usually within 30 minutes to 2 hours after ingesting medication	Minutes to hours depending on degree of abnormal motion	In the morning, often lingering throughout the day at times starting within weeks of conception
Quality	N/A	N/A	N/A	N/A
Quantity	Variable severity	Variable severity	Variable severity depending on degree of abnormal motion	Variable, more than three vomiting episodes/day refer for evaluation of hyperemesis gravidarum
Setting	Recent history of travel, ingestion of tainted food or water	Has taken medication that causes nausea and vomiting within hours	Flying, aboard ship, train, or car	Peaks at 10 to 16 weeks, usually improves or resolves by 20 weeks
Associated symptoms	Diarrhea, abdominal cramping	None	Vertigo	Enlarged uterus
Modifying factors	Usually lasts 24 to 48 hours	Vomiting stops after irritant medication removed. Vomiting continues until serum levels fall of centrally acting drug (several hours)	Can prevent with antihistamines, scopolamine	Small meals help
OBJECTIVE				
	Hyperactive bowel sounds on auscultation	Prescription for agent known to cause nausea	None	Positive pregnancy test
	Usually no abdominal tenderness on palpation	*Local irritant* Nitrofurantoin, tetracyclines, macrolides, NSAIDs		
	Viral most common cause (rotavirus, adenovirus, norovirus)			
	Bacterial causes include *Staphylococci, Campylobacter, E. coli, Salmonella, Shigella* species	*Centrally acting* Opioids		

Medication

Medication is another common cause of nausea and vomiting. Drugs can be local irritants, stimulate specific centers in the brain such as the chemoreceptor trigger zone, or have both mechanisms of inducing emesis. Tetracyclines, nitrofurantoin, macrolide antibiotics, and NSAIDs are common causes of drug-induced irritant nausea and vomiting. Patients have a history of very recent ingestion of the offending agent, and the nausea and vomiting are frequently preceded or accompanied by abdominal discomfort or pain. The initial episode of emesis usually provides relief by removing the medication from the stomach. The incidence of this type of reaction can be reduced by taking the medication with food and/or a full glass of water. Opioids are by far the most common cause of drug-induced centrally mediated vomiting. The symptoms begin as soon as the serum level of the medication is high enough to stimulate the chemoreceptor trigger zone in the brain and continue for hours until the serum levels fall drastically. Vertigo may precede or accompany the nausea and vomiting. This type of nausea can only be prevented by medication such as phenothiazines, which block the effects of the drug on the chemoreceptor trigger zone. Taking narcotics with food or a full class of water has *no* impact on the incidence or duration of drug-induced central nausea and vomiting. Cancer chemotherapy agents cause nausea and vomiting by both mechanisms.

Motion Sickness

In susceptible patients, flying, traveling by ship, or traveling in any moving vehicle such as a train or automobile can cause stimulation of the vestibular apparatus of the inner ear, inducing vertigo, nausea, and eventually emesis. The more severe and disorienting the motion the patient experiences, the more likely the patient will develop motion sickness. The incidence of motion sickness can be reduced by using agents that stabilize the vestibular apparatus such as meclizine, diphenhydramine, and scopolamine.

Nausea and Vomiting of Pregnancy

Seventy to eighty percent of pregnant women will experience "morning sickness" in the first trimester of pregnancy. The term morning sickness is a misnomer since the majority of women who experience it will have the uncomfortable sensations throughout the day. Onset occurs within weeks of conception, peaking at 10 to 16 weeks and resolving by 20 weeks. While the exact cause of the nausea and vomiting of pregnancy is unclear, both human chorionic gonadotropin (hCG) and rising estrogen levels have been implicated. Hyperemesis gravidarum is a condition of severe nausea and vomiting during pregnancy that can lead to excess maternal and fetal morbidity and mortality. Pregnant women who experience three or more episodes of vomiting per day should be quickly referred for definitive diagnosis and treatment. All females of childbearing age who present with nausea and vomiting should be questioned about their last menstrual period (LMP) and have a pregnancy test done.

• POTENTIALLY SERIOUS CAUSES OF NAUSEA AND VOMITING

All patients who present with nausea and vomiting should be screened for the following potentially serious causes (Table 11.3). A careful history and, if possible, physical examination are needed to determine the need for immediate referral. In a community pharmacy, the patient's profile can be quickly reviewed for medications and diagnoses, plus a modified review of systems covering each potential cause can be quickly done.

TABLE 11.3	Typical Presentation of Serious Causes of Nausea and Vomiting
Disease	*Other Symptoms*
CNS	
Migraine	Positive migraine history, severe pulsating headache with or without aura
Meningitis	Headache, fever, stiff neck, disorientation, seizures, nuchal rigidity, photophobia
Trauma/stroke	History of head trauma, headache, neurological deficits, history of diabetes, hypertension, hyperlipidemia, elderly
GI	
Peptic ulcer disease/gastritis	Burning epigastric pain *if bleeding may get hematemesis, coffee ground vomitus, or melena*
Appendicitis	Acute abdominal pain (RLQ), fever, constipation, urinary retention
Cholecystitis/pancreatitis	Severe RUQ/umbilical/epigastric pain
Hepatitis A	History of exposure to tainted food or water, history of travel, jaundice, malaise, myalgia, fever
Intestinal obstruction	Constipation, severe abdominal pain, history of prior abdominal surgery
GU	
Urinary tract infection (UTI)	Dysuria, frequency, fever, flank pain, urgency
Pelvic inflammatory disease (PID)	Abdominal pain, fever, vaginal discharge/bleeding, lower abdominal and/or suprapubic pain
Uremia	History of renal problems or long-standing diabetes or prostate/urinary retention in elderly males
MISC	
Myocardial infarction (MI)	Crushing substernal/epigastric pain ± radiation, diaphoresis
Diabetic ketoacidosis	Dehydration, history of type 1 diabetes

Migraine Headache

The vast majority of patients with migraines experience nausea with or without vomiting. Check for the presence of a pulsating headache, photophobia, phonophobia, aura, or a history of migraine or other vascular headaches. See Chapter 13 for further details.

Trauma/Stroke (CVA)

Patients with a severe headache, recent history of head trauma, a sudden change in vision, or other neurological deficits should be immediately referred. See Chapter 13 for further details.

Meningitis

In addition to nausea and vomiting, patients with meningitis may present with high fever, headache, disorientation, a stiff neck (nuchal rigidity), or photophobia. See Chapter 13 for further details.

Myocardial Infarction

About a fourth of patients with myocardial infarction will experience nausea and/or vomiting. Check for crushing severe substernal or epigastric pain, with the typical radiation and diaphoresis. See Chapter 9 for more complete workup for myocardial infarction.

Peptic Ulcer Disease

One of the risks with peptic ulcer disease (PUD) is that the erosion may induce an upper GI bleed. If a patient with a history of past or current PUD presents with a

132 PART 2 Assessment of Symptoms

recurrence or worsening of symptoms or presents with nausea and or vomiting, the possibility of bleeding from the ulcer needs to be evaluated. Bleeding gastric and duodenal ulcers will produce distinct symptoms. A very large quantity of blood may produce vomitus that consists of bright red blood. This represents a medical emergency and is called hematemesis. If the volume of bleeding is less and it sits in the stomach or small intestine for a period of time before emesis, the vomitus will have the appearance of coffee grounds, which represents partially digested blood. Finally, upper GI bleeding may manifest itself as melena, which are black tarry stools representing significant blood loss from the upper gastrointestinal tract. See Chapters 10 and 25 for further details.

Viral Hepatitis
Early in the course of hepatitis A, nausea and vomiting are common symptoms along with fatigue and flu-like symptoms, including fever. Serum transaminase levels (ALT, AST) are greater than 300 IU/dL. The patient may be jaundiced, have dark urine and elevated bilirubin levels. Elevated IgM anti-HAV antibodies are diagnostic.

Appendicitis
Classical appendicitis presents as RLQ pain. Inflammation may induce the peritoneal reflex, which prevents bowel and bladder emptying. Many cases present with epigastric distress or heartburn and the pain may migrate to the umbilical area before settling in the RLQ. Nausea and vomiting frequently accompany the migration of abdominal discomfort. See Chapter 10 for further details.

Pancreatitis/Cholecystitis
Pancreatitis and cholecystitis can also cause nausea and vomiting. Umbilical pain and tenderness are the hallmark of acute pancreatitis, while right upper quadrant pain is typical in cholecystitis. See Chapter 10 for further details.

Intestinal Obstruction
Intestinal obstruction eventually causes vomiting, often without nausea, along with severe abdominal pain and tenderness. See Chapter 10 for more details.

Pelvic Inflammatory Disease
In females of childbearing age who present with nausea and vomiting, the patient should be queried about a vaginal discharge and recent sexual activity with a new partner, in addition to checking for pregnancy. Most patients with pelvic inflammatory disease (PID) will have a fever plus lower quadrant and suprapubic discomfort or pain in addition to the nausea and vomiting. See Chapter 16 for more details.

Urinary Tract Infection
As above, females of childbearing age presenting with nausea and vomiting should also be asked about dysuria, frequency, fever, urgency and flank pain to rule out acute pyelonephritis (upper urinary tract infection [UTI]). Midstream clean catch urinalysis with large numbers of white cells or bacteria is a quick diagnostic approach. See Chapter 16 for more details.

Uremia
In older patients with long-standing diabetes or prostatic hypertrophy, uremia needs to be ruled out with a urinalysis for protein and/or serum creatinine.

Type 1 Diabetes Mellitus

In patients with Type 1 diabetes mellitus or those with gradual onset of nausea and vomiting, diabetic ketoacidosis needs to be ruled out. Blood tests for plasma glucose and urinalysis for glucose can be quickly used to confirm suspicions of diabetic ketoacidosis.

• KEY REFERENCES

1. Lee NM, Saha S. Nausea and vomiting of pregnancy. *Gastroenterol Clin North Am.* 2011;40:309-334.
2. Metz A, Hebbard G. Nausea and vomiting in adults. *Aust Fam Physician.* September 2007;36:688-692.
3. Scorza K, Williams A, Phillips JD, Shaw J. Evaluation of nausea and vomiting. *Am Fam Physician.* 2007;76:76-84.
4. Getto L, Zeseron E, Breyer M. Vomiting, diarrhea, constipation and gastroenteritis. *Emerg Med Clin North Am.* 2011;29:211-237.

CASE 11.1

Edwin Bourke, a 40-year-old Gulf War veteran presents with a 36-hour history of nausea and vomiting with intermittent abdominal pain. His past medical history is significant in that he received a penetrating abdominal wound from which he fully recovered 15 years ago. He also complains of a headache, chills, and general arthralgias and myalgias. A review of his chart reveals a dental visit 2 days ago, where he received prescriptions for erythromycin 500 mg four times a day, Vicodin one to two tablets every 4 hours for severe pain, and ibuprofen 600 mg one table four times a day for 3 days.

a. List three possible causes for Edwin's problems. Explain your rationale.

_____

_____

_____

_____

_____

b. List four questions, examinations, or laboratory tests you would perform to confirm the diagnosis. Explain your rationale.

_____

_____

_____

_____

_____

TWELVE

Diarrhea and Constipation

1. Accurately identify the most likely etiology when patients present with abnormal bowel function, through history, diagnostic tests, and patient findings on examination to enable recommendation of effective treatment or referral to an appropriate provider.

2. Use the knowledge of the pathophysiology, etiology, and common presentations of diarrhea and constipation as a primary symptom to review prescription orders for appropriateness and to accurately educate patients about their disease and its treatment.

3. Use the knowledge of the pathophysiology, etiology, and common presentation of diseases with diarrhea and constipation as a primary symptom to accurately interpret the diagnostic process to advise regarding the most appropriate prescription therapy.

• BACKGROUND

Diarrhea and constipation are very common presentations in ambulatory and urgent care centers. In the United States, up to 27% of patients have experienced constipation. Similarly, 211 to 375 million cases of diarrhea are reported annually. While there are a variety of definitions for both conditions, normal frequency of bowel movements in most adults range from three times a day to every 3 days. Even though most causes are self-limiting, both can be a symptom of a serious or life-threatening disorder. Because both disorders are so common and generally self-limiting, patients frequently try treatment with nonprescription products prior to seeking medical care. Therefore, screening patients for those more serious forms of these disorders is critical before recommending from the multitude of products available for self-care.

• DIARRHEA

Etiology

Diarrhea, defined as three or more bowel movements within a 24-hour period, can be classified as acute, persistent, and chronic. Acute diarrhea lasts for less than 14 days; persistent diarrhea lasts for more than 14 days; and patients experiencing diarrhea for more than 30 days have chronic diarrhea. Dysentery is usually defined as acute diarrhea in which subjects have frequent watery stools, often with blood and mucous. The most common cause of acute diarrhea is infection with viral pathogens, such as norovirus and rotavirus. Common bacterial causes include *Shigella* and *Salmonella* species along with *Campylobacter jejuni, Clostridium difficile,* and *Escherichia coli* species. *Giardia lamblia, Entamoeba histolytica,* and *Cryptosporidium* species are the most common protozoal causes of diarrhea. Noninfectious causes of acute diarrhea include foods and medication. Inflammatory bowel diseases such as celiac disease, microcolitis, ulcerative colitis, and Crohn's disease all cause chronic diarrhea. Irritable bowel syndrome is a noninflammatory condition that in two versions (diarrhea predominant and mixed) cause chronic diarrhea. Lastly, diabetic gastroparesis, acquired immunodeficiency syndrome (AIDS), and post-gastrointestinal (GI) tract surgery are uncommon causes for chronic diarrhea. While most viral diarrheas are self-limiting (typically lasting 24 to 48 hours) complications such as dehydration are uncommon, except in infants and the elderly. Some bacterial diarrheas produce toxins that result in more serious complications such as toxic megacolon, intestinal perforation, sepsis, and even death. Some parasitic infections can cause persistent diarrhea and some may migrate to other internal organs such as the liver. Unfortunately, causes of diarrhea cannot be easily differentiated by symptoms alone. Therefore, when patients present to the pharmacy for OTC antidiarrheal products, a general rule applies. Any acute diarrheal illness >48 hours in duration should usually be referred for medical evaluation and treatment as indicated. Obviously, any patients with persistent or chronic diarrhea should be referred. Other causes for referral will be discussed under specific disorders.

Diagnosis

Identifying the cause of acute, persistent, and chronic diarrhea requires a careful and complete history. Patients should be questioned about recent travel, hospitalization, antibiotic use, dietary changes, or contact with others with similar symptoms. A history of bloody diarrhea is a cause for emergency referral to medical care. Some disorders, such as irritable bowel syndrome, are generally a diagnosis of exclusion. Physical examination, especially for dehydration, is also important. Examination, culture, and other studies of fecal material are important for the diagnosis of more serious causes of infectious diarrhea. Diagnostic endoscopy and some blood tests can help differentiate among chronic causes of diarrhea. See specific disorders for further details.

Common Causes of Acute Diarrhea (Table 12.1)

Viral Gastroenteritis Viral gastroenteritis can occur as diarrhea alone, but is usually accompanied by nausea and vomiting, fever, cramping abdominal pain, and malaise. Patients have a history of recent travel, exposure to a sick family member, or exposure to other sick people around the patient (nursing home, cruise ship, dormitory), or recent attendance at a potluck, picnic, or other potential sources of spoiled food or contaminated water. Physical examination is usually negative for abdominal tenderness and bowel sounds are usually hyperactive on auscultation. Most viral disease is caused by norovirus or adenovirus, but rotavirus is common in children. Norovirus and adenovirus are also called the "24-hour stomach flu" because of the short duration of symptoms (usually less than 48 hours). The disease is self-limiting in most adults and children, but like all infectious diarrheal diseases, infants under 1 year of age, adults >65 years of age, and immunocompromised patients can rarely have complications such as dehydration or more prolonged diarrhea. Rotavirus usually lasts for up to 1 week, so preventive oral rehydration is recommended because of the greater risk of dehydration.

Usually Self-Limiting Bacterial Gastroenteritis The symptoms of these generally self-limiting bacterial diarrheal diseases are very similar to their viral counterparts, but tend to last up to 7 days, increasing the risk of dehydration and necessitating preventive oral rehydration. *Campylobacter jejuni*, nontyphoid *Salmonella* species, *Shigella,* and *Staphylococcus aureus* are the most common causes. While antibiotic therapy is unnecessary in most cases, patients who are immunocompromised are at risk for systemic spread, sepsis, and death. Patients with high fever >102°F (39°C), those who appear toxic or fail to respond to supportive therapy require further workup and appropriate antibiotic therapy.

Toxigenic Bacterial Diarrhea While most *Salmonella, Shigella, and Escherichia coli* species produce local toxins that cause "travelers' diarrhea," some such as Shiga toxin–producing strains of *E. coli* can cause systemic effects such as hemorrhagic colitis and hemolytic-uremic syndrome, which can be fatal. Bloody stools are a hallmark sign of this dangerous pathogen. Probably the most widespread toxigenic bacterial diarrhea is *Clostridium difficile* or *C. diff.* This organism is a slow growing anaerobic bacteria that is normally held in check by normal GI tract flora. When the patient receives a broad spectrum antibiotic, those normal GI tract flora are killed and *C. difficile* is permitted to grow and cause diarrhea. Symptoms include fever, watery diarrhea with unusual odor, described by some to smell like "horse manure," and some patients will experience abdominal cramping. If untreated, bowel perforation or toxic megacolon can occur, resulting in peritoneal infections and sepsis. One of the biggest problems is that it can be spread from person to person by health care providers. Once outside the body spores can survive on inanimate objects for prolonged periods. Stomach acid generally kills most spores, so patients on acid suppression therapy with PPIs are more susceptible to *C. difficile* transmission. These spores are hardy and can survive even after cleaning inanimate objects. Because of its characteristics, it can cause epidemics in wards, hospitals, and nursing homes.

Parasitic Diarrhea Cryptosporidiosis, giardiasis, and amebiasis are common parasitic-induced diarrheal diseases. These have a longer incubation period and the diarrhea generally lasts more than 1 week. *Cryptosporidium hominis* and other animal species can cause human diarrheal disease. Also known as crypto, cryptosporidiosis is

TABLE 12.1	Common Causes of Acute Diarrhea

A. DIAGNOSTIC SCHEMATA FOR COMMON CAUSES OF NAUSEA AND VOMITING

Viral	Parasitic	Medications
Bacterial	Dietary	

B. DIFFERENTIAL DIAGNOSIS OF COMMON CAUSES OF ACUTE DIARRHEA

SUBJECTIVE	*Viral*	*Bacterial*	*Parasitic*	*Dietary*	*Medications*
Location	N/A	N/A	N/A	N/A	N/A
Onset	6 to 48 hours after ingestion	6 to 48 hours after ingestion	Several days to weeks	Post-bariatric surgery, after ingestion of spicy food or lactose containing foods	Usually within hours to days after ingesting medication
Quality	Varied	Sometimes watery tools	Greasy, foul smelling (*Giardia*)	Burning sensation with spicy food	Varied
Quantity	Variable severity	Variable severity	Variable severity	Variable severity	Variable severity
Setting	Recent history of travel, ingestion of tainted food or water	Recent history of travel, ingestion of tainted food or water. Recent antibiotic use for *C. diff*	Exposure to recreational (lake) water for cryptosporidiosis and giardiasis or daycare for giardiasis or recent travel to Africa, Latin America, India for amebiasis	Exposure to food that can cause diarrhea	Has taken medication that causes diarrhea within last few hours or days
Associated symptoms	Nausea, vomiting, abdominal cramping	Abdominal cramping	Abdominal cramping	May have cramping, nausea, vomiting	May have cramping, nausea, vomiting
Modifying factors	Usually lasts 24 to 48 hours	Lasts up to 7 days	Last more than 1 week	None	Diarrhea stops after last of medication passes through bowel after discontinuation
OBJECTIVE					
	Hyperactive bowel sounds on auscultation	Hyperactive bowel sounds on auscultation	Hyperactive bowel sounds on auscultation	None	Prescription for agent known to cause diarrhea
	Little or no abdominal tenderness on palpation	Little or no abdominal tenderness on palpation	Little or no abdominal tenderness on palpation		*Local irritant* Macrolides, dementia medications, clavulanate
		Stool culture	Stool for ova and parasites		*Indirect* Antibiotics, magnesium, acarbose
		Fever			
	Viral most common cause (rotavirus, adenovirus, norovirus)	*Campylobacter, E. coli, Salmonella, Shigella* species	*Cryptosporidium hominis, Giardia lamblia, Entamoeba histolytica*		

contracted through outdoor water sources as in lakes, rivers, and streams. Patients should be questioned about recent camping trips and water skiing or swimming in recreational water. Because the spores have an outer protective shell, it can be resistant to chlorine disinfection and outbreaks have occurred from city water supplies. In people with normal immune systems complications other than dehydration are uncommon. Specific diagnosis can be made by microscopic stool examination for ova and parasites and a specific antigen test. *Giardia lamblia* is also found in recreational water like *cryptosporidium*. In addition, daycare centers are also sources for the transmission of *Giardia* species. Fecal matter in patients with giardiasis has been described as "greasy" and has a unique foul odor. Diagnosis is also established by microscopic stool examination, culture and/or organism specific serological testing. Both diseases have effective antimicrobial treatments and other than dehydration are usually without sequelae. *Entamoeba histolytica* is uncommon in this country but is common in developing countries especially those with tropical climates where poor sanitation and overcrowding are more common. Travel within a month to Africa, Latin America, or India usually raises suspicion for the potential of amebiasis as a cause of diarrhea. *Entamoeba histolytica* can live in the intestines without causing disease in patients with normal immune systems. However, sometimes even in the face of normal immunity, it becomes invasive and causes diarrhea. It can also spread to other organs to form abscesses, most commonly in the liver, but also in the lungs and brain. Accurate microscopic examination for fecal matter microscopically requires considerable experience and expertise. Tests for antibodies to the organism are accurate in 85% of patients in the United States and are used in addition to microscopic analysis of feces.

Dietary Causes Various changes in dietary habits may also be a cause of diarrhea. Patients with lactase deficiency can have episodic bouts of diarrhea after ingesting dairy products due to osmotic effect of undigested lactose. Bloating and flatulence are also common manifestations due to the lactose fermenting coliform bacteria in the colon, which convert the lactose to carbon dioxide. Milk products are the most common cause and the incidence of symptoms is dose related. In addition, most patients can tolerate fermented cheeses such as sharp cheddar because much of the lactose is converted to lactic acid in the cheese-making process. Some public water systems have high magnesium content, so moving to a new area with higher levels may induce mild diarrhea of several weeks' duration. Eventually, the bowel adjusts to the higher magnesium levels. Spicy food (curry, Thai, Mexican) can also induce diarrhea due to the irritant properties of the spices. Finally, bariatric surgery induces gastric dumping syndrome, which includes diarrhea, in 20% of patients.

Medication Medication is another common cause of diarrhea. Drugs can be local irritants or have pharmacological effects. Overuse of both irritant and osmotic laxatives can be a cause of acute diarrhea. Antacids typically contain high quantities of magnesium salts and even one or two large doses can cause loose stools. Broad spectrum antibiotics can alter intestinal flora, which may cause diarrhea. However, clavulanic acid is a direct irritant and accounts for the higher incidence of diarrhea with amoxicillin/clavulanic acid combination than with amoxicillin alone. Similarly, macrolides, specifically erythromycin, are motilin agonists accounting for the high incidence of diarrhea with these agents. Minerals such as magnesium and occasionally iron salts can also cause diarrhea. Many drugs currently used to treat dementia are parasympathomimetic and diarrhea is a common side effect. Side effects of some oral agents used in the treatment of type 2 diabetes mellitus causes enough diarrhea to limit adherence in many patients. Acarbose and miglitol by their mechanism of action create flatulence and diarrhea, while metformin's irritant effects on the intestine can limit its use in certain patients. While drugs used to treat AIDS have been listed as possible frequent causes of diarrhea, the high background incidence of diarrhea in patients infected with human immunodeficiency virus (HIV) casts doubt on many of the reported rates in the literature. Finally, cancer chemotherapy routinely causes episodes of diarrhea.

Miscellaneous Causes In the early stages of intestinal obstruction, the bowel tries to clear the obstruction by increasing peristalsis, which can temporarily cause diarrhea. However, it is very short lived and quickly followed by signs of intestinal obstruction, e.g., constipation, abdominal pain, bloating, nausea, and vomiting. See Chapter 10 for more detail.

Common Causes of Chronic Diarrhea

Continuous or episodic diarrhea that lasts for more than 30 days usually indicates a systemic disease that requires referral to appropriate medical care. Other than amebiasis and *C. difficile*, infectious causes of diarrhea rarely last for more than 2 weeks. Medications and food intolerances while primarily acute in onset and duration can last for longer than 30 days, but patients usually relate the ingestion of medication or particular foods to the diarrheal episodes. Therefore, patients who present with chronic diarrhea syndromes should be questioned about travel to developing countries, recent hospitalization or antibiotic therapy, and changes in medication or diet in addition to investigating the causes discussed below.

Inflammatory Bowel Disease Over three-fourths of patients with inflammatory bowel disease (IBD) present with chronic intermittent or episodic diarrhea. Microcolitis, ulcerative colitis, and Crohn's disease are the most common forms of IBD. These disorders require endoscopy and biopsy of the intestine to confirm the diagnosis. Microcolitis has been viewed in the past as a precursor or mild form of IBD. Upon endoscopy, the gross appearance of the bowel is normal, but biopsy specimens reveal lymphocytic infiltration and increases in collagen content of the colon wall. Ulcerative colitis and Crohn disease cause gross visible changes in the bowel, are associated with an increased risk of colon cancer, and in the more severe forms can be life threatening. Ulcerative colitis symptoms vary with the extent of the colon affected. Diarrhea or loose stools are common and rectal function can be compromised if the rectum is involved. An urgent need to defecate is also common. Crohn's disease can occur throughout the GI tract, so in addition to ileocolonoscopy, other imaging studies may be required. If Crohn disease is present in the small intestine, then the patient will present with watery diarrhea because of the greater loss of fluid that cannot be compensated for by the colon. Finally, acute exacerbations may mimic appendicitis without the diarrhea due to right lower quadrant pain.

Celiac Disease Celiac disease, also known as celiac sprue or gluten-sensitive enteropathy, is a T-cell-mediated autoimmune reaction to gluten that occurs in about 1% of the population. In one study, less than 21% of patients with celiac disease had been diagnosed. It is more frequent in women than men. The disease is associated with two specific human lymphocyte antigen (HLA) types. Unfortunately, while almost all patients with celiac disease have either or both, 30% to 40% of the general population carries those HLA types. Gluten peptides such as gliadin penetrate between the cells of the epithelium to be deamidated by transglutaminase (tTG). This form binds to HLA, which activates cytotoxic T cells which damage the epithelium and produce antibodies to gliadin and tTG. Manifestations include episodic diarrhea, weight loss, and abdominal distention. Some patients have very little diarrhea but may present with iron-deficiency anemia, osteopenia, or a myriad of other non-GI symptoms. If suspected, immunoglobulin A (IgA) antitissue transglutaminase antibody levels (IgA-anti-tTG antibodies) in the serum are measured. To verify the diagnosis, patients with a positive test for IgA anti-tTG antibodies require a biopsy of the intestinal wall while ingesting gluten to confirm the diagnosis. The condition is easily controlled with a low gluten or gluten-free diet.

HIV Patients with HIV are susceptible to opportunistic infectious diarrhea due to decreased immune system function. Like with other opportunistic infections, elevations of CD4 lymphocyte count with highly active antiretroviral therapy (HAART) restore immunity and reduce the incidence of infectious diarrhea. While the most common cause is parasitic diarrhea, viral and bacterial diarrhea may also occur. In patients with suppressed immune functions, some unusual organisms, not seen in uninfected patients can be involved, including cytomegalovirus (CMV), *Mycobacterium avium* complex (MAC), and *Isospora belli*. These can cause serious infections with serious consequences. In 15% to 46% of HIV patients with diarrhea, no pathogen can be found. HIV infection by itself is associated with HIV enteropathy, which has diarrhea as a predominant symptom. Finally, HAART medications themselves can cause diarrhea.

Irritable Bowel Syndrome Irritable bowel syndrome (IBS) occurs in 10% to 15% of the population. It comes in three major types. First, constipation-dominant IBS is more common in females. Second, diarrhea-dominant IBS is more common in men. Finally, mixed-features IBS presents with short bouts of diarrhea, alternating with longer periods of constipation. Patients experiencing abdominal pain and discomfort at least 3 days a month for the past 3 months accompanied by altered bowel function should be evaluated for IBS. IBS is a diagnosis of exclusion. Serologic tests screening for celiac disease should be done in patients with mixed or diarrhea-predominant IBS. A careful history should be done, looking for alarm signs and symptoms (weight loss, anemia, blood or mucous in the stools, family history of colon cancer). In some cases, the abdominal pain/discomfort is relieved by defecation. The cause of IBS is unknown and probably multifactorial. Postinfectious and small intestine bacterial overgrowth (SIBO), are commonly discussed as potential causes.

• BLOATING/ABDOMINAL DISTENTION

Bloating, abdominal distension, and a sense of fullness are common symptoms that can occur alone or in conjunction with other GI symptoms. They are frequently associated with inflammatory bowel diseases, constipation, food intolerances such as celiac disease and lactase deficiency, and intestinal obstruction. Diabetic gastroparesis is a specific entity that deserves special attention because of pharmacists' frequent involvement in the management of diabetes.

Diabetic Gastroparesis

When managing patients with diabetes, one must screen for a late complication of diabetic neuropathy which is known as diabetic gastroparesis. Patients who develop gastroparesis already have peripheral diabetic neuropathy (numbness, tingling, and/or pain in the feet). The neuropathy then extends to the autonomic nervous system with resultant delay in stomach and bowel emptying. Symptoms include early fullness while eating, bloating, belching, abdominal distension, heartburn, nausea, vomiting, constipation, and in the early stages as the bowel tries to overcome the lack of autonomic control by other physiological means, brief periods of diarrhea.

• CONSTIPATION

Normal frequency of bowel movements ranges from three times a day to every 3 days. Intervals between bowel movement of equal to or greater than every 4 days is considered constipation. Patients over 70 years of age may consider not just frequency of bowel movement, but also straining during defecation and difficulty or incomplete evacuation to be symptoms of constipation. Fecal matter is usually soft, formed, and brown in color due to stercobilin, derived from bilirubin. Color can also vary with the type of food. Red meat darkens stool due to breakdown of heme protein and iron release. Iron tablets can impart a dark green or green black color and a large amount of red chili peppers can color the stool red. Pale or white stools may indicate common bile duct obstruction such as caused by gallbladder disease, or cancer, and may be accompanied by jaundice. Fecal volume varies by the amount of food ingested and the amount of fiber ingested. Men tend to produce larger fecal volumes probably due to greater food intake. Culture and generations can also alter patient's perceptions of "normal." Historically, bowel movements have been viewed as cleansing the body of toxins, so regular daily bowel movements were a sign of health. For that reason, patients over 70 years of age today tend to worry if they do not have a bowel movement every day. "An apple (fiber) a day keeps the doctor away" is a saying that supports that belief. These beliefs have made several older generations frequent laxative users. Those beliefs are declining rapidly with younger generations and subsequently laxative use is declining.

Acute or Rapid Onset Constipation

In the elderly, intestinal obstruction can cause sudden onset or rapidly progressive constipation, which is usually accompanied by associated symptoms such as abdominal pain, nausea, vomiting, and abdominal distention. Similarly, constipation can be a sign of colon cancer. Recent changes in medication such as opioid analgesics can be marked by the sudden appearance of constipation. Stimulation of the protective peritoneal reflex by recent abdominal surgery or inflammation of the intestine due to appendicitis or trauma may induce the effect, which can result in sudden constipation. One of the reasons post-abdominal surgery patients are encouraged to walk early and often is that walking internally indicates normality and helps disengage the reflex more quickly.

Chronic or Intermittent Constipation

There are multiple causes of chronic or intermittent constipation. Medication is a common cause. Opiates, drugs with anticholinergic properties, and calcium channel blockers are prescription medications commonly associated with constipation. Nonprescription drugs such as calcium salts taken for the prevention of osteoporosis and vitamin/mineral preparations are also common causes of constipation. Dehydration is also a common cause especially in patients who move to or visit areas of low humidity such as the Southwestern United States. During pregnancy, issues like calcium supplementation, using maternal fluid to maintain fetal well-being, and physical interference by the growing fetus can combine to make constipation a problem. Females over 50, should have thyroid function tests done since hypothyroidism, a cause of constipation, is more frequent in that population. Similarly, in older females the trauma of multiple childbirths may lead to constipation due to pelvic floor dysfunction. Dietary changes, such decreased fiber or fluid intake, and insufficient exercise can also negatively impact bowel movement frequency or consistency. Less common but potentially more serious is diabetic gastroparesis. Irritable bowel syndrome with constipation should be ruled out.

Patients should be asked about the frequency, color, and consistency. Hard stools may indicate dehydration. Changes in medication, eating, and drinking habits should be queried. Physical examination of the abdomen should be conducted looking for previous surgical scars, abdominal distension, masses, and alarm bowel sounds (high-pitched tinkling sounds found in intestinal obstruction). Associated symptoms are important keys to referral. In patients with constipation plus severe abdominal pain and abdominal distention, and who look sick, intestinal obstruction should be investigated. In patients with long-standing diabetes, constipation accompanied by bloating, belching, and early satiety may indicate diabetic gastroparesis. Elderly patients with cold intolerance, fatigue, loss of energy, and hair loss, plus constipation may be hypothyroid. Patients with any of the above alarm symptoms, failure of laxatives to relieve constipation, potential for drug- or surgery-induced disease, or constipation of 7 or more days duration should be referred for further evaluation.

• KEY REFERENCES

1. Getto L, Zeserson E, Breyer M. Vomiting ,diarrhea, constipation and gastroenteritis. *Emerg Med Clin North Am*. 2011;29:211-237.
2. Pfeiffer ML, DuPont HL, Ochoa TJ. The patient presenting with acute dysentery. *J Infect*. 2012;64: 374-386.
3. Pawloski SW, Warren CA, Guerrant R. Diagnosis of acute or persistent diarrhea. *Gastroenterology*. 2009;136:1874-1886.
4. Du Pont HL. Bacterial diarrhea. *N Engl J Med*. 2009;361:1560-1569.
5. Abraham B, Sellin JH. Drug-induced diarrhea. *Curr Gastroenterol Rep*. 2007;9:365-372.
6. Hammerle CW, Crowe SE. When to consider the diagnosis of irritable bowel syndrome. *Gastroenterol Clin North Am*. 2011;40:291-307.
7. Wenzl HH. Diarrhea in chronic inflammatory bowel disease. *Gastroenterol Clin North Am*. 2012;41:651-675.
8. Kartalija M, Sande MA. Diarrhea and AIDS in the era of highly active antiretroviral theapy. *Clin Infect Dis*. 1999;28:701-707.
9. Fasano A, Catassi C. Celiac disease. *N Engl J Med*. 2012;367:2419-2426.
10. King AR. Gluten content of the top 200 medications of 2008: a follow-up to the impact of celiac sprue on patients medication choices. *Hosp Pharm*. 2009;44:984-992.
11. Leung L, Riutta T, Kotecha J, Rosser W. Chronic constipation: an evidence based review. *J Am Board Fam Med*. 2011;24:436-451.
12. Jamshed N, Lee Z, Olden KW. Diagnostic approach to chronic constipation in adults. *Am Fam Physician*. 2011;84:299-306.

CASE 12.1

Martha Oncedaly, a 72-year-old school teacher who 2 weeks ago retired to Tucson and lives at the Desert Legacy in independent living comes into your store. She asks what is good for this constipation she has had since she arrived here. You remember her because she had complained about the food at Desert Legacy while she was waiting for several prescriptions to be filled 2 weeks ago when she arrived. They include calcium carbonate 500 mg, 3 qd, vitamin D 400 IU qd, Vicodin 2 tablets q6h severe joint pain, and piroxicam 20 mg qd.

What are the two most likely causes of her constipation?

_____

_____

_____

_____

_____

List three questions/examinations/lab tests you would ask/perform to help pinpoint the cause?

_____

_____

_____

_____

_____

CASE 12.2

One year later Martha returns to your pharmacy and asks for something to help her with her diarrhea. You remember that Martha got an extra refill of her medications to take on vacation about a month ago. Martha looks pale and like she is not feeling well. When you note her bending over clutching her stomach, she admits to an occasional cramping RLQ abdominal pain.

List three potential causes for Martha's symptoms.

_____

_____

_____

_____

_____

List six questions/examinations/lab tests you would ask/perform to help pinpoint the cause?

_____

_____

_____

_____

_____

Headache

1. Accurately identify the most likely etiology when patients present with a headache, through history, diagnostic tests, and appropriate patient findings on examination to enable the appropriate recommendation of effective treatment or referral to an appropriate provider.

2. Use the knowledge of the pathophysiology, etiology, and common presentations of headaches as a primary symptom to review prescription orders for appropriateness and to accurately educate patients about their disease and its treatment.

Headaches are very common, with over 95% of patients suffering from at least one headache in their lifetime. Between 250 and 800 workdays/1000 patients in the U.S. are lost due to headaches. Headaches can occur as part of a systemic illness, such as influenza, or as a single symptom. The International Headache Society classification system (ICHD-2) has over 150 pages of concise diagnostic criteria for different types of headaches. In the literature, headaches have been classified in a variety of ways. Primary headaches, the most common, include tension-type headaches, migraine headaches, and cluster headaches. Secondary headaches are by definition all nonprimary headaches and include those due to meningitis, hypertensive emergencies, strokes, temporomandibular joint (TMJ) pain dysfunction syndrome, trauma related, and pseudotumor cerebri. Others have classified them by seriousness or urgency. Acute onset headaches are mostly secondary, are more serious, and can be life threatening, requiring immediate diagnosis and intervention. Chronic or recurrent headaches, which include all the primary headaches and have a much more benign prognosis.

• ETIOLOGY

The causes of headache are multiple and at times complex in pathophysiology. Infectious processes, vascular problems, malignancy, medications, trauma, metabolic disorders, musculoskeletal problems, dental problems, diagnostic procedures, and hypoxia all are etiologic causes of headaches. Even among primary headaches, the exact cause of some may not be known or the exact nature of the pathophysiology is unclear and potentially controversial.

• DIAGNOSIS

There are several ways to classify headaches to facilitate diagnosis. For the purposes of this chapter, headaches will be organized as either primary or secondary.

• COMMON PRIMARY HEADACHES

The three main causes of a primary headache are tension-type headache, migraine headache, and cluster headache. While there are typical symptom patterns with each of the three primary headaches, initially it may be difficult to distinguish between severe tension headaches and some milder forms of migraines. Table 13.1 provides a quick guide to prominent features of the common primary headaches.

Tension-Type Headache
Tension headaches are the most common form of headache. Eighty-six percent (86%) of patients aged 12 to 41 have reported at least one tension headache during a 1-year period. The exact pathophysiology of tension headaches is still unclear. The current theory involves sensitization of dorsal horn neurons due to increased activity of the muscles and nerves in the neck, head, and shoulders.

Tension-type headaches typically present with mild-moderate pain intensity and are described as a bilateral, nonpulsating headache. The pain is constant and typically described as dull, pressure, vise-like, etc. Tension headaches are usually associated with muscle tenderness in the head, neck, and shoulders, which can be elicited by palpation of the muscles and rotation of the head and neck. Precipitating factors include stress, tension, and head/neck movements. Physical activity has little effect on the pain intensity. Neurological examination is normal and the overall physical examination is unremarkable except for some palpable muscle tenderness.

TABLE 13.1	Common Primary Headaches

A. DIAGNOSTIC SCHEMATA FOR COMMON PRIMARY HEADACHES
Migraine Headache
Episodic Tension Headache
Cluster Headache

B. DIFFERENTIAL DIAGNOSIS OF COMMON PRIMARY HEADACHES

SUBJECTIVE	Migraine	Tension	Cluster
a. Location	Unilateral in 60% to 75%. Remaining are global or frontal	Bilateral	Unilateral usually starting around eye or temple
b. Onset	Builds quickly over an hour or so to peak	Relatively sudden onset.	Acute sudden onset over minutes
c. Quality	Pulsating	Dull, squeezing ache like band around head	Piercing, deep
d. Quantity	Severe, incapacitating Lasts 4 to 72 hours	Mild to moderate. May be off and on	More painful than migraine Lasts 30 to 180 minutes
e. Setting	Family history common. More common in females	Stress or mental tension	Occurs in "clusters" daily for several days then remission. More common in males
f. Associated symptoms	20% have aura (classic migraine). Also nausea, vomiting, photophobia, or phonophobia are common	Stiff/painful neck muscles	Ipsilateral (same side as pain) nasal congestion or rhinorrhea, conjunctival injection or lacrimation, eyelid edema, facial sweating, other autonomic signs
g. Modifying factors	Exercise makes it worse, lying down makes it better, dark room makes it better	Analgesics	Physical activity may help

Reasons for referral of tension headaches include more than 15/month, patients with increasing frequency of headaches, those that do not exactly fit the diagnostic criteria, or in whom standard treatments with analgesics are ineffective. Referral is necessary in these patients to eliminate secondary causes such as mass occupying lesions, medication overuse headache, or TMJ pain dysfunction syndrome.

Migraine Headache

Migraine headaches are the second most common primary headache with a prevalence of 23/1000 and they more commonly occur in women in a 3:1 ratio. There are 18 types and subtypes of migraine headaches listed in IHCD-2. The two most common are migraines without aura or common migraines (64%), and migraine with aura or classic migraines (18%). At times, the diagnosis of migraine can be difficult. In one study, 98% of patients with sinus headaches actually had migraine or probable migraine headaches. Regardless of the presence of aura, migraines present with moderate to severe pain that is incapacitating, unilateral, pulsating, or throbbing and is made worse by physical activity. In addition, patients may experience nausea, vomiting, photophobia, or phonophobia. ICDH-2 requires that patients meet two of the four initial criteria and during the headache experience one of the second group of symptoms for the diagnosis of migraine headaches. Ten to thirty percent of patients will have an aura before and/or during the headache, which may consist of flashing lights, scotoma, visual disturbances, paresthesias, or a prodrome of tiredness, fatigue, mood changes, or gastrointestinal symptoms. One of the reasons for the structure of the ICDH-2 migraine criteria is that 20% to 30% of patients with migraines *do not* experience *each* of the *typical* symptoms, i.e., unilateral, pulsating, photophobia, phonophobia, and nausea. Migraine headaches typically last 4 to 72 hours. Many times patients may require a neurologist who specializes in headaches to accurately diagnose and effectively treat migraine headaches. A neurological examination will be normal.

The etiology of migraine headaches has remained controversial for decades. There may be multiple causes that explain the variety of presentations and individual responses to different preventive and treatment regimens. The old theory was that changes in neurotransmitter activity in the brain lead to a vasoconstriction followed by rebound vasodilation in intra- and extracranial blood vessels, which causes headache. While there is evidence to support this older model, most experts now feel that migraines are a gene-based disease, because there is a close family history of migraine headaches found in over 70% of patients newly diagnosed. In these patients, dysfunction in the periaqueductal gray matter causes the loss of inhibition over the cortex of the brain. This results in an electrical wave that causes trigeminovascular neuronal hyperreactivity involving decreased or destabilized serotonin activity in the brain stem. This leads to the release of inflammatory, vasodilator neuropeptides such as CGRP (calcitonin gene-related peptide), PACAP (pituitary adenylate cyclase activating peptide), and nitric oxide (NO). Those neuropeptides cause an inflammation of the vessels and tissue in the midbrain that leads to the pain and eventual vasodilation. Current research efforts are developing drugs that block the activity/release of each of these inflammatory mediators.

Cluster Headache

The last major primary headache, the cluster headache, is relatively uncommon, with a prevalence of 0.5 to 1.0/1000 patients. It occurs primarily in men in a ratio of 5:1. Cluster headaches present with severe pain (worse than migraine pain) in the orbital, supraorbital, or temporal region that is unilateral and pulsating, lasting 30 to 180 minutes if untreated. In addition, attacks occur in clusters from once every other day to eight times/day with headache-free periods lasting days to months. To diagnose cluster headaches, patients must have one or more autonomic symptoms ipsilateral (same side) to the location of the pain. These include nasal congestion or rhinorrhea, conjunctival injection (redness) or lacrimation, miosis and/or ptosis, forehead and/or facial sweating, or eyelid edema. Other than the eye findings, a neurological examination will be normal. Patients with cluster headaches need to be seen by a neurologist or headache specialist for management.

• SECONDARY HEADACHES

Secondary headaches usually have more serious consequences that require immediate intervention. Any patient presenting with what seems like a primary headache but has an abnormal neurological examination requires a workup for a secondary headache. New headaches in patients over 50 or any severe headache requires immediate further diagnostic testing. CT scans are the initial choice and are accurate in identifying acute hemorrhage, trauma to bony structures, and sinus disorders. MRIs are used to rule out infarction, mass occupying lesions, brain abscesses, and craniocervical junction abnormalities. Recently, one author updated a mnemonic for secondary headaches called SNOOP 4. S stands for systemic and includes immunosuppressed patients, infectious meningitis, brain abscess, and metastatic tumor. N indicates neurologic abnormality, which would relate to infarcts or mass occupying lesions. The first O is for sudden onset that indicates cerebrovascular accident (CVA), subarachnoid hemorrhage, or arterial dissection. The second O is for onset of new headache over age 50, which considers temporal arteritis, neoplastic, or vascular issues. Finally, P stands for pattern change with 4 potential causes including progressive headache and papilledema. For the pharmacist, other than tension headaches, patients should be referred for definitive diagnosis and treatment.

Temporomandibular Joint Dysfunction Syndrome

One of the symptoms of TMJ dysfunction can be a headache. Initially, because of associated myofascial pain in some patients it was thought that it caused tension headaches. However, recent literature shows a much stronger link with migraine headaches and chronic daily headaches than tension headaches.

Suspicion of TMJ disorders as a cause of headache can be confirmed with a careful history and limited physical examination. Place the palmar surface of the fingers of both hands over each TMJ. Have the patient open their mouth wide. A palpated clicking sensation or audible click confirms the potential for a TMJ disorder. In addition, simultaneously observe the opening and closing of the mouth. Normally, the jaw opens vertically straight up and down. Any jerky, sideways or angled movement during opening and/or closing may be indicative of TMJ disorder. Patients with TMJ disorder headaches commonly will awaken with their headache and many have a history of bruxism (grinding the teeth at night) or regular jaw clenching. Many patients have occlusal disorders with underbites more common than overbites. In some patients chewing gum is associated with the headache. Patients suspected of headaches secondary to TMJ disorders should be referred to a dentist initially for evaluation of TMJ disorders.

Medication Overuse/OTC Headaches

Medication overuse headache is a relatively new entity. While it occurs in patients with both tension and migraine headaches, patients with episodic migraines and women are the most frequent patients to develop this type of headache. There are three criteria for diagnosis. The first is a chronic daily headache for more than 15 days/month. The second criteria is a 3-month overuse of ergotamine, triptans, opioids, or combination analgesics (including those with butalbital) for more than 10 days/month. Alternatively analgesics or any combination of ergots, triptans, opioid analgesics for more than 15 days/month without overuse also meet the criteria. Finally, there must be a history of recent development or markedly worsened headache during medication overuse. Patients who you suspect of this problem should be referred to a neurologist or headache specialist for diagnosis and treatment. Treatment involves tapering the causative medication or discontinuing it while providing other medication for pain relief. Elimination or marked reduction in headache frequency after 60 days is diagnostic.

Hypertensive Emergency (Malignant Hypertension)

Patients who present with blood pressures >220/120 are at risk for hypertensive encephalopathy, as well as intracranial and subarachnoid hemorrhages. Patients with all three conditions can present with a moderate to severe headache. In hypertensive encephalopathy, cerebral edema occurs, causing the headache and potential changes in behavior and cognitive function. Funduscopic examination of the eye many times reveals papilledema, a swelling and blurring of the optic disc. Treating the blood pressure reduces the risk of those complications and the patient's symptoms including the headache.

Tumor/Mass Occupying Lesion

Tumors of the brain can be either malignant or nonmalignant. Also, they can be primary tumors or metastatic lesions from a primary cancer elsewhere in the body. Patients previously diagnosed with other malignancies that may metastasize to the brain who present with a headache should be immediately referred to their oncologist for further diagnostic evaluation. Headaches, cognitive decline, or behavior changes with focal neurologic deficits are typical presentations. Some tumors such as benign meningiomas are diagnosed during evaluation of a primary headache and can be an incidental finding. Regardless, unexplained headaches, progressive headaches, or new headaches with or without neurological deficits should be immediately referred to a neurologist or headache specialist for further evaluation

Meningitis

Meningitis can be caused by a variety of microorganisms including bacteria, viruses, fungi, and mycobacteria.

Viral meningitis, also known as aseptic meningitis due to the absence of any organism upon Gram stain or culture of the cerebrospinal fluid (CSF), is the most common form of meningitis. Enteroviruses, such as coxsackievirus and echovirus, are the most common causes of viral meningitis. Others include arboviruses herpes simplex, mumps, and HIV. Mumps should be suspected in patients with swollen parotid glands in patients who have not received appropriate vaccination with MMR. In patients at risk, who present with possible symptoms of meningitis, testing for HIV should be done.

Bacterial meningitis in adults is caused primarily by *Streptococcus pneumoniae* or *Neisseria meningitidis*. *Listeria monocytogenes* should be suspected in patients who are pregnant, over 50 years of age or immunocompromised. Mycobacterial meningitis should be suspected in areas where tuberculosis is endemic and in immunocompromised patients such as those with HIV.

Fungal meningitis is usually found in immunocompromised patients. *Cryptococcus* and *Aspergillus* species are the most common infecting agents. *Candida* species also cause meningitis especially in hospitalized patients. In areas where systemic fungal infections are endemic, e.g., coccidioidomycosis in the San Joaquin Valley in California and the Sonoran Desert of Arizona and Northern Mexico should be included in any differential diagnosis of patients suspected to have meningitis.

While presenting symptoms vary in severity and by microorganism, they generally include some combination of headache, fever, neck stiffness (nuchal rigidity), altered mental status, photophobia, nausea/vomiting, seizures, focal neurological deficits, and a skin rash, in addition to generalized fatigue, malaise, arthralgias, and myalgias. The Kernig and Brudzinski signs, once the gold standard for meningeal irritation, have proven to be of limited usefulness (positive predictive level of 27%), because now patients tend to present earlier in the course of the disease. Testing for nuchal rigidity also is only marginally better as a positive predictive sign. Also, the classic triad of fever, neck stiffness, and altered mental status is found in only two-thirds of adults diagnosed with bacterial meningitis. If headache is added as a fourth manifestaion, then 95% of patients with two of the four signs or symptoms were diagnosed with bacterial meningitis.

Confirmation of the cause of meningitis depends on examination of the CSF. Table 13.2 provides a guide to the CSF findings in the common forms of meningitis. Generally, CSF pressure, number and type of white blood cells, amount of protein, and glucose levels or ratio of serum to CSF glucose are used. Gram staining the CSF sample

TABLE 13.2	CSF Differential Diagnosis: Meningitis			
Examination	Bacterial	Viral	Fungal	Mycobacterial
Opening pressure	Elevated	Usually normal	Variable	Variable
White blood cell count	>1000/mm³	20 to 500/mm³	Variable	Variable
Predominant WBC type	PMN	Lymphocytes/monocytes	Lymphocytes	Lymphocytes
Protein	>100 mg/dL	100 to 500 mg/dL	50 to 200 mg/dL	100 to 500 mg/dL
CSF-serum glucose ratio	<0.6 (<40 mg/dL)	>0.5 (normal)	decreased	<40 mg/dL
Other	Lactate > 4.2 mmol/L	PCR		
	Serum procalcitonin >0.5 ng/mL			
	Peripheral WBCs >10,000+ >80% PMNs			

will reveal bacteria in 60% to 80% of patients with bacterial meningitis. CSF and blood samples are also sent for culture and susceptibility. Nucleic acid amplification tests such as PCR assays are rapid and are used primarily to detect viral species, mycobacteria, and some fungi and have been used to identify specific bacterial species. Current PCR assays are being more frequently used as costs decline.

Pseudotumor Cerebri (Idiopathic Intracranial Hypertension)

Pseudotumor cerebri is a rare disorder (<1.0/100,000) typically seen in overweight females of childbearing age. It is due to an imbalance between the production and reabsorption of CSF, resulting in increased intracranial pressure and headache. If left unchecked, permanent visual changes can occur. In addition to headache, visual disturbances and papilledema can occur. The reason that it is important to pharmacists is that it can be caused or exacerbated by medications. For example, both minocycline (also other tetracyclines) and isotretinoin have been implicated. Of particular importance is that when filling a new prescription for oral isotretinoin, the pharmacist needs to make sure that the patient stops their minocycline before starting the isotretinoin to reduce the risk of the combination inducing the condition. Women returning for the initial refill should be questioned about new onset headaches and visual problems and the pharmacist should verify that they have stopped any tetracycline.

Acute Trauma/Post-Trauma Headache

A new moderate to severe headache occurring within 12 to 24 hours after closed-head trauma should be referred to urgent/emergent care for evaluation of subarachnoid or intracerebral bleeding. In particular, special attention should be given to patients on drugs that interfere with normal coagulation, e.g., aspirin, clopidogrel, warfarin, regular NSAID use, chronic long-term phenytoin use (due to higher INR due to enzyme induction of vitamin K metabolism).

Post-trauma headaches (post-concussion headaches) can last for weeks after the injury. They can present like all three types of common primary headaches although tension-type headaches are the most common manifestation. Patients with headaches that might be due to a recent history of trauma to the head or neck and shoulders should be referred to the care of a neurologist for evaluation and follow-up.

Cerebrovascular Accident (Stroke)

The role of a pharmacist in the management of patients with diabetes, hypertension, dyslipidemia, and oral anticoagulant therapy for patients with atrial fibrillation or prosthetic heart valves is well established in the medical literature. All the above conditions contribute directly or indirectly to a markedly increased risk of stroke (CVA). Therefore, the pharmacist must use their assessment skills at every visit to ascertain whether or not the patient is suffering from this complication of their chronic diseases. In addition, as part of patient education efforts, the pharmacist needs to familiarize the patient with the signs and symptoms of stroke, because successful or optimal prevention of permanent sequelae is dependent on early self-detection and treatment.

Etiology Traditionally, acute cerebrovascular events are divided into two major categories: stroke or CVA and transient ischemic attack (TIA). Previously, a TIA was characterized as a cerebrovascular event without infarction, leading to focal neurological signs and symptoms that lasted less than 24 hours and left no residual effects. TIAs have also been called reversible ischemic neurological deficit (RIND), which is consistent with the older definition. A stroke or CVA was defined as focal neurological signs and symptoms that lasted greater than 24 hours and involved infarction of brain tissue. Recent evidence has shown that this classic 24-hour distinction is misleading in that many patients with transient (<24 hours) symptoms actually have a cerebral infarction. A task force of the American Heart Association has recommended that the 24-hour distinction between TIA and CVA should be removed based on a review of the literature. Instead the differentiation of CVA and TIA should be defined in terms of tissue damage (infarction). The task force recommended that the definition of TIA be changed to *a transient neurological dysfunction caused by focal brain, spinal cord, or retinal ischemia, without acute infarction.* No time frame was attached to *transient.* The definition of stroke was changed to *an infarction of central nervous system tissue.* Further, they recommended that analogous to acute coronary syndrome the spectrum of neurovascular events affecting the brain be called acute neurovascular syndrome. Therefore, past comparisons of TIA to angina pectoris and CVA to myocardial infarction are no longer considered correct or applicable. However, they did not go so far as to define the elements of the spectrum as has been done with chest pain (STEMI versus NSTEMI versus unstable angina). We have known that these multiple *silent infarctions* or *ministrokes,* (up until now classified as TIAs) have been implicated as the etiology of the largest group of patients with dementia, i.e., multi-infarct dementia. In addition, evidence shows as many as 20% to 25% of high-risk patients with a TIA will have a stroke within the next 90 days, most likely during the week after the TIA. Therefore, any signs or symptoms potentially indicative of any acute cerebrovascular event require immediate referral for a comprehensive workup and definitive care.

Acute cerebrovascular events have two major causes: ischemic and hemorrhagic. Ischemic events (80% to 88%) are primarily due to atherosclerosis or embolism. The atherosclerotic process is the same as for myocardial infarction, and is associated with a gradual accumulation of intra-arterial plaque. If the plaque is unstable, it may eventually rupture initiating a platelet-based clot, which may progress to decreased circulation and a subsequent infarct. Embolic strokes are due to clots that form in the heart in patients with atrial fibrillation or prosthetic cardiac devices such as a heart valve. A portion of the clot becomes dislodged and ultimately travels to a part of the circulatory system of the brain, which is too narrow for it to pass through. The result is obstruction of the circulation to tissue past that point. Hemorrhagic strokes (12%

to 15%) are due to a ruptured aneurysm or blood vessel. Uncontrolled hypertension and a combination of hypertension and atherosclerosis are the primary etiologies in hemorrhagic strokes.

Diagnosis While this evidence-based change in definition does not impact the pharmacist's role in the early detection of symptoms or control of predisposing conditions such as dyslipidemia, hypertension, and diabetes, it does change the urgency with which patients with those symptoms need to be referred. It also increases the importance of patient education in self-recognition of potential acute neurovascular syndrome symptoms and the need for immediately seeking care when they occur.

Manifestations of acute neurovascular syndrome include impaired speech or language, visual disturbances, double vision or visual loss, facial drooping, trouble swallowing, weakness or numbness/tingling on one side of the body, impaired coordination of limbs or gait dysfunction, vertigo, dizziness, stiff neck, headache, sudden change in behavior (often recognized by people other than the patient), seizure, syncope, confusion, or cognitive impairment. One simple aid that may help in teaching patient self-recognition skills of the more apparent signs and symptoms of stroke is the mnemonic FAST.

F = Face   Face drooping and/or asymmetry when patient smiles.
A = Arms   Patient may not be able to raise both arms evenly.
S = Speech   Patient may slur words and may not be able to repeat a simple sentence correctly.
T = Time   If the patient has any of these, call 911 immediately.

Specific physical findings to confirm the dysfunction could include dysarthria (trouble speaking), cranial nerve deficits, unilateral weakness, unilateral loss of sensation, cerebellar dysfunction, and abnormal pupil examination. The dysfunction may be of short duration if it is a small infarction or it may continue in the case of a larger infarction.

A diffusion weighted imaging MRI (MRI-DWI) is the test of choice due to its sensitivity to detect small infarctions and distinguish between new and old lesions, and even between ischemic and hemorrhagic stroke. The MRI should be done as soon as possible, at least within 24 hours even if the dysfunction lasts less than 2 hours. Transcranial and carotid Doppler ultrasonography, CT or MR angiography, or CT scan are alternative imaging tests if MRI-DWI is not readily available.

Roughly one-third of patients referred for a stroke workup do not have a stroke. Alternative diagnoses may include seizures, sepsis, encephalopathy, mass occupying lesion, syncope, delirium, dementia, migraine, subdural hematoma, hypo- or hyperglycemia, benign paroxysmal positional vertigo, psychogenic/functional cases, and cervical or lumbar spine disorders. Many of these causes can be established (thereby ruling out stroke) by history, physical examination, routine laboratory tests, and brain imaging.

• SUMMARY

The pharmacist's role in preventing acute cerebrovascular events focuses on the control of comorbid conditions such as hypertension, diabetes, dyslipidemia, and anticoagulation that can lead to TIA and/or stroke. In addition, pharmacists can play a major role in educating patients with those disorders to readily recognize signs and symptoms of acute neurovascular syndrome and if present to seek immediate help. At every visit for these comorbid disorders, the pharmacist needs to probe for typical symptoms and via neurological examination probe for typical signs. By doing this at every visit, it reinforces the patient's understanding of self-recognition.

• KEY REFERENCES

1. Crystal SC, Robbins MS. Epidemiology of tension-type headaches. *Curr Pain Headache Rep*. 2010; 14:449-454.
2. Bendtsen L, Jensen R. Tension type headaches. *Neurol Clin*. 2009;27:525-535.
3. Bartleson JD, Cutrer M. Migraine update: diagnosis and treatment. *Minn Med*. 2010;93:36-41.
4. Van Kleef M, Lataster A, Narouze S, Mekhail N, Geurts JW, van Zundert J. Cluster headache. *Pain Pract*. 2009;9:435-442.
5. Martin VT. The diagnostic evaluation of secondary headache disorders. *Headache*. 2011;51:346-352.
6. Clinch CR. Evaluation of acute headaches in adults. *Am Fam Physician*. 2001;63:685-691.
7. Goncalves DAG, Camaris CM, Speciali JG, et al. Tempomandibular disorders are differentially associated with headache diagnosis: a controlled study. *Clin J Pain*. 2011;27:611-615.
8. Evers S, Marziniak M. Clinical features, pathophysiology and treatment of medication-overuse headaches. *Lancet Neurol*. 2010;9:392-401.
9. Chadwick DR. Viral meningitis. *Br Med Bull*. 2006;75-76:1-14.
10. Lin AL, Safdieh JE. The evaluation and management of bacterial meningitis: current practice and emerging developments. *Neurologist*. 2010;16:143-151.
11. McArthur KS, Quinn TJ, Walters MR. Diagnosis and management of transient ischaemic attack and ischemic stroke in the acute phase. *BMJ*. 2011;342:1938.
12. Cucchiara B, Kasner SE. In the clinic: transient ischemic attack. *Ann Intern Med*. 2011; 154(1):ITC11-15.
13. Easton JD, Saver JL, Albers GW, et al. Definition and evaluation of a transient ischemia attack. *Stroke*. 2009;40:2276-2293.
14. Rhoney DH. Contemporary management of transient ischemic attack: role of the pharmacist. *Pharmacotherapy*. 2011;31(2):193-213.

CASE 13.1

Edith Coiner is a 54 year-old-patient with type 2 diabetes mellitus who you see regularly in clinic. Today, during her regular follow-up visit Edith mentions that she has had four severe headaches in the last month and is concerned.

Problem List		Medication
1988	Allergic rhinitis	Loratadine 10 mg qd
1992	Diabetes mellitus type 2	NPH 70/30 insulin
1997	Proteinuria	24 units q AM
2001	Neuropathy	12 units q PM
1992	Hypertension	Chlorthalidone 25 mg q AM
		Enalapril 20 mg bid
1992	Hyperlipidemia	Atorvastatin 40 mg q PM

List three possible causes for Edith's headaches. Explain your rationale.

_____

_____

_____

_____

_____

List six diagnostic tests, physical examinations, or questions you would order, perform, or ask to evaluate Edith's headaches. Explain your rationale.

_____

_____

_____

_____

_____

FOURTEEN

Inflamed (Red) Eye

1. Accurately identify the most likely etiology when patients present with an inflamed, red eye and/or other eye symptoms, through history and patient findings on examination to enable the appropriate recommendation of effective treatment or referral to an appropriate provider.

2. Use the knowledge of the pathophysiology, etiology, and common presentations of common eye complaints as a primary symptom to review prescription orders for appropriateness and to accurately educate patients about their disease and its treatment.

• INTRODUCTION

Patients presenting with redness in the visible portion of the eye is a common symptom in primary and urgent care practice. Nearly 6 million cases of acute conjunctivitis also known as "pink eye" are reported annually in the United States. Approximately 15% of adult patients suffer from allergic ocular conditions. Patients routinely present to the pharmacy with eye complaints. However, minority of causes of red eye can be treated with nonprescription products so the primary role of the pharmacist is referral to either primary, emergent, or specialty care. The most common specific causes of a red eye are (1) infectious (viral or bacterial); (2) allergic; and (3) "nonspecific," which includes irritative. There are other conditions that can be confused with conjunctivitis, including some that need urgent or emergent management.

• RELEVANT ANATOMY

Location of the redness can be important so a brief review of eye anatomy is important. The term conjunctivitis means inflammation of the conjunctiva (singular) or conjunctivae (plural). The conjunctiva is usually described as having three parts, all of which are thin, transparent layers of mucous membrane. The most external and easily observable portion is that which overlies the white portion (sclera) of the eyeball itself. This is called the bulbar or ocular conjunctiva. It covers the entire sclera, but it does not cover the central anterior portion of the eyeball (the cornea). That is, it extends onto the eyeball up to, but not beyond, the limbus. The limbus is the union of the cornea and the sclera and a conjunctivitis limited to the limbus is an important clue to more serious cause of a red eye. When the bulbar conjunctiva is normal (not inflamed), it cannot be differentiated from the sclera beneath it, because it is clear. Another portion of the conjunctiva, visible if the eyelids are inverted, covers the inner linings of both upper and lower eye lids (the palpebrae). This portion of the conjunctiva is called the palpebral or tarsal conjunctiva. There is a third portion of the conjunctiva that is difficult to visualize, because of its anatomic location. This portion is located at the fornix, which is the communication between the palpebral and bulbar conjunctivae. In practical terms, conjunctivitis can be bulbar (the lining over most of the eyeball) or palpebral (the linings inside the eye lids) or both. The pink or red coloration is due to increased visualization of blood vessels in the conjunctivae due to vasodilation of the vessels. There are numerous possible causes of this increased vasodilation, but in general it is usually due to either irritation or inflammation. Inflammation of the surface of the cornea is known as keratitis and keratoconjunctivitis is inflammation of both the conjunctiva and the corneal surface.

• DIAGNOSIS

Elements of Evaluation of Eye Conditions That Indicate Urgent or Emergent Referral

Since there are few eye conditions that can be successfully treated with over-the-counter (OTC) products, the pharmacist will end up referring most patients. More importantly some patients present to the pharmacy to attempt to self-treat eye problems that may cause permanent loss of vision without immediate referral and treatment. Therefore, it is very important that pharmacists are aware of signs and symptoms that indicate serious eye problems. The following findings should *always* be a reason to advise the patient to see an eye-care specialist, usually on an emergent basis. These are

TABLE 14.1	Symptoms in Inflamed Eye Requiring Immediate Referral (May incur visual loss if not seen immediately)
Pain in the eyeball itself (true eyeball pain)	
Significant change in vision (decreased visual acuity)	
Photophobia (extreme sensitivity to light)	
Severe foreign body sensation	
Limbal or ciliary flush	
Any corneal irregularity	
History of trauma to the eye	
Cutaneous vesicular eruption on the face or near the eye	
Soft tissue swelling near the eye or eyelids	
Hyphema or hypopyon	
Contact lens wearers	

findings that are *not* caused by simple conjunctivitis or other non-sight-threatening conditions (Table 14.1).

1. **Pain in the eyeball itself** Pain in the eyeball itself is far worse than the gritty sensation some patients with common forms of conjunctivitis have. Any suggestion of true eyeball pain is a reason for emergent referral. This symptom indicates a severe vision-threatening problem regardless of etiology.

2. **Significant change in vision** (not corrected by removal of any episodic discharge) This is mostly a subjective manifestation, but may be partly objective if a crude visual acuity test can be done having the patient read newsprint at arm's length, presuming the patient's baseline ability to do this is known. True visual impairment is an indication of a severe, possibly vision-threatening problem.

3. **Photophobia** (extreme sensitivity to light) Significant, severe, or persistent photophobia is another warning symptom. However, due to the primarily subjective nature of this complaint, it is more difficult to evaluate. Photophobia is extreme light sensitivity. Most people dislike a flashlight suddenly shone into their eyes and a typical reaction is to close the eyes, look away, or otherwise shield the eyes. However, when the patient is continuously bothered by the usual amount of ambient light present indoors in most homes and businesses, this is abnormal. However, even when this is present to a pathologic degree, removal of the light, that is, moving the patient to a darkened room, will alleviate the discomfort. In the darkened setting, the patient will be able to open the eyes and keep them open. True photophobia is usually an indication of serious uveal tract or possibly other serious ophthalmic disorder. The uveal tract consists of the iris, ciliary body, and choroid. Its structures extend from the iris, just under the cornea (near the anterior pole of the globe) to near the optic nerve at the posterior pole of the globe. A rather long list of potentially serious, vision-threatening problems can cause inflammation of the uveal tract (uveitis). Patients demonstrating this symptom should be referred to an eye-care specialist immediately. Not infrequently these conditions accompany an autoimmune arthritis such as rheumatoid arthritis.

4. **Severe foreign body sensation** (eye shielded even without light shining in) Eye problems that cause a significant amount of foreign body sensation may be

associated with corneal inflammation due to irritation, infection, or damage. This corneal inflammation, known as keratitis, has both subjective and objective components. The most helpful symptom that suggests keratitis is a severe foreign body sensation. The patient will complain of the feeling of "something in the eye" and as a result, will have difficulty opening and especially, keeping open the affected eye. The eyelids will be squeezed together, so as to close the eye. The patient will usually complain of severe discomfort, and perhaps express it as true pain. The eye will remain closed even in a darkened room. The patient may appear to shield the affected eye from light, but even when placed in a darkened room, they are reluctant to open the eye. The patient will generally resist even gentle attempts to open the eye by separating the lids. If the eye can be opened slightly in a darkened environment, shining a light into the eye usually does not worsen the situation, unless the patient is also experiencing photophobia. Appreciate that severe foreign body sensation is distinct from true photophobia. Objectively, there may be a small scratch or ulcer, which is not always visible on inspection with a penlight. However, it may have progressed to a defect in the cornea that is visible. Also if the cornea is anything except completely clear, there is some abnormality present. To confirm the presence of corneal damage, infection, inflammation, or ulceration, a fluorescein stain is conducted. Either an eye drop or an impregnated strip is placed in the eye. Then allow the dye to distribute over the corneal surface. The external eye is then examined with a blue light (cobalt blue or Wood lamp) via a magnifying binocular slit lamp. Lesions in the cornea clearly stand out as blue to green images. Figure 14.1 shows the typical dendritic pattern lesion of herpes simplex keratitis outlined by fluorescein stain. There are numerous possible causes of keratitis, all of which require referral, to an eye-care specialist, on an emergent basis.

5. **Limbal or ciliary flush** (Figure 14.2) This is an objective finding, but requires only simple inspection of the eye, without any direct patient contact. The limbus is the border between the cornea and the sclera. It is usually devoid of visible vessels or redness. When a problem causes inflammation of either the cornea (keratitis)

FIGURE 14.1 Herpes simplex keratitis. A large dendritic lesion after fluorescein staining. The patient had been diagnosed with "pink eye" in a prior visit. Source: photo contributor: Kevin J. Knoop, MD, MS. Reproduced with permission from Knoop KJ, Stack LB, Storrow AB, Thurman, RJ. *The Atlas of Emergency Medicine*, 3rd ed. McGraw-Hill, Inc; 2010. Fig. 2-37. Copyright © McGraw-Hill Education LLC.

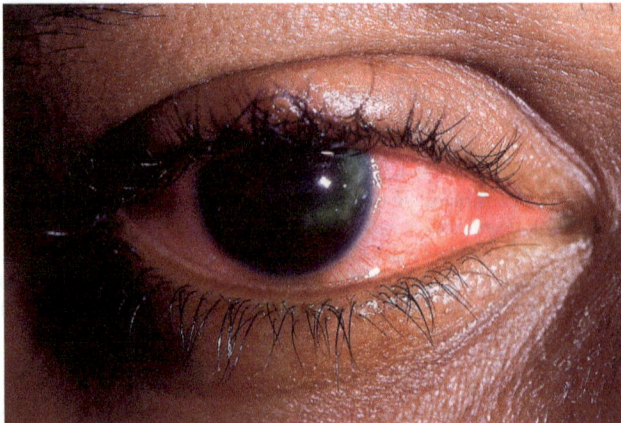

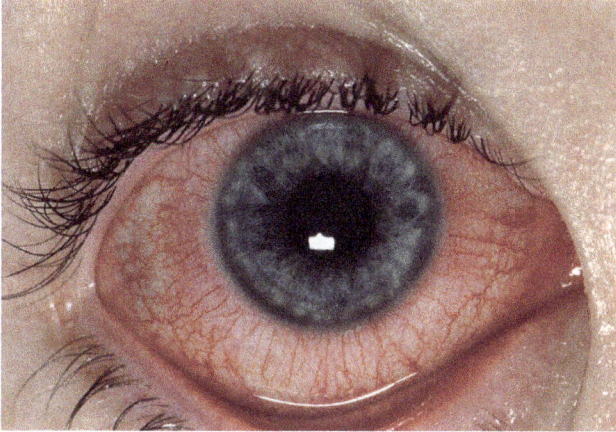

FIGURE 14.2 Anterior uveitis. Marked conjunctival injection and perilimbal hyperemia ("ciliary flush") are seen in this patient with recurrent iritis. Source: photo contributor: Frank Birinyi, MD: Reproduced with permission from Knoop KJ , Stack LB, Storrow AB, Thurman RJ. *The Atlas of Emergency Medicine*, 3rd ed. McGraw-Hill, Inc; 2010. Fig. 2-27. Copyright © McGraw-Hill Education LLC.

or the anterior portion of the uveal tract (iritis), a limbal flush occurs. The *flush* means that there are visible (dilated) blood vessels concentrated at the border of the cornea and the sclera (limbus), and often the area immediately surrounding the limbus is deep pink or red.

6. **Any corneal irregularity** (i.e., anything except a perfectly clear cornea)

7. **Any history of trauma or obvious evidence of trauma to the eye**

8. **Cutaneous vesicular distribution on the face or near an eye** Cutaneous vesicular distribution on the face or near an eye indicates the potential of either herpes simplex or herpes zoster eye infections. Both can cause permanent visual impairment by damaging the cornea. Herpes zoster ophthalmicus is shingles involving ocular structures. This is especially true if the ophthalmic (the most superior) branch of cranial nerve 5 is affected. Hutchinson's sign, presence of vesicles on the nose can be indicative of ocular involvement.

9. **Any soft tissue swelling near the eye** (dacryocystitis, orbital cellulitis, preseptal cellulitis) Swelling and inflammation (cellulitis) of one or both eyelids and/or other structures immediately surrounding the eye may indicate a serious bacterial infection. If orbital cellulitis is present there is usually some abnormality of extra-ocular movement (EOM). Adults may have a history of trauma (including surgery) preceding development of any of the problems.

10. **Hyphema/hypopyon** Under normal circumstances fluid is not visible in the anterior chamber. A visible meniscus of blood, cloudy fluid or purulent material in the anterior chamber is an ocular emergency. Blood in the anterior chamber due to trauma or over-anticoagulaltion is called a hyphema, while cloudy or purulent fluid is a hypopyon, (Figure 14.3) caused by inflammation or infection of the internal structures of the eye. In addition, most patients will also usually have other cardinal signs, i.e. visual impairment, eyeball pain, photophobia, limbal flush.

11. **Contact lens wearers** Another special situation involves patients who regularly use contact lenses, or whose intermittent use of contact lenses immediately preceded the onset of the acute condition for which they have sought care. Contact lens

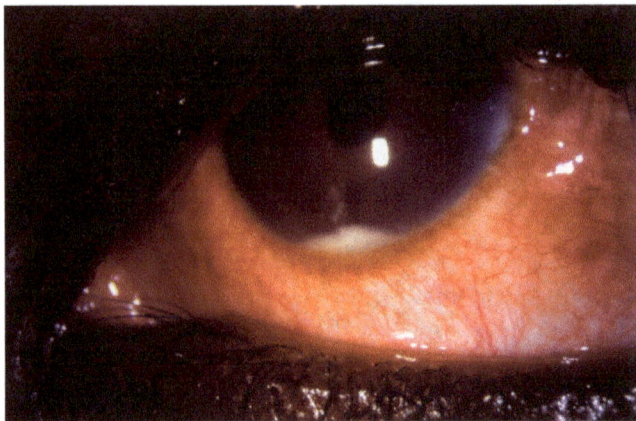

FIGURE 14.3 Hypopyon in acute anterior uveitis (iritis). (Reproduced with permission, from Riordan-Eva P, Cunningham ET, eds. *Vaughan & Asbury's General Ophthalmology.* 18th ed. McGraw-Hill, Inc; 2011:60. Fig. 3-4. Copyright © McGraw-Hill Education LLC.)

wearers may have a more serious disorder than is initially suspected due to infections with unusual organisms, keratitis, or corneal abrasion. It is prudent to recommend referral to an eye-care specialist for virtually all patients who have used contact lenses recently and have developed a new eye or vision complaint. This is true even if they seem to have only an irritative, allergic, or viral or bacterial conjunctivitis.

Common Causes of Inflamed, Red Eyes

The three most common causes of red eye are allergic, viral, and bacterial conjunctivitis (Table 14.2). Their relative incidence is in the order as listed. That is, allergic conjunctivitis is the most common, and may affect up to 40% of the US population. The infectious causes of conjunctivitis are, as a group, second to allergic causes. The most common types of infectious conjunctivitis are those caused by viruses. The next most common are those due to bacteria. Irritative conjunctivitis is another common cause of redness in the eye and is due to exposure to wind, dust, or swimming pool chlorine. The other three are usually not completely manageable in the community pharmacy setting. However, meaningful service can be provided by a screening/triage function, and, where appropriate, by recommendation of initial management suggestions in the form of nonpharmacological modes or OTC medications.

Irritative Conjunctivitis

Chlorine from swimming pools, smoke, intense light (snow blindness), dry windy conditions are common causes of conjunctival inflammation, redness, and irritation. Usually bilateral, these conditions are all best treated by avoidance of the irritant and preventive measures (wearing goggles or sunglasses), but topical OTC products may provide temporary relief until preventive measures can be fully implemented. The patients should be queried about specific details of recent exposure to any of the common irritants, use of prescription eye drops, recent changes in eye cosmetics, or contact lens solutions. Patients with new or long-term glaucoma medication, contact lens wearers, and suspected allergic reactions to eye products should be referred to an eye-care specialist.

TABLE 14.2	Red Eye

A. DIAGNOSTIC SCHEMATA FOR THE DIAGNOSIS OF A RED EYE

Allergic Conjunctivitis
Viral Conjunctivitis
Bacterial Conjunctivitis
Vernal, Atopic, and Giant Papillary Keratoconjunctivitis
Herpes Simplex and/or Herpes Zoster Keratoconjunctivitis
Gonococcal and/or Chlamydial Conjunctivitis

B. DIFFERENTIAL DIAGNOSIS OF RED EYE

SUBJECTIVE	Allergic Conjunctivitis	Viral Conjunctivitis	Bacterial Conjunctivitis	Vernal/Atopic/Giant Papillary Keratoconjunctivitis	Herpes Simplex/Zoster Keratoconjunctivitis	Gonococcal/Chlamydial Conjunctivitis
Location	Bilateral	Unilateral initially, but spreads to other eye	Usually bilateral	Usually bilateral but can be unilateral occasionally	Usually unilateral	Unilateral or bilateral
Onset	Acute	Acute	Acute	Chronic	Acute	Acute
Quality	Itching	Mild, irritating foreign body sensation	Mild, irritating foreign body sensation	Severe foreign body sensation, plus Severe itching	Simplex may mimic viral conjunctivitis,	Severe foreign body sensation
Quantity	Episodic	N/A	N/A	N/A	N/A	N/A
Setting	SAC at specific times of the year, PAC, year-round	Others have it	Others have it	VKC common in males age 4 year to puberty. AKC young adult to fifth decade. GPC in contact lens users, postsurgery	N/A	May have genital form of the infection as well. Treat systemically
Associated symptoms	Watery discharge, allergic rhinitis, asthma	Variable discharge from usually clear to mucopurulent. Viral cold symptoms. Eye matting	Purulent discharge, eye matting in the AM	Photophobia. Atopic dermatitis on face and eyelids in AKC. VKC—stringy discharge	Photophobia, decreased visual acuity, vesicular skin lesions around eye. Typical shingles prodromal symptoms	Copious hyperpurulent discharge in gonococcal. Also photophobia, blurred vision. *Chlamydia* mimics viral conjunctivitis. May have mucoid discharge
Modifying factors	Antihistamines make it better, exposure to allergen makes it worse	N/A	N/A	N/A	N/A	N/A
OBJECTIVE	Usually mildly inflamed or injected	Mild to moderate inflammation. Periauricular lymphadenopathy may be present	Usually moderate to severe inflammation with a purulent eye discharge	GPC—upper lid palpebral papillae. Papillae in VKC and AKC	Visible cutaneous herpetic lesions around an eye or with cranial nerve 5 distribution. Dendritic pattern on fluorescein stain with slit lamp for herpes simplex	Eyelid swelling, periauricular lymphadenopathy in gonococcal

AKC = atopic keratoconjunctivitis; GPC = giant papillary conjunctivitis; PAC = perennial allergic conjunctivitis; SAC = seasonal allergic conjunctivitis; VKC = vernal keratoconjunctivitis.

Allergic Conjunctivitis

Allergic conjunctivitis characteristically presents as an acute episode of allergy affecting the eyes. Often, however, it becomes either frequently recurring or chronic. There are two basic types: seasonal allergic conjunctivitis (SAC) and perennial allergic conjunctivitis (PAC). These differ by the types of allergens causing symptoms. SAC is most typically caused by seasonal plant pollens, whereas PAC is usually caused by allergens to which the patient is exposed year-round (most commonly the house dust mite, animal dander, and components of the cockroach). These two basic types of allergic conjunctivitis parallel the system of categorizing the types of allergic rhinitis. In fact, allergic conjunctivitis commonly coexists with allergic rhinitis and less frequently with other atopic diseases (asthma and/or atopic dermatitis). While PAC is sometimes thought of as chronic, most patients present with episodes of acute exacerbations, as opposed to having symptoms constantly. SAC can even be chronic during the patient's "season," which may extend for up to 6 months. However, with SAC, there is clearly an extended period of time (months) when the patient is virtually without allergic conjunctivitis symptoms. The most common symptoms of allergic conjunctivitis, whether it is SAC or PAC, are itching of the eye, watering of the eye, and redness of the conjunctiva. These manifestations are usually bilateral. The itch can be intense. The wateriness is characterized by predominantly being clear, rarely mucoid, but never purulent. Rarely does the wateriness obstruct vision to any significant degree. The redness is variable, but usually mild to moderate and generalized throughout the visible bulbar and palpebral conjunctivae (Figure 14.4). Sometimes there is a mild foreign body sensation in the eye.

There are three subtypes of allergic conjunctivitis that warrant special mention. All three may involve the cornea (cause keratitis), and progression could cause serious, possibly vision-threatening damage to the cornea. These three conditions are vernal keratoconjunctivitis (VKC), atopic keratoconjunctivitis (AKC), and giant papillary conjunctivitis (GPC). Therefore, patients suspected of having any one of these three *should be referred to an eye-care specialist*. They are best recognized by their severity and chronicity compared to simple SAC or PAC and additional symptoms of keratitis or photophobia. All three have in common with SAC and PAC, the symptom of itch. However, VKC, in particular, may cause very intense itching. They are distinct from SAC and PAC in that they are chronic and are often associated with a stringiness to the ocular discharge. Photophobia, while common in VKC is less common in AKC and GPC. VKC is common in male children with other atopic diseases and begins from ages 4 to 10 years and disappears after puberty. AKC occurs most often in young adult males and continues into the fifth decade. The presence of atopic dermatitis on the eyelids and face is very common. GPC occurs predominately in contact lens users, but can occur following surgery as a reaction to sutures. If anything suggests these more serious forms, or the patient does not respond to continued use of an OTC product or nonpharmacological mode of management that has been suggested, the patient should be referred.

Viral Conjunctivitis

Viral conjunctivitis is, by far, the most common of the infectious causes of conjunctivitis (up to 80%). While there is considerable overlap in the manifestations of viral and allergic conjunctivitis, there are some differences. Viral conjunctivitis usually begins on one side, but may spread to the other eye, whereas allergic conjunctivitis is almost always bilateral (unless a load of antigen is deposited into one eye, perhaps, by rubbing the eye after touching an allergen). The discharge in viral conjunctivitis varies considerably ranging from a thin, clear, watery discharge to a mucoid and/or

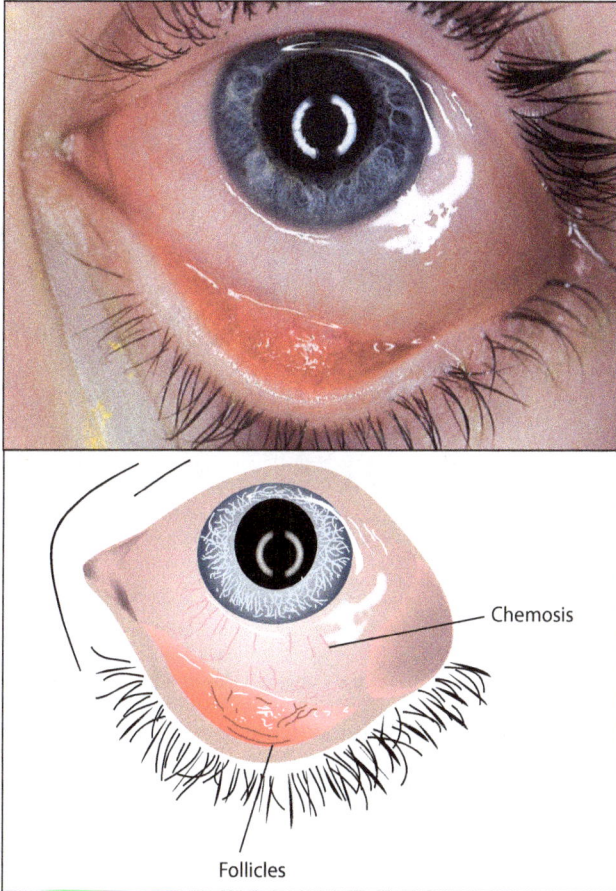

FIGURE 14.4 Allergic conjunctivitis. Conjunctival injection, chemosis, and a follicular response in the inferior palpebral conjunctiva in this patient with allergic conjunctivitis secondary to cat fur. Source: photo contributor: Timothy D. McGuirk, DO. Reproduced with permission from Knoop KJ, Stack LB, Storrow AB, Thurman, RJ. *The Atlas of Emergency Medicine*, 3rd ed. McGraw-Hill, Inc; 2010. Fig. 2-8. Copyright © McGraw-Hill Education LLC.

mucopurulent discharge, overlapping in appearance with the discharges of both allergic conjunctivitis and bacterial conjunctivitis (Figure 14.5). Viral conjunctivitis may be associated with other symptoms of upper respiratory viral infectious disease, such as rhinitis, scratchy or mildly sore throat, mild malaise, possibly a low-grade fever, and possibly cough. If itch is associated with viral conjunctivitis, it is much less marked than that associated with allergic conjunctivitis. The degree of redness varies and is not a useful differential feature. One of the most unique features of viral conjunctivitis is that it may be associated with lymphadenopathy, particularly in the periauricular area. Positive findings favor viral conjunctivitis, but their absence does not rule out other possibilities. Follicles, especially on the palpebral conjunctivae, may occur with either viral or allergic conjunctivitis, although most sources indicate that they are more common with allergic disease. Their presence can be determined with minimal

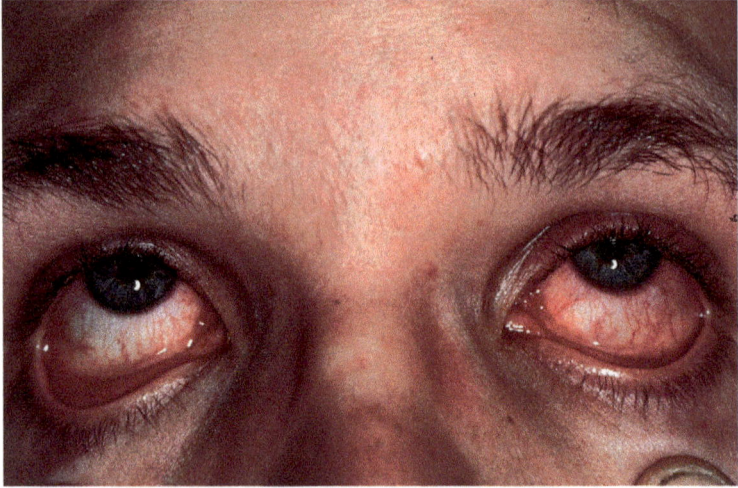

FIGURE 14.5 Viral conjunctivitis. Note the characteristic asymmetric conjunctival injection. Symptoms first developed in the left eye, with symptoms spreading to the other eye a few days later. A thin watery discharge is also seen. Source: photo contributor: Kevin J. Knoop, MD, MS. Reproduced with permission from Knoop KJ, Stack LB, Storrow AB, Thurman, RJ. *The Atlas of Emergency Medicine*, 3rd ed. McGraw-Hill, Inc; 2010. Fig 2–4. Copyright © McGraw-Hill Education LLC.

patient contact, by slight downward traction on the lower lid, so as to expose the palpebral conjunctiva.

The majority of viral conjunctivitis is caused by one of the adenoviruses. There is no pharmacologic therapy that is effective for this entity. This is unfortunate, as the infection is highly communicable. The incubation period ranges from 5 to 12 days and the period of communicability ranges from 10 to 12 days, continuing while the eye is red and symptomatic. Patients, especially children, with adenoviral conjunctivitis remain infectious during the symptomatic phase of the disease, regardless of whether or not they are being treated with an ocular anti-infective. Because of the difficulty of easily distinguishing between viral and bacterial conjunctivitis most patients with pink eye are started on a broad spectrum anti-bacterial agent and told that they will no longer be infectious after 24 to 48 hours of use of that anti-bacterial agent. However, if in fact the patient has a viral conjunctivitis, they will remain infectious, despite anti-bacterial therapy. It is an unfortunate fact that many school policies allow a child to return to school after having been on an anti-bacterial agent for 24 to 48 hours, despite the fact that most of them have a viral conjunctivitis for which the anti-bacterial has absolutely no effect. This certainly contributes to the frequency of viral conjunctivitis among children in such school systems.

While the pharmacist cannot recommend any curative therapy, some advice for symptomatic treatment can be suggested. In fact, except for the two specific types of viral conjunctivitis discussed below, there is no effective anti-viral therapy available. However, some patients will derive some symptomatic relief from cold compresses, topical wetting agents (artificial tears), possibly the topical OTC antihistamine/mast cell stabilizer (ketotifen), and even topical decongestants. As usual, the pharmacist is wise to advise the patient to seek medical care for symptoms that worsen at any time, or for symptoms that do not improve in 3 to 4 days.

Two specific types of viral conjunctivitis deserve separate mention. These are viral conjunctivitis due to herpes simplex virus or herpes zoster virus. Fortunately, these two viruses comprise a small minority of the various viral causes of conjunctivitis. Cutaneous vesicles on the face or near an eye are a common manifestation of viral infectious disease due to herpes simplex and herpes zoster. Initially, symptoms of herpes simplex conjunctivitis may be limited to irritation or pain in the eye, watery discharge, and visual blurring. Herpes simplex virus can cause a progressive, serious, and potentially sight-threatening type of viral conjunctivitis. It usually includes involvement of the cornea, making it a viral keratoconjunctivitis or pure viral keratitis (Figure 14.1). Symptoms often include significant irritation (severe foreign body sensation), photophobia, in addition to redness, watery discharge, and visual blurring. In some cases, vesicles occur on the skin of the eyelids or around the eye. If vesicles are present on or near the eyes in a patient with other manifestations of a red eye, especially if there is any corneal abnormality, a limbal flush or any of the four findings that indicate referral (eye pain, visual impairment, photophobia, or severe foreign body sensation), suspect herpes simplex keratitis and refer the patient to an ophthalmologist immediately. Herpes zoster ophthalmicus (HZO) is the other potentially sight-threatening cause of viral conjunctivitis or keratoconjunctivitis. HZO is a type of shingles. The prodrome of stinging, burning, and sometimes itching occurs before the development of any visible lesions. The initial lesion is a vesicle, which progresses through the stages of pustule, ulcer, and crust. Both the signs and symptoms of HZO occur in the pattern of a dermatome. When the trigeminal (fifth cranial) nerve is affected, facial lesions will occur. When the most superior (ophthalmic) branch of the trigeminal nerve is affected, ocular involvement is likely. Some sources mention Hutchinson's sign, which is the presence of a vesicle on or near the tip of the nose. Supposedly, this increases the chance of corneal involvement. Any suggestion of HZO, by symptoms (including eye pain, visual disturbance, photophobia, severe foreign body sensation) or a dermatomal distribution of lesions on the face or near the eye or nose, should warrant immediate referral to an ophthalmologist.

Bacterial Conjunctivitis

Bacterial conjunctivitis is the least common of the three conditions that are the emphasis of this chapter (Figure 14.6). It may also be the easiest to differentiate from the

FIGURE 14.6 Bacterial conjunctivitis. Mucopurulent discharge, conjunctival injection, and lid swelling in a 10-year-old with *H. influenzae* conjunctivitis. Source: photo contributor: Frank Birinyi, MD. Reproduced with permission from Knoop KJ, Stack LB, Storrow AB, Thurman, RJ. *The Atlas of Emergency Medicine*, 3rd ed. McGraw-Hill, Inc; 2010. Fig. 2-2. Copyright © McGraw-Hill Education LLC.

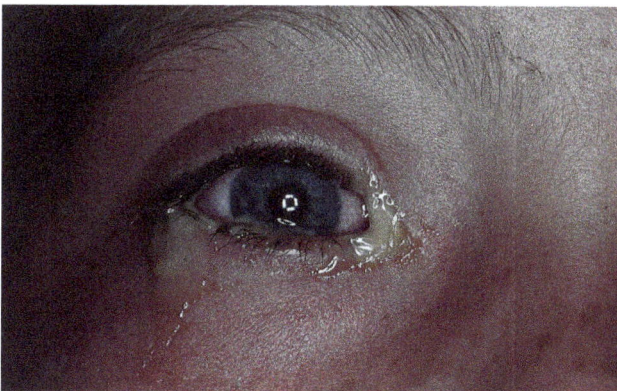

other two common types of conjunctivitis (allergic and viral). The most useful differential feature is the nature of the ocular discharge. Some sources indicate that bacterial conjunctivitis commonly causes matting of the eyelids, especially upon awakening in the morning. While it is true that if this feature is present, it suggests bacterial conjunctivitis, if it is not present, the entity cannot be ruled out. Depending on the way the patient may express their symptoms, some cases of allergic and many cases of viral conjunctivitis may also be associated with a degree of eyelid matting. Another commonly cited differential feature is that the discharge is usually purulent, at least more often so than allergic or viral conjunctivitis. Again, while this is useful if found, a lack of purulence cannot be relied on to rule out bacterial conjunctivitis. Similar to viral conjunctivitis, bacterial conjunctivitis most often begins in only one eye. However, it usually becomes bilateral, probably because of autoinoculation. In fact, bilateral involvement with bacterial conjunctivitis is more likely to occur than with viral causes. A useful differential feature is the relative lack of associated symptoms with bacterial conjunctivitis. It is not associated with other manifestations of upper respiratory infection. Manifestations are usually limited to the eye(s). Another possible differential feature is the lack of ocular itching, which usually occurs in allergic and sometimes in viral conjunctivitis. Due to the purulent nature of the discharge, bacterial conjunctivitis is more likely than allergic or viral causes to create some visual blurring. However, this blurring should clear completely with removal or cleansing of the discharge from the eye. There should be no permanent visual disturbance from bacterial conjunctivitis. If visual abnormalities persist after cleaning the discharge from the eye, some complication, such as a keratitis, should be suspected and the patient immediately referred. In children, the most common etiologic bacteria are *S. pneumoniae, H. influenzae,* and *M. catarrhalis*, although *Staphylococcus* sp may be involved. In adults, *S. aureus* is most common, followed by *S. pneumoniae, H. influenzae*, and possibly coagulase negative *Staphylococcus* sp. Any specific therapy for what is truly a bacterial conjunctivitis will require a primary care provider's prescription. That is, all patients suspected of having a true bacterial conjunctivitis should be referred to a primary care provider. The urgency of referral might depend most on duration and severity of symptoms. Most cases of bacterial conjunctivitis are not sight threatening, and as such not an urgency. However, significant discomfort can arise from the symptoms, and it is best to have the patient seen as soon as possible. The best thing a pharmacist could suggest other than referral would be warm compresses for the discomfort.

Two special types of bacterial conjunctivitis deserve brief mention. Both of these two special types of bacterial conjunctivitis can occur in newborns, although these patients would be unlikely to be initially presented to a pharmacist. Both are most often unilateral, but may become bilateral due to autoinoculation. Both would require immediate referral. The first is hyperpurulent or hyperacute conjunctivitis and the second is inclusion conjunctivitis. In adults, both are usually sexually transmitted illnesses (STIs). Hyperpurulent or hyperacute conjunctivitis is usually due to *N. gonorrhoeae.* The hyperpurulent term simply means that the discharge is unmistakably purulent, copious, and continuous. Almost as soon as the discharge is cleared, it reaccumulates. Other symptoms are similar to the more common types of bacterial conjunctivitis, albeit perhaps more severe. In addition, eyelid swelling, conjunctival edema (chemosis), and periauricular lymphadenopathy may occur. Untreated, this process can quickly progress to cause corneal ulceration and perforation. Any indication of photophobia or severe foreign body sensation may be an indication that this corneal involvement has already begun. In all cases, immediate referral is indicated, usually for systemic therapy of gonorrhea. The patient should be advised that sexual contacts are at risk of some type of gonococcal infection.

Inclusion conjunctivitis is due to certain serotypes of *Chlamydophila trachomatis.* The presentation is much less dramatic than hyperpurulent conjunctivitis. In fact, inclusion conjunctivitis appears more like viral conjunctivitis. The redness may be somewhat more pronounced than typical viral conjunctivitis, and there may be follicles on the palpebral conjunctiva. The discharge is mucoid and usually not profuse, but can progress to have a more purulent nature. Itch is not a common feature. However, there may be a rather significant degree of foreign body sensation. If this disease is even suspected, immediate referral should be advised. This is necessary for both appropriate systemic anti-microbial therapy and contact follow-up (as it is also usually an STI in adults).

Miscellaneous Eye Conditions

The following conditions are not commonly sight or vision threatening, and rarely in need of emergent care. However, there is little that the pharmacist can suggest, other than appropriate (nonurgent, nonemergent) referral to a primary care or eye-care provider and possibly initial symptomatic (nonpharmacologic or OTC) care. Some of these conditions can accompany or coexist with one of the three more common causes of conjunctivitis (allergic, viral, bacterial). However, some are entirely separate entities, and will often be recognizable as such. They will only be briefly defined and characterized. The interested reader is referred to other sources for more detail.

> *Blepharitis* is inflammation of the eyelids, usually manifest as redness and swelling of the margins (outer edges) of the eyelids. It may be allergic or bacterial in etiology. It may occur along with allergic conjunctivitis.

> *Chalazion* is chronic inflammation due to plugging of a meibomian gland in an eyelid. It is a benign process, which is often asymptomatic, except for the patient noticing a lump on the eyelid.

> *Hordeolum* (or stye) is an acute inflammation due to plugging of one of several different glands in the eyelid. Many become acutely infected usually with bacteria from the skin.

> *Pingueculum* is a degenerative process of the conjunctiva. It is relatively common, benign, usually asymptomatic, and consists of a white or yellowish deposit of hyaline on the bulbar conjunctiva, at the 3- and/or 9-o'clock positions relative to the cornea. Commonly occurs in patients exposed to dry windy conditions.

> *Pterygium* is similar to a pingueculum in appearance but can grow over the cornea, and has different pathological origins. It may partially obstruct vision. (Figure 14.7)

> *Subconjunctival hemorrhage* is due to a broken or leaking vessel in the conjunctiva, which results in deposition of a contiguous area of blood under the conjunctival membrane. It is asymptomatic. Most commonly, it is caused by rubbing the eye, especially in response to itching. However, it may be due to a sudden sneeze or cough. Patients usually become aware of the process by seeing their eye in a mirror, or by having somebody else point it out to them. It is a self-limiting, completely benign process that resolves in several days.

> *Entropion and ectropion* are abnormal inward and outward (respectively) folding or turning of the (usually lower) eyelid. Entropion can result in corneal irritation and even abrasion. Ectropion is less symptomatic, but may be associated with increased tearing, due to decreased tear retention, along with resultant dry eyes. Long-term use of irritative ophthalmic solution for glaucoma can cause ectropion.

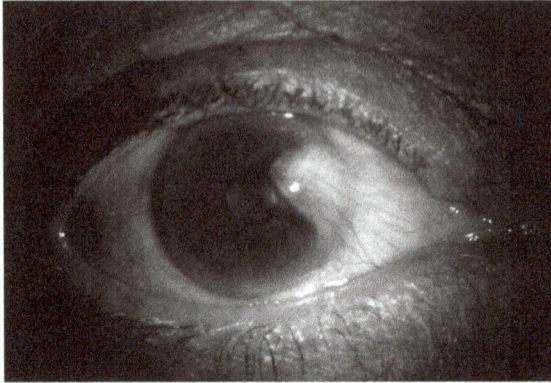

FIGURE 14.7 Pterygium encroaching on the cornea and invading the visual axis. Source: Reproduced with permission from Riordan-Eva P, Cunningham ET, eds. *Vaughan & Asbury's General Ophthalmology*, 18th ed. McGraw-Hill, Inc; 2011:106. Fig. 5-32. Copyright © McGraw-Hill Education LLC.

• KEY REFERENCES

1. Cronau H, Kankanala RR, Mauger T. Diagnosis and management of red eye in primary care. *Am Fam Physician*. 2010;81:137-144.
2. Sethuraman U, Kamat D. The red eye: evaluation and management. *Clin Pediatr*. 2009;48:588-600.
3. Seth D, Kahn FI. Causes and management of red eye in pediatric ophthalmology. *Curr Allergy Asthma Rep*. 2011;11:212-219.
4. Deibel JP, Cowling K. Ocular inflammation and infection. *Emerg Med Clin North Am*. 2013;31:387-397.
5. Azari AA, Barney NP. Conjunctivitis—a systematic review of diagnosis and treatment. *JAMA*. 2013;310:1721-1729.
6. Visscher KL, Hutnick CML, Thomas M. Evidence-based treatment of acute infective conjunctivitis— breaking the cycle of antibiotic prescribing. *Can Fam Physician*. 2009;55:1071-1075.
7. Leonardi A, Bogacka E, Fauquert JL, et al. Ocular allergy: recognizing and diagnosing hypersensitivity disorders of the ocular surface. *Allergy*. 2012;67:1327-1337.
8. Kari O, Saari KM. Diagnostics and new developments in the treatment of ocular allergies. *Curr Allergy Asthma Rep*. 2012;12:232-239.
9. American Academy of Opthalmology Corneal/External Disease Panel. *Preferred Practice Guidelines. Conjunctivitis*. San Francisco, CA: American Academy of Ophthalmology; 2013. www.aao.org/ppp. Accessed 2014, June 15.

![CASE 14.1]

Rick O'Shea comes to your pharmacy to pick up a refill on his fluticasone inhaler. He also asks what is good for his bloodshot eyes. Pertinent history includes his love of dirt biking in the desert, which he does every evening after work, plus his nightly swim at the YMCA. He also complains of a recent onset of joint pain in his hands. Upon observation you notice mild diffuse inflammation of both conjunctivae, no discharge, and small yellowish patches at the 3- and 9-o'clock positions in both eyes.

1. List two possible causes for Rick's bloodshot eyes. Explain your rationale.

   _____

   _____

   _____

   _____

   _____

2. List three questions that you would ask to help determine the cause of Rick's inflamed eyes. Explain your rationale.

   _____

   _____

   _____

   _____

   _____

3. List three questions you would ask to make sure this was not a vision-threatening condition that required immediate referral.

   _____

   _____

   _____

   _____

   _____

FIFTEEN

Musculoskeletal Symptoms and Disorders

LEARNING OBJECTIVES

1. Accurately identify the most likely etiology when patients present with a musculoskeletal symptom, through history, diagnostic tests, and appropriate patient findings on examination to enable the appropriate recommendation of effective treatment or referral to an appropriate provider.

2. Use the knowledge of the pathophysiology, etiology, and common presentations of musculoskeletal complaints as a primary symptom to review prescription orders for appropriateness and to accurately educate patients about their disease and its treatment.

3. Use the knowledge of the pathophysiology, etiology, and common presentation of diseases with musculoskeletal complaints as a primary symptom to accurately interpret the diagnostic process to advise regarding the most appropriate prescription therapy.

• ETIOLOGY

Musculoskeletal complaints are among the most frequently encountered primary care visits. Trauma, either acute or overuse, to muscles, ligaments, tendons, bones, or joints is a common cause for symptoms involving the musculoskeletal system. Other diverse etiologies such as autoimmune diseases, vitamin deficiencies, infections, disordered metabolism or clearance, and medication also have to be considered when a patient presents with musculoskeletal symptoms.

• DIAGNOSIS

The diagnosis of specific musculoskeletal complaints requires an organized approach. Eliciting a history of trauma is essential. A positive reply will send the diagnostic process toward traumatic injuries, such as overuse or sports injuries. A negative response directs the inquiries toward nontraumatic causes. Location is the second most important diagnostic clue. Many times different diseases are associated with different locations, e.g., rheumatoid arthritis occurs primarily in the metacarpophalangeal (MCP) joints and proximal interphalangeal (PIP) joints of the hands, whereas osteoarthritis (OA) is predominantly a disease of the weight bearing joints, such as the knee and hip. OA may also affect distal interphalangeal joints (DIP). Whether the pain is in the joint, over a bone, or in a muscular area also helps differentiate etiology. Numbness and tingling or blue, pale discoloration in an extremity are symptoms requiring immediate referral. Finally, physical examination helps confirm the diagnosis. Swelling, decreased or increased range of motion, increased pain on movement, redness, heat, and fever all help discriminate among specific problems.

• COMMON INJURIES RELATED TO TRAUMA/OVERUSE

Plantar Fasciitis

Plantar fasciitis is an overuse injury in runners and walkers; the pain is located on the medial aspect and bottom of the heel. Many times it becomes severe enough to prevent continuation of running for up to 12 months. To avoid the pain, patients tend to walk on the ball and lateral side of the foot. On physical examination, there is pain upon palpation of the medial calcaneal tubercle, passive dorsiflexion of the foot, eversion of the foot, and active dorsiflexion of the big toe. Patients complain of pain in the morning that is worse with the first few steps, or when starting activity with it getting better as they continue to walk or run. It needs to be aggressively treated at the first sign. Continued running will worsen the condition and lead to longer times for healing. Immediate treatment includes ice, but rest, and eventually stretching and strength exercises are the treatments of choice.

Ankle Sprain

Grade 1 sprains include mild swelling, little or no decrease in range of motion, point tenderness over the ligament but no bruising. Grade 2 sprains have moderate swelling, marked decrease in range of motion, and a bruise over the ligament. Grade 3 sprains present with severe swelling, extensive bruising, and severely decreased range of motion. Immediate treatment involves ice, elevation, and rest from 7 days for grade 1 to 4-6 weeks for grade 3.

Tennis and Golfer Elbow (Epicondylitis)

"Tennis elbow" is caused by the repeated use of one-handed backhands. Patients present with tenderness upon palpation just distal to the *lateral* epicondyle and on resisted extension of the wrist or finger or when the thumb and forefinger are actively opposed like grabbing a tea cup. Two-handed backhands are effective at preventing the initial and any reinjury. Golfer elbow presents with pain upon palpation just distal to the *medial* epicondyle and resisted flexion of the wrist. Rest should be followed by exercises to stretch and strengthen associated muscles and tendons.

Carpal Tunnel Syndrome

Carpal tunnel syndrome is caused by continuous pressure on the median nerve by the flexor retinaculum along with the other muscles and tendons that form the carpal tunnel that cross the median nerve in the wrist. It was originally thought to be caused by repetitive use of the hands and wrists. It was considered an occupational hazard for typists, barbers, and assembly line workers. However, current evidence has shown that the most important factor is a congenitally narrow carpal tunnel. Overuse of the hands and wrists then contribute to the development of the condition. Patients present with numbness, tingling, or pain in the thumb, first two fingers, and the thumb of the third finger. The opposite side of the third finger and the little finger are not impacted because they are innervated by the ulnar nerve. Diagnosis is confirmed by a positive Tinel sign, which puts pressure on the medial nerve by pressing or tapping over the carpal tunnel. The Phalen test is done by having the patient hold their forearms upright and parallel to the floor, then pointing the fingers down and pressing the backs of the hands firmly together for 1 minute. Positive tests are a duplication of the symptoms.

Knee Injuries

The most common acute knee injuries involve the four primary ligaments of the knee and the meniscus, the layer of cartilage between the tibia and the femur. The ligaments can be strained and sprained (torn). Ligament tears and meniscus damage may have to be repaired surgically to regain full function.

Regardless of the injury, swelling usually occurs. If it occurs immediately, it suggests a ligament tear or fracture of the knee cap. If swelling occurs over a period of hours, then meniscus damage is most likely. In addition, pain upon weight bearing and difficulty bending the knee may also occur. Unfortunately, injuries may involve more than one structure or may not present in a typical fashion. Knees that "give way" or are unstable are usually associated with ligament injuries, while grinding in the knee and the knee that cannot be straightened ("locking") are typical of meniscus injuries. Injuries to the anterior cruciate (ACL) or posterior cruciate (PCL) ligaments can be tested using *drawer tests* or versions of classical drawer tests such as the Lachman, which is the most sensitive for PCL injuries. Make sure to test the good knee first for more accurate comparison. Medial collateral (MCL) and lateral collateral (LCL) ligament tears are also detected using drawer tests. Drawer tests put stress on the specific ligament. Excessive movement in a particular direction is diagnostic. Meniscus damage is tested with the McMurray and Apley tests. Any clicking or popping is indicative of meniscus damage. X-rays and MRIs of the knee may be needed to confirm specific diagnoses.

Back Injuries

Most common back injuries involve the lower back and may be fractures, disc injuries, or muscle injuries. The important thing is to recognize symptoms that require immediate medical attention. The most frequent injury involves the muscles of the lower back due to excessive use. These injuries tend to manifest themselves 24 to 48 hours after the inciting incident. Usually, the pain subsides after 72 to 84 hours. Any low back pain that is not getting better after 72 hours needs immediate medical attention. Injuries to the disc are mostly herniated discs (aka protruding, bulging, or ruptured disc). Pain usually is first noticed at the time of injury or immediately thereafter. Sciatica or radiculopathy is nerve pain that shoots down the hip and back of the leg like an electric shock, or numbness and/or tingling in one or more lower extremities and warrants immediate referral for evaluation. If persistent pain occurs in the elderly or is insidious in onset, fractures due to osteoporosis or systemic diseases such as ankylosing spondylitis need to be ruled out. Lack of attention can lead to permanent nerve damage and/or muscle weakness. CT scans, MRIs, x-rays of the spine may be required to confirm suspected diagnoses.

• COMMON ARTHRITIDES

Causes of joint pain include repetitive overuse, repeated trauma, immunologic, metabolic, and infectious disorders. There are several keys to accurate diagnosis including the number and location of joints involved, acute versus insidious onset, other symptoms such as serious eye disease, skin rash, patterns of the discomfort, plus fatigue and malaise.

If the pain is of acute onset and only occurs in a single joint (monoarticular), then traumatic and overuse disorders such as bursitis, tendonitis, sprains, and fractures should be suspected. A careful history regarding overuse or trauma is important in ruling out this cause. In particular, in elderly patients, fracture due to osteoporosis and/or falls should be suspected and ruled out. Infectious causes like septic arthritis and osteomyelitis, should be also suspected. CT scans, MRIs, and arthrocentesis (aspiration of synovial fluid from the affected joint) may be required for diagnosis. The presence of cloudy fluid, white or red blood cells, and bacteria are abnormal findings. Aspirated synovial fluid will be cultured. A CBC will show a typical bacterial infection white count (>10,000 WBC, > 80% mature and immature PMNs) in septic arthritis. Arthrocentesis is also indicated if gout or pseudogout is suspected. Classically associated with the big toe, gout can occur in any joint in the lower body plus hands and wrists. Typically the joint is exquisitely painful, swollen, and warm to the touch. High-plasma uric acid levels due to overproduction or undersecretion are usually present. Synovial fluid contains urate crystals upon microscopic examination. Pseudogout presents in the knee joints of elderly patients with gout-like symptoms. However, the synovial fluid contains precipitated calcium pyrophosphate dihydrate rather than urate crystals.

Acute onset, migratory polyarthritis is most likely gonococcal arthritis or post-streptococcal acute rheumatic fever. Other polyarthritides such as rheumatoid arthritis (and its variants) and systemic lupus erythematosus (SLE) can present acutely but are typically more insidious in onset. Lastly, acute onset polyarthritis occurring in large joints, such as the knees, in young males may indicate Reiter syndrome an autoimmune arthritis associated with conjunctivitis and urethritis.

Joint pain occurring in multiple joints with a chronic, intermittent, or insidious onset is associated with noninflammatory arthritis such as OA, autoimmune arthritides such as SLE, and rheumatoid arthritis and its variants. Table 15.1 presents key features used in the differential diagnosis of these common disorders.

Osteoarthritis (Degenerative Joint Disease or DJD)

The most frequently occurring arthritis is OA. Nearly 27 million patients suffer from the disease in the United States including 70% of those over 65 years of age. OA is generally regarded as a noninflammatory arthritis, and is associated with aging, repetitive trauma, and obesity. However, recent research into genetics and synovial fluid markers has brought new information regarding the type and role of inflammation and potential

TABLE 15.1	Differential Diagnosis of Chronic Polyarticular Arthritis		
Parameter	**OA**	**RA**	**SLE**
Joint location	Weight bearing (knees, hips, ankles)	Hands and feet (MCP, PIP, MTP)	Can mimic both RA and OA
Symmetrical	No	Yes	Variable
Diagnostic lab tests	None	Rheumatoid factor, ACPA	LE Prep, ANA
Morning stiffness	Variable	Yes	Variable
Autoimmune inflammation	No	Yes	Yes
Joint swelling	No	Yes	Yes
Associated symptoms	Uncommon	Ulnar deviation Rheumatoid nodules	Joint pain may not be primary problem. May present as skin rash, or problems with kidneys, heart, lungs, or CNS

genetic links to biostructural issues. OA primarily affects the larger weight bearing joints such as the knees, hips, and ankles, but can involve any previously injured or overused joint including those of the shoulder, spine, and hands. The most common cause is excessive load caused by obesity and/or repetitive overuse. Also deficiencies in biostructure (cartilage, bone, muscle, ligaments), but with a normal load can cause OA.

Diagnosis is primarily a clinical one. Pain and decreased range of motion are primary findings. Crepitus or grinding sensations can be felt over the joint when flexion and extension of the joint occur. Point tenderness on palpation is not uncommon. The degree of pain varies with severity of the disease. In the early stages pain is worse after rest, with the pain disappearing in minutes upon movement. In the later stages pain may be constant and weight bearing activity increases in pain are common. There is generally little swelling, and no associated symptoms, systemic manifestations, or abnormal laboratory tests as there are in autoimmune arthritides such as rheumatoid arthritis. Occasionally, x-ray of the joints reveals degenerative changes, especially joint space narrowing.

Rheumatoid Arthritis

Rheumatoid arthritis (RA) is an autoimmune, inflammatory, erosive arthritis that affects 1.5 million people per year. Two times as many women as men are diagnosed with RA. A systemic disease, early symptoms may include primarily fatigue and malaise with intermittent bouts of joint pain. Multiple small joints are involved usually the MCP, PIP, wrist, metatarsophalangeal (MTP), and ankle joints. The disease tends to be symmetrical, occurring in both the hands and toes but not necessarily the same joints on both hands. It is a naturally cyclical disease, where patients with active disease complain of morning stiffness lasting up to 1 hour. Affected joints are swollen, hot, and painful with decreased range of motion. If untreated the disease progresses with joint erosion and loss of function to cause deformities. As the disease progresses, other joints can become involved. Ulnar deviation of the fingers is common if untreated. The disease can also impact other organs in the body including the heart and lungs. Patients with RA present with elevated erythrocyte sedimentation rate (ESR) due to large quantities of immune complexes in the plasma, and elevated high-sensitivity C-reactive protein (hs-CRP). Unfortunately, these acute phase reactants are not specific for RA. The rheumatoid factor (RF), usually measured as an IgG or IgM autoantibody. Titers of >1:160 are diagnostic. Similarly, anticyclic citrullinated peptide antibodies (ACPA) are more specific for RA and can be found before clinical signs and symptoms of disease are present. Antinuclear antibodies (ANA) are usually absent. Because of the intermittent cyclic nature of the disease and its insidious onset in 90% of the cases, the diagnosis of early disease can be difficult. Serologic diagnosis is complicated by the small percentage of patients with RA who will have positive ANA as well as patients with other autoimmune diseases such as SLE who may have positive RA titers. To aid in the diagnosis of RA, the American College of Rheumatology developed a scoring guideline (Table 15.2).

Treatment is centered on stopping the autoimmune-mediated joint destruction. In managing patients with RA, a combination of symptoms set forth in various scoring systems (ACR-20, disease activity score-28, and simplified disease activity index), radiological changes, and acute phase reactants (ESR and hs-CRP) are used to monitor efficacy of drug treatment. Successful treatment is indicated by falling titers of acute phase reactants, no radiographic changes, and decreasing symptom scores.

Common Rheumatoid Arthritis Variants

There are several common arthritides that are variants of RA. Presentation is similar but with specific additional associated symptoms. Felty's syndrome is RA with leukopenia, and occasionally anemia or thrombocytopenia and/or splenomegaly. Sjogren syndrome is RA plus conjunctiva sicca (dry eyes) and xerostomia (dry mouth). Psoriatic arthritis occurs in about 10% of patients with psoriasis.

Systemic Lupus Erythematosus

SLE is a systemic disease that can present with joint pain that can mimic both RA and OA. The number of patients with SLE is similar to that of RA. Eighty-five percent of patients with SLE are women and initial diagnosis occurs between the ages of 15 and 45. If untreated, the disease is commonly fatal. Sixty years ago the 5-year survival rate was less than 50%. Today the 15-year survival rate is over 80%. Because of its systemic nature, diagnosis should be suspected if patients present with two or more common systemic symptoms. Those include skin rash, photosensitivity, arthritis, renal damage,

TABLE 15.2	Criteria for the Diagnosis of Rheumatoid Arthritis
Criteria	**Score**
Joint involvement	
1 large joint	0
2 to 10 large joints	1
1 to 3 small joints	2
4 to 10 small joints	3
>10 small joints	5
Serology	
Negative RF and ACPA	0
Low positive RF and ACPA	2
High positive RF and ACPA	3
Acute phase reactants	
Normal C-reactive protein (CRP) and erythrocyte sedimentation rate (ESR)	0
Abnormal CRP and ESR	1
Duration of symptoms	
<6 weeks	0
>6 weeks	1
Six (6) or more points diagnostic of rheumatoid arthritis	

pulmonary symptoms, cardiac symptoms, CNS symptoms such as seizures or psychosis, hematological abnormalities, and constitutional symptoms such as fatigue, malaise, fever, or weight loss. Laboratory tests historically included LE Prep, a test using blue dye to detect SLE antibodies. This test has been replaced due to its limited accuracy by ANA which is diagnostic. Over 90% of patients with active SLE will have elevated titers. Double-stranded ANA is specific for SLE, but is present in less than half of the patients. Anti-Smith antibodies are also more specific than ANA titers. About 50% of patients will have low complement levels (C3 and C4). Patients suspected of SLE need urinalysis and renal function tests, LFTs, CBC to help identify specific organ system involvement and monitor disease progression. Treatment with immunosuppressives helps to prevent multiorgan damage and eventually death.

Other Autoimmune Arthritides

There are two other autoimmune arthritides of interest. Ankylosing spondylitis occurs in males with HLA B27 antigen. It causes inflammation of the spine, which eventually leads to ossification of the discs and surrounding connective tissue, leading to vertebral fusion. Scleroderma occurs primarily in females and involves an inflammatory process that increases the deposition of collagen in many tissues especially blood vessels. It causes an autoimmune vasculitis, leading to Raynaud's phenomenon, plus a tightening and thickening of the esophagus and skin of the finger and face. Eventually it can involve the thyroid, intestinal tract, heart, lungs, and kidneys. Scleroderma is also known as progressive systemic sclerosis.

• BONE DISEASES THAT CAN BE CONFUSED WITH JOINT PAIN

Osteopenia is a generalized term describing the loss of bone mineral from trabecular portions of bones. Generally, the presence of osteopenia is detected by dual energy x-ray absorptiometry (DEXA) of the hip bones. DEXA results are expressed as T scores, which estimate bone mineral density. T scores are based on the number of standard deviations from the mean of healthy 30-year-old women of the patient's ethnicity. Normal is a score of –1.0 or higher. A T score of –1.0 to –2.5 is osteopenia and a T score >–2.5 (more negative) is considered diagnostic of osteoporosis. Ultrasound of the heel bone is not as accurate as DEXA because the test measures cortical rather than trabecular or porous bone.

There are two primary types of osteopenia. Osteomalacia is due to vitamin D deficiency and involves *bone mineral density only*. Patients with lactase deficiencies, those on enzyme-inducing anticonvulsants, and/or who have little or no sun exposure are at higher risk for developing osteomalacia. In children, it is called rickets. The bones soften and become misshapen because the cartilaginous matrix is still in place but without the stiffening influence of calcium and phosphate. Therapy with vitamin D and calcium and sometimes vitamin K restore bone mass and strength. In adults, there is no misshapen bone structure and symptoms include dull, unrelenting, aching pain with widespread distribution. When asked to point to where the pain is located, patients will point to the long bones of the forearms and legs rather than the joints. The pain is usually not relieved by NSAIDs. Most will have serum 25-OH vitamin D levels well below 20 ng/mL. Bone scans will reveal Looser's lines, small linear microfractures in the bone.

The other causes of osteoporosis is age and postmenopausal status. Osteoporosis, rather than being a vitamin D deficiency, is due to a disorder of bone turnover. Normally, there is a balance between osteoclast activity, which breaks down bone tissue, and osteoblast activity that rebuilds bones. Osteoporosis is an imbalance of osteoclast/osteoblast activity where osteoclast activity dominates, causing *bone mineral loss as well as loss of cartilaginous bone matrix.* This is most harmful to the more porous trabecular bone that contains the marrow. Cortical or dense bone is less affected. Therefore, the complication of osteoporosis is fractures of bone that is primarily trabecular, i.e., spinal vertebrae, hip, and wrist. After onset of osteoporosis, the patient, regardless of treatment, can never completely regain all lost bone mass due to the loss of matrix.

• KEY REFERENCES

1. Kiriakidou M. Systemic lupus erythematosus. *Ann Intern Med.* 2013;159(7):ITC4-1.
2. Aletaha D, Neogi T, Silman AJ, et al. 2010 Rheumatoid arthritis classification system: an American College of Rheumatology/European League Against Rheumatism collaborative initiative. *Ann Rheum Dis.* 2010;69:1580-1588.
3. Bijlsma JWJ, Berenbaum F, Lafeber FPJG. Osteoarthritis: an update with relevance for clinical practice. *Lancet.* 2011;377:2115-2126.
4. Sinusas K. Osteoarthritis: diagnosis and management. *Am Fam Physician.* 2012;85:49-56.
5. Jackson JL, O'Malley PG, Kronke K. Evaluation of acute knee pain in primary care. *Ann Intern Med.* 2003;139:575-588.
6. Grover M. Evaluating acutely injured patients for internal derangement of the knee. *Am Fam Physician.* 2012;85:247-252.
7. Sembrano JN, Polly DW. How often is low back pain not coming from the back? *Spine.* 2008;34:E-27-E32.
8. Czajka CM, Tran E, Cai AN, DiPreta JA. Ankle sprains and instability. *Med Clin North Am.* 2014;98:313-329.
9. Rosembaum AJ, DiPeta JA, Misner D. Plantar heel pain. *Med Clin North Am.* 2014;98:339-352.

CASE 15.1

You are on rotation at Posada Del Diablo Convalescent Center. All new patients have their records reviewed and are interviewed by the pharmacy student to evaluate potential drug-related problems and make any recommendations for changes in the therapeutic regimen. Samantha Roanhorse, a 58-year-old Native American, was admitted last night and it is your job to review her records and interview her.

Problem List	*Medication*
1960 Gran mal epilepsy due to severe head trauma	Phenytoin 400 mg q hs
	Phenobarbital 120 mg q hs
1972 Alcoholism	
1980 Schizophrenia	Risperidone 4 mg q hs
2001 Diabetes mellitus type 2	Metformin 500 mg bid
ALLERGIES: milk, penicillin, aspirin	

Sam's chart has not caught up with her, but the discharge summary from the psychiatric hospital reveals she was admitted for exacerbation of her schizophrenia. During her stay she was switched to risperidone with good results. The nurse tells you that her counterpart at the hospital called to tell her that the hydrocortisone cream that was sent back with the patient is for a rash on her face, neck, and elbows. During your interview, Sam's biggest complaint is about pains in her arms and legs that are poorly relieved by acetaminophen. When asked, she complains of pains in her hands, wrists, forearms, shins, knees, and toes. She also makes a vague reference to a recent fall that upon further questioning she denies.

Given her medical history, list three likely causes of Sam's aches and pains. Explain your rationale.

_____
_____
_____
_____
_____

List six questions you would ask, examinations you would perform, and/or diagnostic tests that you would order to better determine the cause of her pain. Explain your rationale.

_____
_____
_____
_____
_____

SIXTEEN

Dysuria and Vaginal Discharge

LEARNING OBJECTIVES

1. Accurately identify the most likely etiology when patients present with a chief complaint of dysuria or vaginal discharge, through history, diagnostic tests, and patient findings on examination to enable the pharmacist to appropriately recommend effective self-treatment or refer the patient to an appropriate provider.

2. Use knowledge of the pathophysiology, etiology, and common presentation of dysuria and vaginal discharge to review prescription orders for appropriateness and to accurately educate patients about their disease and its treatment.

3. Use knowledge of the pathophysiology, etiology, and common presentation of dysuria or vaginal discharge to accurately interpret the diagnostic process to enable the pharmacist to advise providers regarding the most appropriate prescription therapy.

Nearly 5% of patients seen in emergency departments present with complaints related to the genitourinary system. Dysuria (painful urination) and vaginal or urethral discharge are the most common complaints. There are three major causes of dysuria: vaginitis, sexually transmitted diseases (STDs), and urinary tract infections (UTIs). Pharmacists are often asked for advice regarding potential self-care of dysuria and vaginal discharge with nonprescription medication. Therefore, understanding major causes and how to determine if the patient's symptoms are appropriate for self-care are important skills. In addition, when counseling patients on the use of medications, understanding the symptoms and complications of the disease allows the pharmacist to provide necessary information. Finally, to evaluate the appropriateness of therapy or to advise a prescriber on appropriate therapy, the pharmacist needs to understand the process of differential diagnosis for dysuria and vaginal discharge.

• GENERAL APPROACH TO THE PATIENT WITH DYSURIA

Since dysuria is a prominent symptom of three separate disorders, providers (including pharmacists) need to take a structured approach to assessing which disorder is the most likely cause of the patient's dysuria. There are some key initial questions that will help the provider narrow his/her diagnostic focus and make the decision whether the patient is a candidate for self-treatment or needs to be referred (Table 16.1). Unfortunately, other than vaginitis, there are few genitourinary disorders that lend themselves to self-treatment, so positive responses to most questions require referral. For example, if a patient has a vaginal discharge and dysuria, it is possible, but unlikely that they have a UTI, and further questioning as to the specific cause of the vaginal discharge is warranted. Similarly, urethral discharges are usually representative of STDs. Dysuria, plus urinary frequency or urgency point to lower tract UTIs, whereas dysuria, plus systemic signs (nausea, vomiting, fever, abdominal or flank pain, and rigors) point to an upper UTI (acute pyelonephritis). A vaginal discharge plus systemic symptoms point

TABLE 16.1	Initial Questions for Patients With Chief Complaint of Dysuria
Question	**Positive Response Points to:**
Vaginal discharge?	Vaginitis, STD
Urethral discharge?	STD
Internal dysuria?	UTI, STD
External dysuria?	Vaginitis
Unprotected sex with new or multiple partners?	STD
Previous history of STD?	STD
Urinary frequency, urgency?	UTI
External blisters/lesions?	STD
Fever, abdominal/flank pain, rigors nausea, vomiting?	UTI (pyelonephritis)/pelvic inflammatory disease (PID)
Rapid onset?	UTI
Slower onset?	STD, vaginitis
Feminine hygiene products/vaginal contraceptive products?	Irritant/allergic contact dermatitis
Condom use?	STD
OTHER	
Immunocompromised	Refer
Colicky sharp back pain	Refer (urolithiasis)
Perineal discomfort in males	Refer (prostate problem)
Trouble starting urine stream in males	Refer (prostate problem)

to possible pelvic inflammatory disease (PID). Positive answers to these questions do not automatically make the diagnosis, but point to a diagnosis more likely than a UTI. Multiple positive answers frequently force the diagnostician to do a complete workup for all three common causes to arrive at a diagnosis.

• VAGINITIS/VAGINAL DISCHARGE

Classically, vaginal infections are characterized by the presence of an excessive or unusual vaginal discharge. Other vaginal symptoms can include odor, vulvovaginal irritation, pruritus, and painful intercourse. The primary urethral symptoms that can accompany a vaginal discharge are dysuria and urethral discharge. With a careful history, dysuria can be described by patients as internal or external. Internal dysuria is described as occurring at the beginning of voiding (where the urethra meets the bladder) and throughout the length of the urethra, due to inflammation and infection of the bladder and/or the entire urethra. Patients with UTIs and STDs tend to describe their dysuria as internal. Patients with vaginitis tend to describe their dysuria as external, e.g., not occurring until the labia or the outer 25% of the urethra. While not in itself diagnostic, it can be a valuable clue to distinguishing between causes of dysuria. While women with one of the common causes of vaginitis often present with dysuria and vaginal discharge, a large percentage may be asymptomatic initially. High-risk women (new or multiple sex partners or previous history of STD) require screening for chlamydia and gonorrhea, which usually requires a pelvic examination. While males who present with gonorrhea or chlamydia typically have a purulent urethral discharge, women may present with cervicitis as a primary finding in chlamydial and gonococcal infections or PID. Cervicitis is a purulent or mucopurulent discharge or bleeding after gentle passage of a cotton swab into the cervical os, during examination with a vaginal speculum. There are three common causes of vaginitis: bacterial vaginosis (BV), vulvovaginal candidiasis (VVC), and trichomoniasis. Table 16.2 lists the subjective and objective characteristics used in the differential diagnosis of vaginal discharge. Classically, one drop or sample of the vaginal discharge, from the pelvic examination, is placed on two slides for microscopic examination. Next, to one slide a drop of saline is added and to the other a drop of 10% KOH is added (Table 16.3). Today there are newer and more accurate office diagnostic tests available. However, they are more expensive than the classic approach and most recommend their use, if the diagnosis is not clear.

Bacterial Vaginosis

BV is not an STD, but there can be an association with sexual activity. Also, technically BV is not a vaginitis. However, it is the most frequently diagnosed cause of vaginal discharge in sexually active women. While the exact pathophysiology is not clearly understood, it appears that it is a disruption in the normal bacterial flora caused by the secretions and/or ejaculates of normal sexual activity raising vaginal pH. This leads to a predominance of several species including *Gardnerella vaginalis*, as well as *Prevotella, Peptostreptococcus,* and *Bacteroides* species. Fifty percent of women with BV are asymptomatic. The most common symptom is a fishy odor. The lack of odor makes BV unlikely, as does a normal pH, both of which are more typical of VVC. Upon pelvic examination, there is an off-white or gray vaginal discharge that adheres to the vaginal wall. The pH of the discharge is always above 4.5 and a normal pH (3.8 to 4.2) virtually eliminates BV as a cause. When a sample of the discharge is mixed with a 10% KOH solution, it gives off a strong fishy odor (whiff test). Microscopically, more than 20% of the epithelial cells have gram-negative coccobacillus (*Gardnerella vaginalis*) attached, i.e., clue cells. There is a more specific test that measures vaginal fluid sialidase activity

TABLE 16.2	Differential Diagnosis of Vaginal Discharge				
SUBJECTIVE	Candida	Bacterial Vaginosis	Trichomonas	Chlamydia	Gonorrhea
Causative agent	Candida albicans, a yeast	Overgrowth of an-aerobic bacteria most commonly Gardnerella vaginalis	A flagel-lated protozoa Trichomonas vaginalis	Chlamydia trachomatis	Neisseria gonorrhoeae
Vaginal discharge	White cottage cheese like	Off-white—gray milky that coats vaginal walls	Frothy white watery	Scant to absent	Scant to absent
Odor	None	Strong fishy odor	Mild	None	None
Itching	++++	±	+	None	None
Other	External dysuria, plus associated genital skin rash typical of candida	External dysuria	External dysuria	Internal dysuria	Internal dysuria
				Urethral discharge ± in males primarily	Urethral discharge ± in males primarily
Sexually transmitted	Atypically	Atypically	+	+	+
Precipitating factors	Pregnancy, BCP, diabetes, recent broad-spectrum antibiotic, menopause, corticosteroid use	Frequent sexual activity	None	Sexual activity with new partner	Sexual activity with new partner
OBJECTIVE					
Microscopic	Branching hyphae with KOH	Positive whiff test with KOH	Mobile flagellates with saline	None	Intracellular gram-negative diplococci
		Clue cells with saline			
Other		Sialidase test	Trichomonas Rapid test (NAATs)	Amplicor CT/NG test (NAATs)	Amplicor CT/NG test (NAATs)

that has >90% specificity and sensitivity, but due to its cost it may be reserved for situations where a specific diagnosis cannot be made by traditional methods.

Candida

VVC is the second most common cause of vaginal discharge. More than 75% of women will experience one episode of VVC in their lifetime. Intense itching is the predominant symptom and the lack of itching makes the diagnosis of VVC unlikely. Typically, there is a lot of inflammation and redness internally and externally on the labia. Red satellite lesions that are pathognomonic of candidal skin infections may be seen on the external genitalia and surrounding areas. While the discharge is typically described as white and cottage cheese like, many times it does not have the *typical* appearance, but may be seen as white plaques or patches on the vaginal wall. Microscopically, a sample of the discharge when mixed with 10% KOH will reveal branched hyphae

TABLE 16.3	Testing Vaginal/Urethral Discharge Samples

Microscopic Examinations

Wet prep (add saline)

Clue cells (epithelial cells with multiple adherent *Gardnerella*) indicate BV

Motile flagellates indicate trichomoniasis

10% KOH

Whiff test—strong fishy odor indicates BV

Branched candidal hyphae indicates VVC

Gram stain of urethral or vaginal discharge

Gram-negative intracellular diplococci indicate gonorrhea

Gram-negative coccobacillus attached to epithelial cells (clue cells) indicates BV

Other Examinations

Culture

Gonorrhea

pH

≥4.5 indicates BV or trichomoniasis

<4.5 indicates VVC

Nucleic acid amplification tests (NAATs) (>90% specificity and sensitivity)

Trichomonas vaginalis

Neisseria gonorrhea

Chlamydia trachomatis

typical of *Candida* species. Vaginal fluid pH is usually normal, but not greater than 4.5. Patients usually have one or more predisposing factors present. Since estrogens increase the susceptibility to VVC, women who are pregnant or on oral contraceptives are at increased risk. Similarly, high levels of glucose in vaginal fluid and urine promote the rapid growth of candida, so suboptimally controlled diabetes mellitus predisposes women to VVC. *Candida albicans* is normal vaginal flora, but their growth is held in check by the low vaginal pH created primarily by *Lactobacillus* species. Broad spectrum antibiotic therapy markedly reduces the number of *Lactobacillus* and allows the pH to rise, creating a vaginal environment that encourages candidal proliferation.

Since VVC is the only vaginitis that is amenable to self-care, the pharmacist needs to question the patient carefully before recommending any product. Patients amenable to self-care will present with several of the following symptoms: external dysuria, intense itching, red, irritated external genital area with potential satellite lesions, and have one or more of the predisposing factors. The patient with a vaginal discharge is best referred if there is a fishy or musty odor, internal dysuria or an absence of itching.

Recurrent VVC or VVC that does not respond to self-care products should prompt a referral. Many times VVC is the first sign of diabetes seen in women. In addition, while the vast majority of VVC is caused by *Candida albicans,* recurrence or resistance may represent VVC caused by nonalbicans *Candida* species such as *Candida glabrata,* which are historically more resistant to imidazole-containing vaginal products.

Trichomoniasis

Trichomonas vaginitis (TV) is caused by a motile flagellate protozoan *Trichomonas vaginalis*, and is the least frequently seen cause of vaginitis. It is seen more commonly in women over 40 years of age and in women of African American descent. The signs and symptoms are not as specific as with BV or VVC, and many women are asymptomatic. The discharge is described as frothy, thin and watery, and white with occasional yellow or greenish tinges. Generally, the odor is mild to nonexistent and the pH of the discharge is greater than 4.5. Microscopically, a wet prep (saline) reveals motile flagellates slightly larger than a leukocyte. Microscopically examining a spun urine sample increases the identification of *Trichomonas vaginalis* compared with the wet prep alone. There is a nucleic acid amplification test (NAAT) for *Trichomonas vaginalis* that, due to cost, may be reserved for situations where the diagnosis is unclear.

Chlamydia

Chlamydial genital infections are the most frequently reported infectious diseases in the United States. Chlamydia is most prevalent in patients 25 years of age and under, and it is commonly asymptomatic. Since complications in women include PID, ectopic pregnancy, and infertility, both CDC and USPSTF recommend that all sexually active women 25 years of age and under and older women with new or multiple sex partners be tested annually. Concomitant infection with gonorrhea is common; therefore, patients diagnosed with chlamydia and their partners should be treated for both diseases. Diagnosis is made using NAATs that are specific for *Chlamydia trachomatis*. The test is accurate for urine, urethral discharge, plus endocervical, vaginal, and rectal swabs. Patients testing positive for *C. trachomatis* should also be tested for gonorrhea, syphilis, HIV, and hepatitis B.

Gonorrhea

Gonorrhea is the second most common bacterial STD. A majority of infections caused by *Neisseria gonorrhoeae* are diagnosed in males because the painful urethral discharge causes them to seek medical attention. Among women, gonorrhea can be asymptomatic. Complications of gonorrhea are similar to chlamydia in women. While gram-negative diplococci, found within neutrophils, are diagnostic in male urethral discharge, the yield in women is much lower. Negative Gram stains, however, do not rule out gonorrhea. Like in chlamydia, NAATs are the diagnostic test of choice in women. They are accurate using urine, plus vaginal, endocervical, rectal and urethral swabs. Concomitant infection with chlamydia is common; therefore, patients diagnosed with gonorrhea and their partners should be treated for both diseases. Patients testing positive for *N. gonorrhoeae* should also be tested for chlamydia, syphilis, HIV, and hepatitis B.

Noninfectious Causes

There are other noninfectious causes of vaginal discharge that make up roughly 10% of patients seen with vaginal discharges. Leukorrhea, a small amount of serous discharge containing vaginal debris, is not unusual and is normal particularly during pregnancy and in women on oral contraceptives. Allergic or irritant contact dermatitis to feminine hygiene products, latex condoms, or topical contraceptive creams/foams can cause vaginal symptoms including discharge. In perimenopausal women atrophic vaginitis should be considered. Retained tampons or other foreign bodies can also be a cause of vaginal odor, discomfort, and discharge.

• URINARY TRACT INFECTIONS

UTI is the most common bacterial infection in women, accounting for 8.6 million ambulatory care visits annually in the US. Half of all women will experience at least one UTI in their lifetime. UTIs are classified in a variety of ways. First is to use anatomical locations. Lower tract UTIs are those primarily involving the bladder and urethra. Cystitis is the term most frequently used to describe lower tract infections. Upper tract UTIs are infections in the kidney(s), and pyelonephritis is the term commonly used to describe upper tract UTIs. UTIs can also be described as complicated and uncomplicated. An uncomplicated UTI is one that occurs in healthy premenopausal women who are not pregnant and have no functional or structural abnormalities in their urinary tract. All others, in addition to pregnant women and patients with functional urinary tract abnormalities, are termed complicated. Other complicated UTIs are those in children, males, patients with diabetes, and patients with indwelling catheters. Recurrent infections and relapsed UTIs are also termed complicated. Complicated infections require longer antibiotic therapy or prophylactic measures. Recurrent UTIs are defined arbitrarily as two infections within 6 months or three to four in 12 months, and each episode is caused by a different organism. Relapsed UTIs are recurrent infections, usually with the same organism, and typically occur in patients with structural abnormalities in their urinary tract.

Eighty to ninety percent of UTIs occur in sexually active females. The short, straight urethra plus the trauma of sexual intercourse force motile coliform bacteria from the introitus (labia and entrance to vagina) into the urethra and bladder. From there, the bacteria may migrate up the ureters and into the kidneys, causing an upper tract UTI. There are multiple other predisposing factors for UTIs. During pregnancy, as the uterus enlarges, it creates temporary structural abnormalities in the urinary tract, predisposing pregnant women to upper and lower tract UTIs, which can lead to miscarriage and other complications. Also as the uterus grows, the pressure on the bladder increases urinary frequency and urgency, potentially masking signs of a UTI. In addition, upper tract disease is frequently asymptomatic in pregnancy. Detection of asymptomatic pyelonephritis is the rationale for pregnant women to have urine cultures done at the first prenatal visit, at 12 to 16 weeks and in the third trimester. Suboptimally controlled diabetes mellitus is a risk factor because higher plasma glucose levels increase glucose in the urine, which provides stimulus for bacterial growth. In addition, plasma glucose levels $\geq$ 200 mg/dL reduce neutrophil activity, reducing the ability to fight bacterial infections. Urinary tract instrumentation, especially indwelling catheters, facilitate invasion of bacteria. Males with prostate problems may not fully void, leaving residual urine in the bladder that promotes bacterial growth.

Diagnosis of a UTI requires a careful history and some laboratory testing (Table 16.4). It is sometimes difficult to accurately diagnose a UTI based on symptoms alone. Patients with cystitis present with dysuria (internal), frequency, urgency and possibly hematuria and may have suprapubic pain near completion of voiding. In the absence of a vaginal discharge, these symptoms are 90% predictive of a UTI. As previously discussed, the provider needs to rule out STDs and common causes of vaginal discharge, usually by history. While the symptoms of cystitis point to a bladder infection, 50% of *cystitis* patients also have what is called silent pyelonephritis or an asymptomatic upper tract UTI. Classical pyelonephritis presents with fever, nausea, vomiting, flank pain, and/or abdominal pain with or without cystitis symptoms. However, large percentages of pregnant women and children may be asymptomatic and still have upper tract disease. The causative bacteria in UTIs are usually normal GI flora that contaminate the introitus due to its close proximity to the anus and fecal matter. In 75% to 85% of uncomplicated UTIs, the infecting organism is a gram-negative coliform bacteria, *Escherichia coli*. *Staphylococcus saprophyticus*, the second leading cause of UTIs, is a gram-positive organism and is found in 10% to 20% of cultures. The remaining causative organisms are also fecal flora, usually other coliforms or enterococcus.

Classically, all patients got a midstream clean catch urinalysis with culture and susceptibility (MSCCUA with C&S) if a UTI was suspected. Now, with newer technology and increased clinical evidence, the culture and susceptibility portion is limited to specific situations, which will be discussed later. The purpose of the MSCCUA

TABLE 16.4	Urine Testing for Urinary Tract Infections
Midstream clean catch urinalysis (MSCCUA)	
Purpose	To avoid contamination from labia, urethra, and prostate. The first 10 ml represents labial/urethral contamination. The last 10 ml represents prostatic sample.
Dipstick tests	
Leukocyte esterase	Tests for presence of PMNs. False positives possible from vaginal discharge
Nitrite	Gram-negative bacteria that cause UTIs convert nitrate in urine to nitrite. False negatives if bacteria do not convert nitrate. (Gram-positive organisms represent 20% of UTI causes.)
Spun urine microscopic evaluations	
WBC	≥10/HPF consistent with UTI
RBC	≥5/HPF consistent with UTI
Potential false-positive results due to contamination in patients with vaginitis or who are menstruating	
Bacteria—not reliable due to normal introital flora, poor hygiene, or vaginitis	
Interpretation of culture results from a MSCCUA	
≥10^5 CFU/ml gram negative bacteria is a positive culture indicating a UTI	
≥10^2 CFU/ml pure culture any organism is a positive culture indicating a UTI	
More than one organism is considered contamination.	

is to avoid contamination from the labia, urethra, and prostate. The first 10 to 20 ml of urine flow contains any bacteria in the urethra and on the labia. The last 10 ml in males potentially has bacteria from the prostate. The method for the MSCCUA is very specific. Wash the labia with soap and water, rinse with water, and pat dry with sterile 4 × 4 gauze pads. While holding the labia apart, start the urine stream, stopping after 10 to 20 ml. Place the sterile collection container in front of the urine stream and collect 20 to 100 ml of urine. Stop the stream and remove the cup from the stream, then finish emptying the bladder into the toilet. During the study that established parameters for interpreting the MSCCUA culture, nurses' aides went into the restroom with the patient, washed the external genitalia with Tincture of Green Soap, rinsed it off with a squeeze water bottle, and ensured the process was done correctly. In actual practice not all of those steps are followed correctly, so most specimens are not true MSCCUAs. Today, patients are given a *kit* and frequently, with little or no instruction, are asked to go into the restroom and urinate into the jar found in the kit. Not surprisingly, there have been multiple problems with interpreting MSCCUA culture results. The *gold standard* for diagnosing a UTI is >10^5 CFU/ml (colony-forming units) and was developed from the study where the clean catch process was religiously followed. However, at the time, coliform bacteria were thought to be the only cause of UTIs, so pure cultures of gram-positive organisms, such *S. saprophyticus or enterococcus*, were considered contamination! If unable to process the urine sample quickly, the standard procedure is to place the urine container in a refrigerator to prevent coliform bacteria from overgrowing at room temperature and invalidating the sample. Unfortunately, gram-positive pathogens are fastidious and may die with exposure to cold, so cultures from infections due to gram-positive organisms were many times mislabeled as no growth. Also in cystitis, the frequent emptying of small amounts of urine from the bladder does not allow the bacteria any time to reproduce, resulting in counts of less than 10^5 CFU/ml. More recent studies, comparing cultures from sterile needle suprapubic aspiration of infected urine from the bladder to those obtained with an MSCCUA clearly demonstrated that any culture of a single organism with ≥10^2 CFU/ml was diagnostic for a UTI. Cultures with multiple organisms regardless of the count are considered contamination, and the specimen and analysis needs to be repeated with proper instruction or assistance.

In addition to culturing the urine specimen, it is spun down and several drops of the sediment are examined under the microscope. The remaining urine is tested for the presence of glucose, ketones, and protein. The most important part of the microscopic examination is counting the number of red blood cells (RBCs), white blood cells (WBCs), and epithelial cells per high power field (hpf). The number of epithelial cells per hpf is indicative of the "cleanness" of the MSCCUA. Less than five or *a few* epithelial cells confirms that the correct procedure for the MSCCUA was followed. Results that list TNTC (too numerous to count) or greater than 10/hpf suggest procedures were poorly followed and results need to be interpreted in that light. In a well-collected MSCCUA, greater than 10 WBCs/hpf is consistent with a UTI. Similarly, inflammation in kidney tissue and the bladder may result in hematuria. More than 5 RBCs/hpf is consistent with a UTI. Finally, the finding of any bacteria in an unspun urine specimen is consistent with >10^5 CFU/ml and is diagnostic for a UTI.

Currently, the laboratory diagnostic gold standard in suspected UTI is still the MSCCUA with microscopic analysis of the spun specimen. The availability of dipstick diagnostic strips for the presence of leukocyte esterase (LE) and nitrite and evidence from clinical studies has markedly reduced the indication for the use of culture and susceptibility testing of the MSCCUA. Urine dipsticks for office use are now available that test for both LE and nitrite. LE is produced by neutrophils that release esterases as part of their defense against bacterial infections. They are also used to detect bacteria in amniotic and ascites fluids. Most common gram-negative bacteria that cause UTIs convert nitrate to nitrite. Positive LE and nitrite tests in a urine sample are diagnostic of a UTI in a patient with typical UTI symptoms. However, each test has its limitations. Since 20% of UTIs are caused by gram-positive organisms, the nitrite test will be negative in those cases, as will UTIs caused by *Pseudomonas* species. LE can give false-positive results especially if a vaginal discharge is present and MSCCUA procedures are not carefully followed. Both may be negative in a patient who has severe frequency and urgency since the levels of bacteria and WBCs in the small volumes of urine may not be high enough to detect either nitrite or LE.

Urine cultures are used to confirm UTIs and provide specific information about their antibiotic susceptibility. When should urine be cultured? Most guidelines and experts agree. All patients with complicated UTIs should have culture and susceptibility testing on their MSCCUA (children, males, structural abnormalities, pregnancy). Also included are patients suspected of acute pyelonephritis, those with diabetes mellitus or who are immunosuppressed, patients with suspected relapse or treatment failures, and those with an unclear diagnosis from the history and physical examination. The main problem with urine cultures and susceptibilities is that it takes 48 hours to get the results, so regardless of the results almost all antibiotic therapy of UTIs is initially empiric.

Given our knowledge of the limitations of laboratory diagnostic testing, two basic approaches to the diagnosis and treatment are used in healthy sexually active women with symptoms of uncomplicated acute cystitis. First, empiric antibiotic therapy, usually short course (3 to 5 days), is implemented after a careful history eliminates other causes. Several studies have shown that in women with recurrent cystitis self-diagnosis and treatment with an on-hand antibiotic is highly effective and reduces the need for laboratory tests. Second, in addition to a careful history, an MSCCUA is obtained and dipstick testing for LE and nitrite is done to confirm the presence of a UTI before short-course antibiotics are prescribed. Finally, if the history does not point to a more specific cause, then a complete pelvic examination accompanied by testing for STDs and vaginitis plus MSCCUA are required to accurately diagnose the cause of dysuria.

In patients with a UTI, if the causative bacteria are susceptible to the empiric antibiotic therapy that is prescribed, the symptoms of dysuria, frequency, urgency, and suprapubic pain will quickly abate in as little as several hours. Systemic symptoms of acute pyelonephritis may take 24 hours to markedly improve. When counseling patients on antimicrobial medication for a UTI, the pharmacist should advise them that if the symptoms are not much better within 24 hours or totally gone by 48 hours, they should call the provider. Similarly, if a patient has been given oral antibiotics for a UTI, the pharmacist should inquire about potential nausea and vomiting due to acute pyelonephritis, which might interfere with oral therapy. Patients with nausea and/or vomiting are usually given a single injection of a long-acting antibiotic and instructed to wait for 24 hours before starting the oral therapy. If the patient received an antibiotic injection, the pharmacist should verify that the patient is to wait 12 to 24 hours (until the nausea disappears) to begin oral therapy. In patients with nausea and vomiting who have not received an injection, the provider should be notified of the potential problem before dispensing.

• KEY REFERENCES

1. Bremnor JD, Sadovsky R. Evaluation of dysuria in adults. *Am Fam Physician.* 2002;65:1589-1596.
2. Hainer BL, Gibson MV. Vaginitis: diagnosis and treatment. *Am Fam Physician.* 2011;83:807-815.
3. Ilkit M, Guzel AB. The epidemiology, pathogenesis and diagnosis of vulvovaginal candidosis: a mycological perspective. *Critic Rev Microbiol.* 2011;37:250-261.
4. Donders G. Diagnosis and management of bacterial vaginosis and other types of abnormal vaginal flora: a review. *Obstet Gynecol Survey.* 2010;65:462-473.
5. McClosky CR. Updated office testing skills for vaginal infections. *Nurse Pract.* 2010;35:46-52.
6. Mylonas I, Bergauer F. Diagnosis of vaginal discharge by wet mount microsopy: a simple and underated method. *Obstet Gynecol Survey.* 2011;66:359-368.
7. Borhart J, Bimbauer DM. Emergency department management of sexually transmitted infections. *Emerg Med Clin North Am.* 2011;29:587-603.
8. Anonymous. Sexually transmitted diseases treatment guidelines, 2010. *MMWR.* 2010;59:1-109, RR-12.
9. Lane DR, Takhar SS. Diagnosis and management of urinary tract infection and pyelonephritis. *Emerg Med Clin North Am.* 2011;29:539-552.
10. Hooton TM. Uncomplicated urinary tract infection. *N Engl J Med.* 2012;366:1028-1037.

CASE 16.1

Doris Daye, a 52 year-old patient, presents to clinic with a chief complaint of dysuria and vaginal discharge. She also has a nonspecific rash over a large area around her groin. She takes Lo-Ovral, an oral contraceptive. Her recent medical history includes type 2 diabetes mellitus, and since she was divorced last year, she has had multiple sexual encounters with different partners.

a. List three potential causes for her dysuria and vaginal discharge. Explain your rationale.

_____

_____

_____

_____

_____

b. List six questions/examinations or lab tests you would ask/conduct/run to determine the cause of her symptoms. Explain your rationale.

_____

_____

_____

_____

_____

c. You ordered several tests for which results have now returned. Interpret the test results. Explain your rationale. How does this change your original assessment?

Microscopic UA   *Culture and Susceptibility of Urine*
Epi   1 to 2/hpf
WBC   TNTC   >10^2 *Staphylococcus saprophyticus*
Glucose   4+
Protein   2+
Vaginal Discharge
Wet mount—negative for clue cells/motile flagellates
KOH prep—multiple hyphae present

_____

_____

_____

_____

_____

CASE 16.2

"All the way" Mae llovtuparti, a 24-year-old fourth-year student pharmacist, presents with a chief complaint of dysuria.

a. List three likely causes of her complaint.

_____

_____

_____

_____

b. List six initial lab tests/physical examinations and/or questions you would *most* like to ask Mae to evaluate the nature of her complaint. Explain your rationale.

_____

_____

_____

_____

c. Mae's urine report comes back as follows:

UA   Culture
Epi—neg   >10^3 E. coli
WBC—10 to 12/hpf
RBC—neg
Glucose—neg
Ketones
What is the likely diagnosis? Explain your rationale.

_____

_____

_____

_____

d. Interpret the following urinalysis/urine culture report if it was Mae's. Explain your rationale.

UA   Culture
Epi—many   >10^2 E. Coli
WBC—TNTC   >10^2 Serratia marcescens
RBC—TNTC   >10^2 Staphylococcus epidermidis
Glucose—3+

_____

_____

_____

_____

CHAPTER

SEVENTEEN

Common Skin Disorders

LEARNING OBJECTIVES

1. Accurately identify the most likely etiology when patients present with a skin rash or other dermatological condition, through history, diagnostic tests, and patient findings on examination to enable the pharmacist to appropriately recommend effective self-care treatment or referral of the patient to an appropriate provider.

2. Use the knowledge of the pathophysiology, etiology, and presentation of common dermatological diseases to review prescription orders for appropriateness and to accurately educate patients about their disease and its treatment.

3. Use the knowledge of the pathophysiology, etiology, and presentation of common dermatological diseases to enable the pharmacist to advise providers regarding the most appropriate prescription therapy.

• INTRODUCTION

There are little data on the prevalence of dermatological disorders in various populations. Estimates and extrapolation of survey results reveal that anywhere from 12% to 31% of visits to physicians involve dermatological problems, depending on location, age, ethnicity, and type of medical provider. Pharmacists are routinely asked for assistance with diagnosis and treatment of many common skin conditions. Therefore, it is important for pharmacists to recognize common skin disorders, so they can make appropriate recommendations about self-care and referral.

• GLOSSARY

Macule	Colored spot <1.5 cm
Patch	Colored spot >1.5 cm
Papule	Bump <1.5 cm
Nodule	Bump >1.5 cm
Pustule	Papule or nodule filled with pus seen in folliculitis, acne vulgaris
Vesicle	Papule or nodule filled with serous fluid seen in allergic contact dermatitis
Bullae	Vesicle >2 cm
Plaque	Raised patch usually seen in psoriasis
Wheal Urticaria Hive	Raised, itching, red areas seen in IgE-mediated allergic reactions
Crust	Dried residue of serum/pus/blood
Scale	Dry flakes of skin
Lichenification	Thickened skin with lots of wrinkles indicating a chronic dermatosis
Atrophy	Tissue paper thin skin, with highly visible arterioles and capillaries—an adverse effect of prolonged topical corticosteroid use
Excoriation	Scratched

• ECZEMATOUS DISORDERS

Eczema is a general term to describe any lesion that is red, and has unclear margins and dry flaky skin. Severe cases can present with widespread lesions including cracks in the skin (fissures), weeping, and excoriation. Chronic forms of eczematous conditions become lichenified (thick, wrinkled skin) with multiple lesions.

Atopic Dermatitis (Atopic Eczema)

Atopic dermatitis is one of the most common skin conditions. It has several common characteristics that make the diagnosis relatively simple in most cases. First, it is associated with other allergic disorders. Most patients have a personal or family history of allergic rhinitis, asthma, or atopic dermatitis (aka atopic disease). Fifty percent of patients have allergic rhinitis, 60% have asthma, and 75% to 80% have a positive family history for one of the three disorders. In roughly 80% of patients, the atopic dermatitis is primarily IgE mediated and their complete blood count will reveal an eosinophilia. The second characteristic is intense itching, which many times precedes the appearance of the eczematous lesions. It is known as the "itch that rashes." The intense itching causes patients to scratch their lesions, leading to an increased incidence of bacterial skin infections. The third characteristic is a common pattern of distribution, which varies by age. Lesions are symmetrical and in infants and toddlers the cheeks and face are the most common site. Many of the cute red-cheeked babies actually have atopic dermatitis (Figure 17.1). In children and many adults, the lesions are located in the fossae, cubital (inside of elbow), and popliteal (back of the knee) (Figure 17.2). Mild cases appear as dry, flaky, and pink skin. In patients with dark complexions, it may appear as lighter patches of skin that itch. Papules are a manifestation of moderate disease. Fortunately, most cases are mild and are amenable to successful treatment with nonprescription emollients and/or topical corticosteroids ointments.

Irritant Contact Dermatitis
Irritant contact dermatitis is an accurate description of the raw, red, dry skin caused by prolonged contact with irritating/drying substances such as urine, feces, soapy water, or irritating chemicals. Diaper rash and "dishpan hands" are examples of common causes of irritant contact dermatitis (Figure 17.3). Protecting the skin from the irritating substance with zinc oxide ointment, frequent diaper changes, or the use of rubber gloves is very effective in preventing irritant contact dermatitis.

Allergic Contact Dermatitis
In contrast to atopic dermatitis, allergic contact dermatitis (ACD) is a T-cell-mediated immune reaction to a contact with specific substances. The appearance of the lesions varies from eczematous and papular red to vesicular lesions as seen with poison, oak, ivy, and sumac (*Rhus* or *Toxicodendron*). Chronic ACD appears

FIGURE 17.1 An infant with atopic dermatitis on the face that has become superinfected. Source: Reproduced from Usatine RP. A baby with pink cheeks. *West J Med.* 2000;172(4):226. With permission from BMJ Publishing Group Ltd.

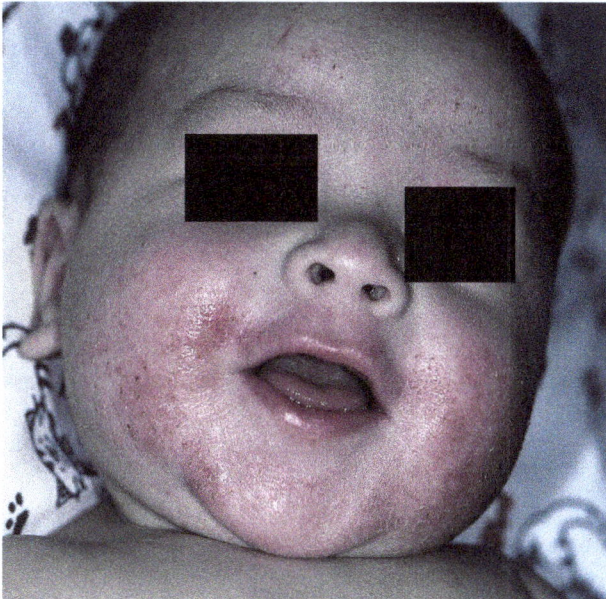

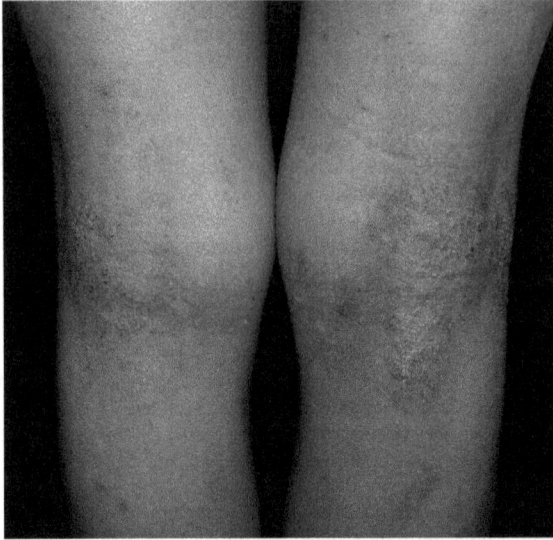

FIGURE 17.2 A 20-year-old young woman with severe chronic atopic dermatitis showing lichenification and hyperpigmentation in the popliteal fossa. (Used with permission of Richard P. Usatine, MD. From Usatine RP, Smith MA, Mayeux EJ, Jr, Chumley H. *The Color Atlas of Family Medicine.* 2nd ed. McGraw-Hill, Inc; 2013.)

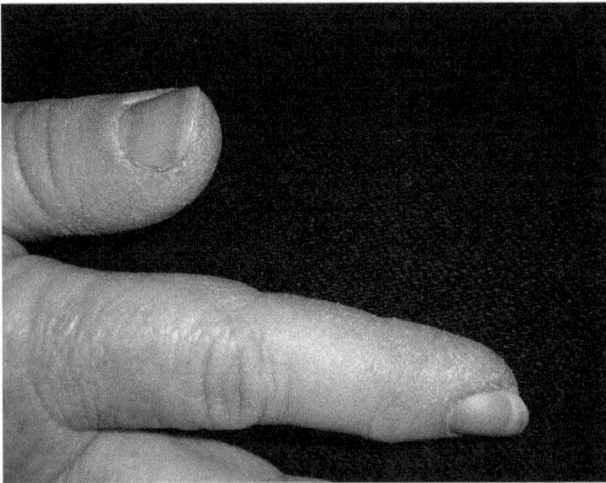

FIGURE 17.3 Occupational irritant contact dermatitis in a woman whose hands are exposed to chemicals while making cowboy hats in Texas. (Used with permission of Richard P. Usatine, MD. From Usatine RP, Smith MA, Mayeux EJ, Jr, Chumley H. *The Color Atlas of Family Medicine.* 2nd ed. McGraw-Hill, Inc; 2013.)

as red lichenified areas. What is unique and diagnostic about ACD is the pattern of the rash is limited to the area of the skin that has been in contact with the allergens. ACD due to laundry detergent is limited to places that sweat or have forced contact (armpits, neck/chest, belt/underwear lines). Nickel is a common cause of

ACD and since it is commonly found in jewelry the lesions occur where earrings, bracelets, or necklaces are worn (Figure 17.4). Also, leather is a common allergen and lesions are found only where the leather makes contact with the skin, i.e., the lesions of ACD due to leather watch bands are limited to a narrow area of the wrist (Figure 17.5 shows ACD to shoe leather). Latex is another common allergen causing ACD. Lesions are limited to areas of contact with latex such as waistbands of underwear, upper portions of men's socks, and outline of latex gloves. ACD secondary to *Rhus* species can be linear where the plant touched the patient's skin as they

FIGURE 17.4 Patient moved up his ring to show the allergic contact dermatitis secondary to a nickel allergy to the ring. (With permission from Milgrom EC, Usatine RP, Tan RA, Spector SL. *Practical Allergy*. Philadelphia, PA: Elsevier; 2004. Copyright Elsevier.)

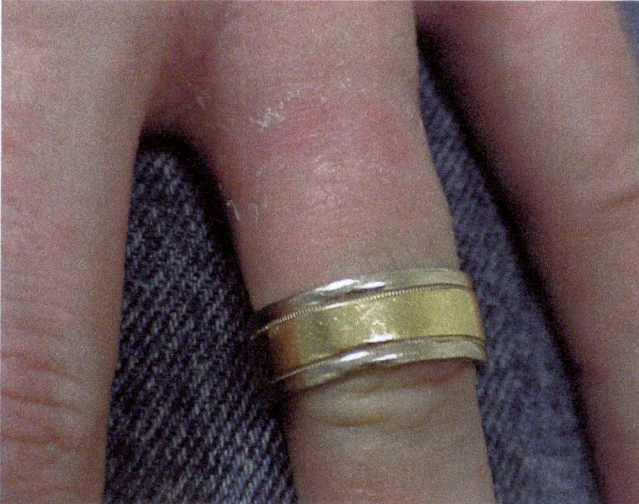

FIGURE 17.5 Allergic contact dermatitis from new shoes. This is the typical distribution found on the dorsum of the feet. (With permission from Milgrom EC, Usatine RP, Tan RA, Spector SL. *Practical Allergy*. Philadelphia, PA: Elsevier; 2004. Copyright Elsevier.)

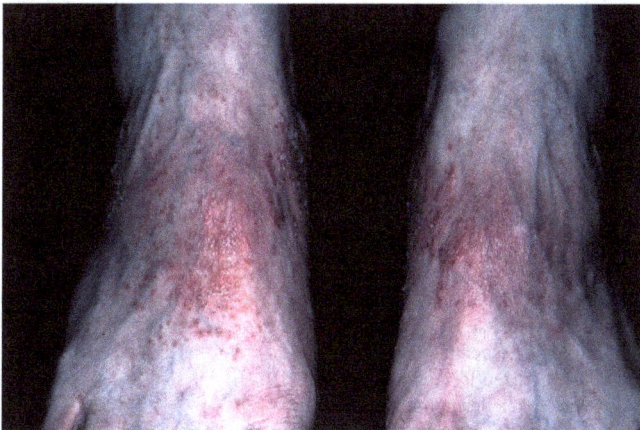

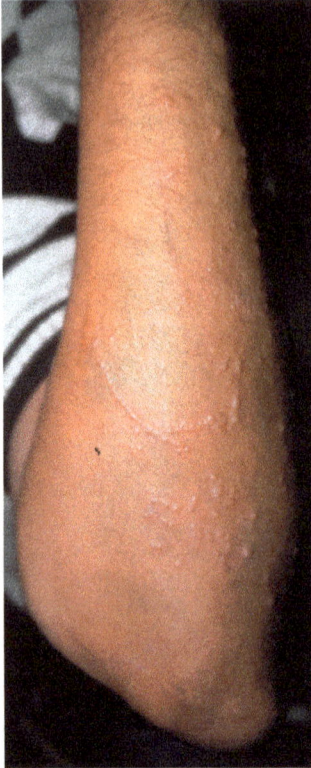

FIGURE 17.6 Multiple lines of vesicles from poison oak on the arm. (With permission from Milgrom EC, Usatine RP, Tan RA, Spector SL. *Practical Allergy*. Philadelphia, PA: Elsevier; 2004. Copyright Elsevier.)

walked by (Figure 17.6). Finally, avoid recommending topical medications that cause ACD. Benzocaine, neomycin, and topical diphenhydramine can cause ACD in up to 25% of patients who use them. Since they do not impact the common skin flora (neomycin) or have very limited efficacy (diphenhydramine and benzocaine), use more effective and useful alternatives.

• SCALY DERMATOSES

Xerosis, also known as dry flaky skin, is easily treated with emollients. In *keratosis pilaris* old skin cells in hair follicles get stuck, forming a scaly, horny plug that is sometimes darker than surrounding skin or may be red in dry weather conditions. It occurs primarily on the outer aspects of the upper arms and occasionally the thighs and cheeks. It is easily treatable with several weeks of a mild keratolytic containing 5% to 12% lactic acid.

Seborrhea/Seborrheic Dermatitis

Both disorders are a result of a local immune reaction to substances produced by a yeast known as *Malassezia furfur* (previously known as *Pityrosporum ovale*). Seborrhea, aka dandruff, produces scales in the scalp. Seborrheic dermatitis appears as yellow, greasy scales over an eczematous-like lesion (Figure 17.7). The lesions occur primarily along the scalp line, nasolabial fold, eyebrows, eyelashes, ears, and over the sternum. It is associated with patients with Parkinson disease. These disorders are not curable, but can be easily controlled with shampoos and topical preparations containing selenium sulfide or zinc pyrithione. Shampooing the hair with selenium sulfide or zinc pyrithione at least weekly maintains remission. More severe cases of seborrheic dermatitis may require topical corticosteroids in addition to the antimalassezia products.

Psoriasis

Psoriasis is a complex immunological reaction involving T-cell proliferation and cytokine release. It presents with raised plaques with sharp margination. Many lesions have adherent silver/white scales that bleed if pulled off (Figure 17.8). The most common sites are the elbows and knees, but can occur anywhere on the body. As many as 10% of patients have an accompanying arthritis (psoriatic arthritis). Recently, psoriasis was found to be associated with an increased risk of cardiovascular disease. Only single, small, coin-sized lesions are potentially amenable to self-care. Most patients should be referred to a dermatologist for definitive therapy.

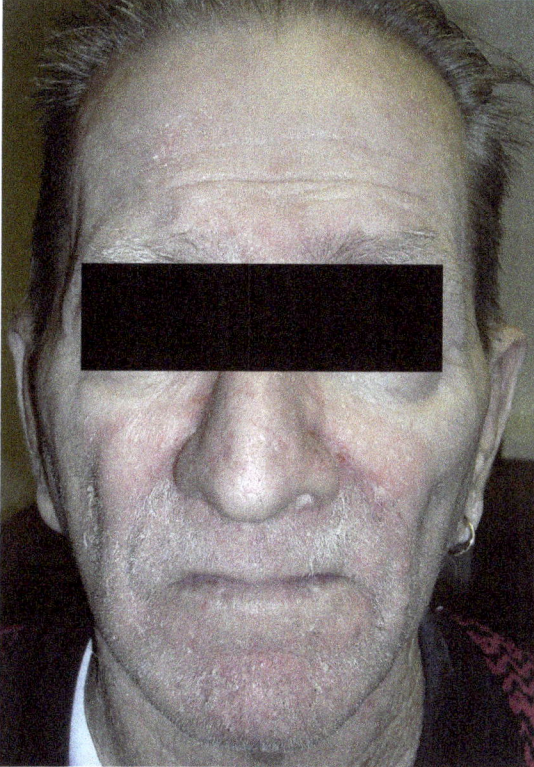

FIGURE 17.7 Seborrheic dermatitis following the typical distribution on the face of a 59-year-old man. Note the prominent scale and erythema on his forehead, glabella, and beard region. (Used with permission of Richard P. Usatine, MD. From Usatine RP, Smith MA, Mayeux EJ, Jr, Chumley H. *The Color Atlas of Family Medicine*. 2nd ed. McGraw-Hill, Inc; 2013.)

• BACTERIAL INFECTIONS

Bacterial infections of the skin usually involve normal skin flora. Normal flora include β-hemolytic *Streptococcus pyogenes*, several staphylococcal species including *S. epidermidis, S. aureus,* and the more antibiotic-resistant community-acquired methicillin-resistant *Staphylococcus aureus (CA MRSA)*. Bacterial infections of the skin require a break in the skin to allow the opportunistic normal flora to gain entrance. Insect bites, minor trauma, lacerations, and abrasions, plus conditions favorable for bacterial growth are all that is required for a bacterial infection to start. Drastically lowering the bacterial count by immediate vigorous and thorough cleaning of even the smallest break in the skin with soap and water drastically reduces the incidence of bacterial infections. While many bacterial infections have separate and sometimes confusing names, even the most superficial infection, like impetigo, can progress to a larger infection involving surrounding soft-tissue known as cellulitis. Bacterial cellulitis is characterized by four to five symptoms. Lesions are *swollen*, very warm or *hot* to the touch, *red* in color, *painful,* and sometimes are associated with *purulent* material or pus (neutrophils used to fight the bacterial infection). Also they tend to spread or grow

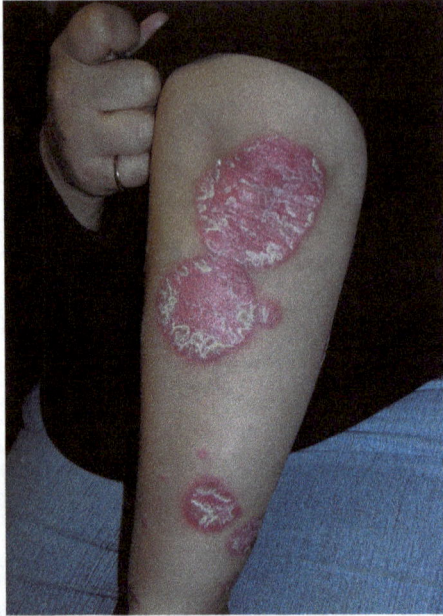

FIGURE 17.8 Typical plaque psoriasis on the elbow and arm. (Used with permission of Richard P. Usatine, MD. From Usatine RP, Smith MA, Mayeux EJ, Jr, Chumley H. *The Color Atlas of Family Medicine*. 2nd ed. McGraw-Hill, Inc; 2013.)

if untreated (Figure 17.9). Most bacterial skin infections require systemic antibiotic therapy. Bacterial skin infections can be confirmed with a complete blood count where the white blood cell differential count shows greater than 10,000 WBCs with more than 80% of the total WBC count consisting of mature and immature neutrophils (PMNs).

FIGURE 17.9 Cellulitis of the foot of a diabetic person in which there is possible necrosis and gangrene of the second toe, requiring hospitalization and a podiatry consult. (Used with permission of Richard P. Usatine, MD. From Usatine RP, Smith MA, Mayeux EJ, Jr, Chumley H. *The Color Atlas of Family Medicine*. 2nd ed. McGraw-Hill, Inc; 2013.)

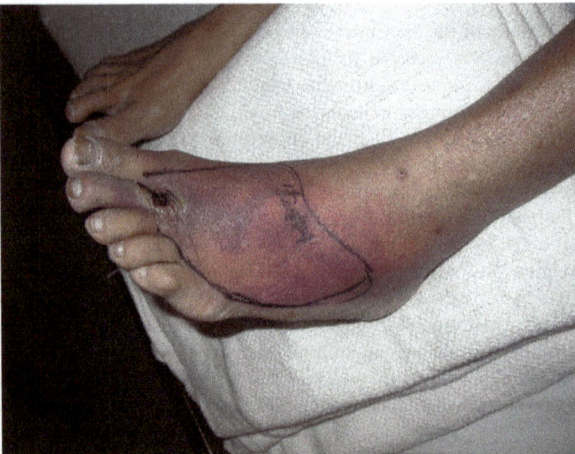

Cellulitis can also be confirmed by marking the outer borders of the red swollen area with ink. If the red swollen area expands outside ink lines, then high likelihood of bacterial cellulitis exists.

Impetigo

Impetigo is a superficial bacterial infection primarily caused by group A β-hemolytic *Streptococcus pyogenes (GABHS)*. The role of staphylococcal species in classical impetgo is a controversial issue. It usually presents with a yellow or honey-colored crust of serosanguineous fluid (Figure 17.10).

Bullous Impetigo

Bullous impetigo is also a superficial lesion that presents with vesicles and bullae. *Staphylococcus aureus* is the causative agent (Figure 17.11).

Folliculitis

Folliculitis is a mildly infected hair follicle with little or no cellulitis. It presents primarily as a pustule surrounding a single hair follicle (Figure 17.12, looks like bacterial folliculitis). Generally, these do not require systemic treatment.

Furuncle

A furuncle, also known as a "boil," is a local cellulitis, arising from a single hair follicle (a folliculitis gone wild), usually caused by *Staphylococcus aureus* (Figure 17.13). Some furuncles are abscess like, with a purulent center and relatively avascular core. Most furuncles do not require systemic antibiotics, but should be surgically drained or "lanced" (opening the avascular core to let the pus drain out) to clear up the infection.

FIGURE 17.10 Typical honey-crusted plaque on the lip of an adult with impetigo. (Used with permission of Richard P. Usatine, MD. From Usatine RP, Smith MA, Mayeux EJ, Jr, Chumley H. *The Color Atlas of Family Medicine*. 2nd ed. McGraw-Hill, Inc; 2013.)

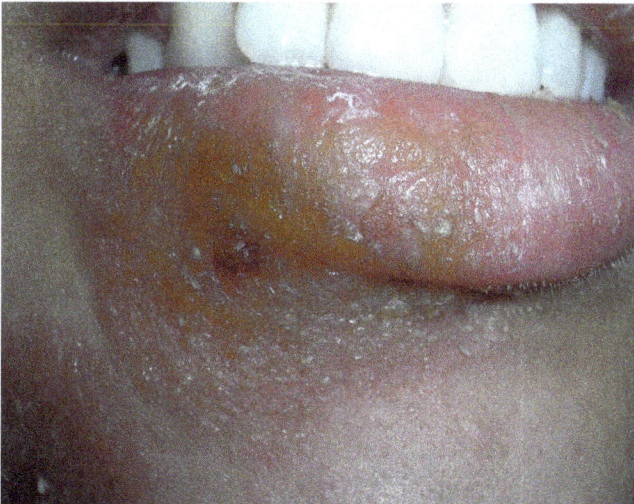

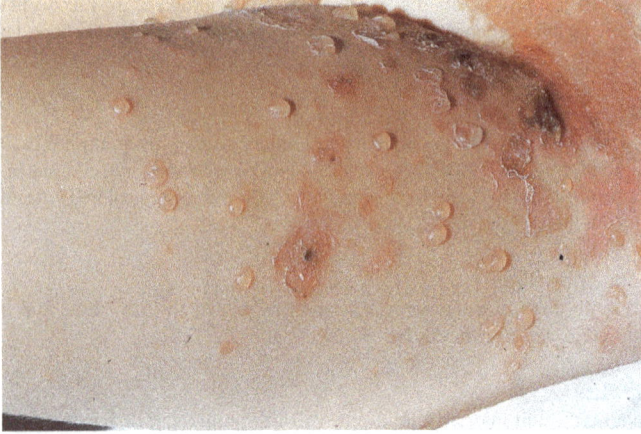

FIGURE 17.11 Bullous impetigo secondary to methicillin-resistant *Staphylococcus aureus* (MRS) on the leg of an 11-year-old child. Note the surrounding cellulitis. Source: Reproduced with permission from Wolff KA, Johnson RA, Saavedra AP, eds. *Fitzpatrick's Color Atlas and Synopsis of Clinical Dermatology*. 7th ed. New York: McGraw-Hill, Inc; 2013. Fig. 25-12. Copyright © McGraw-Hill Education LLC.

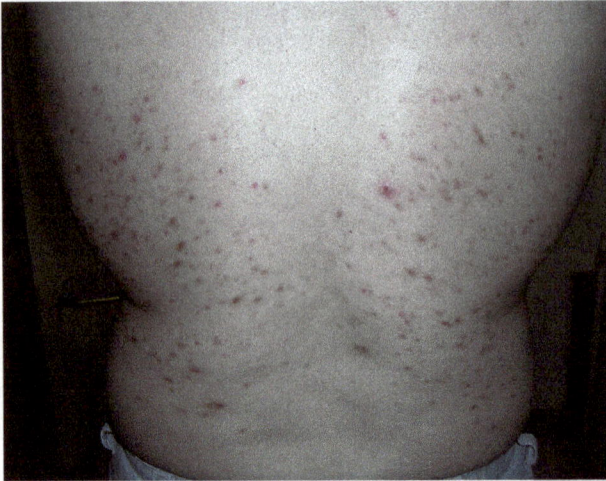

FIGURE 17.12 Eosinophilic folliculitis on the back of an HIV-positive man. (Used with permission of Richard P. Usatine, MD. From Usatine RP, Smith MA, Mayeux EJ, Jr, Chumley H. *The Color Atlas of Family Medicine*. 2nd ed. McGraw-Hill, Inc; 2013.)

Carbuncle

A carbuncle is a large furuncle with a larger area of local cellulitis that involves multiple hair follicles with connecting sinus tracts between follicles. Surgical drainage can be effective but depending on the size and location of the carbuncle, systemic antibiotic therapy may be required.

While the term cellulitis is a generic term for a soft tissue bacterial infection, several have been given specific names due to unique characteristics.

Paronychia is a minor cellulitis around a cuticle.

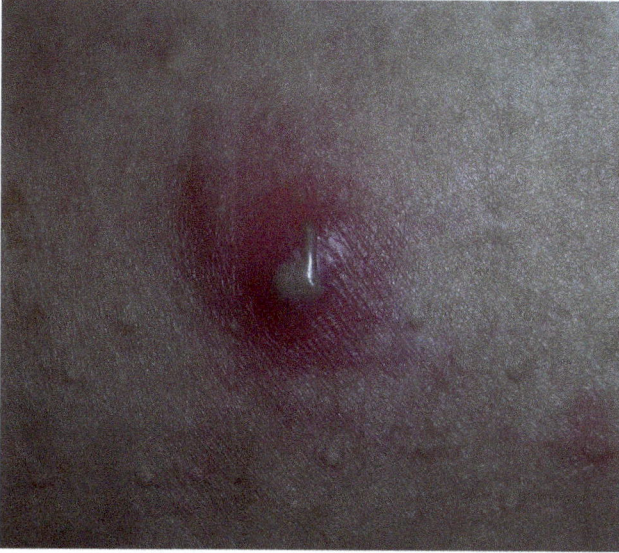

FIGURE 17.13 Isolated single furuncle in an adult woman. (Used with permission of Richard P. Usatine, MD. From Usatine RP, Smith MA, Mayeux EJ, Jr, Chumley H. *The Color Atlas of Family Medicine.* 2nd ed. McGraw-Hill, Inc; 2013.)

Erysipelas is a cellulitis on the face, which moves very rapidly along the fascia due to production of hyaluronidase produced by the causative agent group A β-hemolytic *Streptococcus pyogenes*. It produces little or no purulent material and is a medical emergency due to the close proximity of tracts near the eyes that provide a relatively easy access into the brain.

Necrotizing Fasciitis
Also known as "flesh-eating bacteria," it is usually a multiorganism, mixed aerobe/anaerobe infection including group A β-hemolytic *Streptococcus* pyogenes but can be caused by GABHS alone. GABHS, which produces hyaluronidase allows the infection to move along the fascia, quickly destroying surrounding soft tissue. Failure to quickly identify and appropriately treat this condition can result in permanent loss of large amounts of soft tissue and extremities and may even be fatal. Immunocompromised patients and those with poor peripheral circulation such as patients with poorly controlled diabetes mellitus and a "diabetic foot" are most susceptible (Figure 17.14).

Acneiform Lesions
Acne is defined as an inflammatory, follicular, papular, and pustular eruption involving the pilosebaceous apparatus. The term pustular implies bacterial etiology, hence its inclusion under bacterial infections. In reality, bacterial involvement in acneiform lesions is almost always secondary.

Acne Vulgaris Acne vulgaris is the technical name for typical teenage acne. While the primary pathological driver is testosterone, bacteria (*Propionibacterium acnes*) are a significant part of the overall pathological process and are one target in the treatment of this common disorder. It is a disease involving the vellus hair follicle, where the hair remains invisible inside the follicle. Comedone formation, plugging of

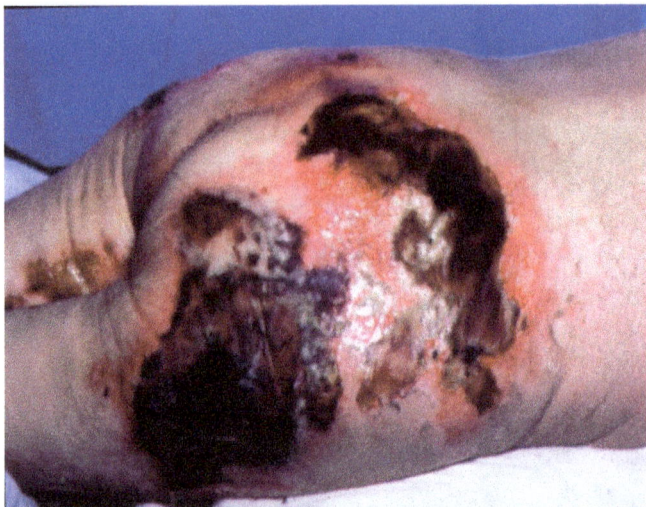

FIGURE 17.14 Necrotizing fasciitis with gangrene. Even with a radical hemipelvectomy this patient did not survive. (Used with permission of Fred Bongard, MD.)

the hair follicle, is an integral step in the pathological process (Figure 17.15 shows an advanced case of acne).

FIGURE 17.15 Severe nodulocystic acne with scarring in a 16-year-old boy. (Used with permission of Richard P. Usatine, MD. From Usatine RP, Smith MA, Mayeux EJ, Jr, Chumley H. *The Color Atlas of Family Medicine*. 2nd ed. McGraw-Hill, Inc; 2013.)

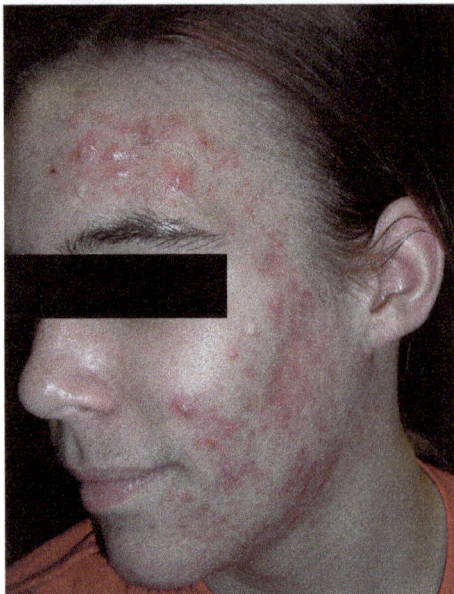

Acne Rosacea Acne rosacea, preferably called rosacea, occurs primarily on the face in adults. One version, the papulopustular type, has papular lesions and tiny pustule-like pimples, but its pathogenesis is totally different than acne vulgaris. It was thought to be a form of acne vulgaris because it responds to the same antibiotics that work in acne vulgaris; hence, it is still incorrectly classified as an acne. While the exact cause is unknown, it is an abnormality of the immune system that causes an inflammatory reaction. It occurs exclusively in adults and has two major presentations. The erythematotelangiectatic version presents as persistent erythema of the central face, with prolonged flushing, burning, or stinging,

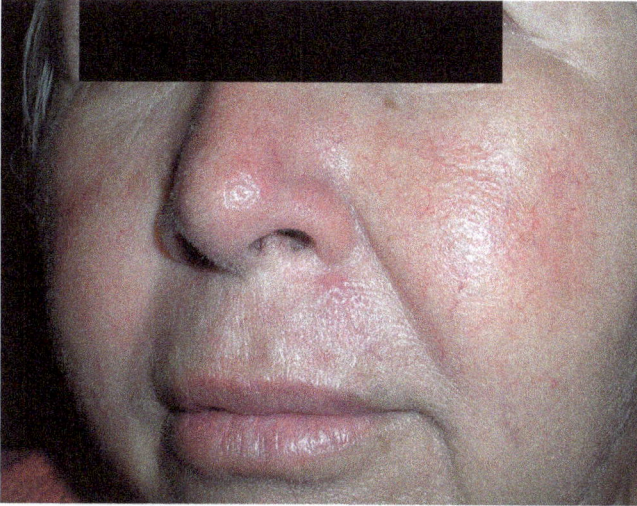

FIGURE 17.16 Erythematotelangiectatic subtype of rosacea in a middle-aged Hispanic woman. (Used with permission of Richard P. Usatine, MD. From Usatine RP, Smith MA, Mayeux EJ, Jr, Chumley H. *The Color Atlas of Family Medicine*. 2nd ed. McGraw-Hill, Inc; 2013.)

and is the most resistant to treatment (Figure 17.16). The papulopustular version mentioned above responds well to 1/10th of the dose of doxycycline used to treat acne vulgaris due to its anti-inflammatory properties. Rosacea symptoms are aggravated by exposure to sunlight, ingestion of ethanol, or exposure to windy conditions. It is more common in women and the pattern of the lesions usually differs by gender. The male pattern is more frequently vertical (forehead, nose, chin), while the female pattern tends to be more horizontal (cheeks under eyes, nose). Untreated rosacea can lead to excessive tissue growth around the nose (rhinophyma) (Figure 17.17).

• VIRAL INFECTIONS

Verrucae (Warts)

Viral in etiology there are two main types of warts, both of which present as external growths of skin above the normal surface. Common warts can occur anywhere, are nonpainful, and are easily treated with nonprescription remedies (Figure 17.18). Plantar warts occur on the bottom of the foot, have significant tissue below the skin surface, can be painful, and are very resistant to treatment, usually requiring referral to a dermatologist or podiatrist (Figure 17.19).

Herpes Simplex

Herpes simplex episodically presents as painful vesicles located on the lips and face (type 1, fever blister, cold sore) (Figure 17.20) or on the genitals (type 2). It is usually a chronic, recurrent condition, with acute episodes occurring periodically and lasting 7 to 10 days. In between acute episodes, the virus resides asymptomatically in local sensory nerves. Multiple physical and emotional stresses are associated with acute attacks. The disease is contagious and can be transferred to others by contact with visible lesions.

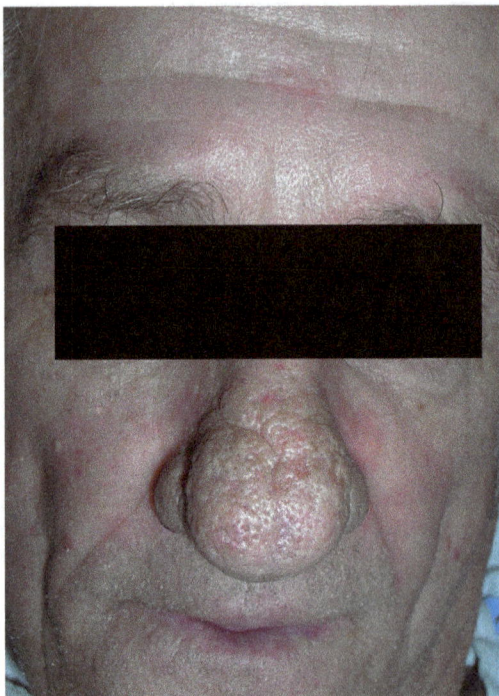

FIGURE 17.17 Rhinophymatous rosacea in an older man who does not drink alcohol. Although this is often called a WC Field nose, it is not necessarily related to heavy alcohol use. (Used with permission of Richard P. Usatine, MD. From Usatine RP, Smith MA, Mayeux EJ, Jr, Chumley H. *The Color Atlas of Family Medicine.* 2nd ed. McGraw-Hill, Inc; 2013.)

FIGURE 17.18 Common warts on the hands of an 11-year-old girl. These periungual warts are particularly difficult to eradicate. (Used with permission of Richard P. Usatine, MD. From Usatine RP, Smith MA, Mayeux EJ, Jr, Chumley H. *The Color Atlas of Family Medicine.* 2nd ed. McGraw-Hill, Inc; 2013.)

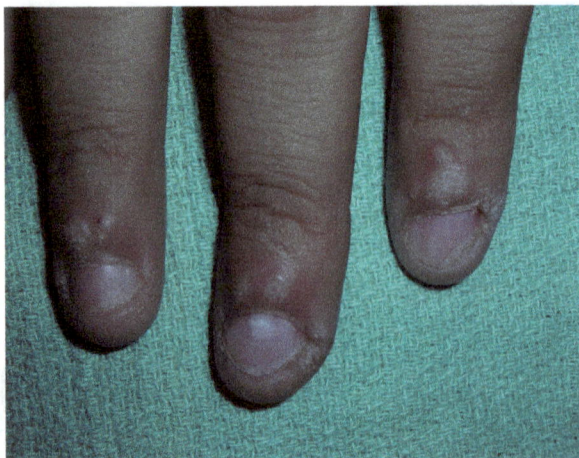

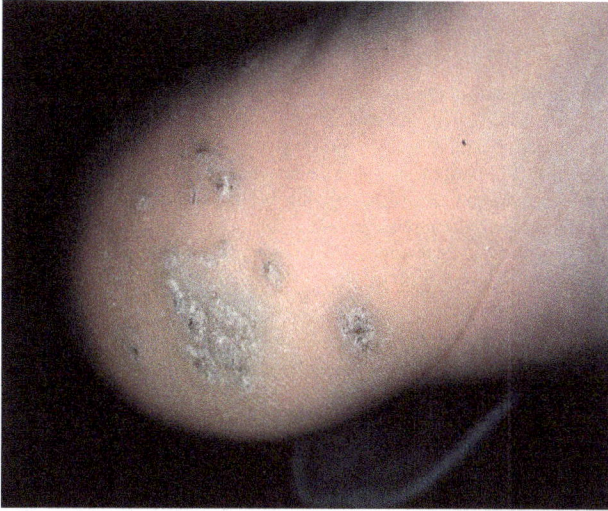

FIGURE 17.19 Plantar warts. Note small black dots in the warts that represent thrombosed vessels. Large plantar warts such as these are called *mosaic warts*. (Used with permission of Richard P. Usatine, MD. From Usatine RP, Smith MA, Mayeux EJ, Jr, Chumley H. *The Color Atlas of Family Medicine.* 2nd ed. McGraw-Hill, Inc; 2013.)

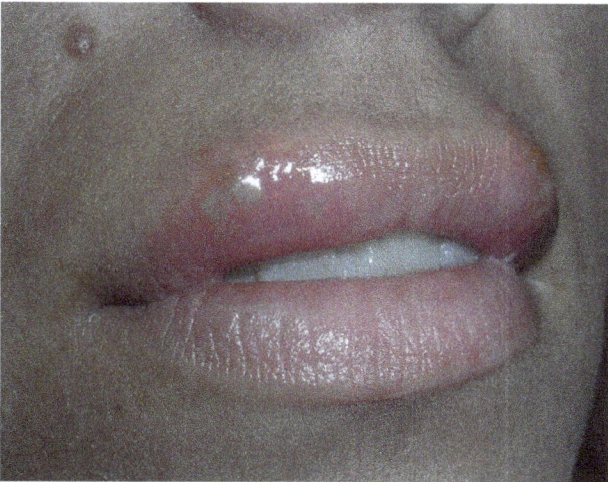

FIGURE 17.20 Orolabial herpes simplex virus in an adult woman showing deroofed blisters (ulcer). (Used with permission of Richard P. Usatine, MD. From Usatine RP, Smith MA, Mayeux EJ, Jr, Chumley H. *The Color Atlas of Family Medicine.* 2nd ed. McGraw-Hill, Inc; 2013.)

Herpes Zoster

Herpes zoster causes chicken pox in children and a much more devastating disease, shingles in older adults. Once a patient has chicken pox as a child, the body's immune system walls it off in sensory nerves. Any reduction in the immune control of the virus will result in the appearance of typical painful vesicular lesions. In shingles, rather than occurring in random patterns, the lesions appear in a linear fashion along skin dermatomes (Figure 17.21). The vesicular eruption is generally preceded by a pro-drome involving pain and itching lasting several days. Shingles is predominantly a disease of patients 60 years of age or older. If untreated, lesions can last up to 5 to 8 weeks. The major complication with shingles is postherpetic neuralgia (PHN), which can last for months or even become permanent. Up to 40% of patients with shingles develop PHN. In about 10% of patients, it lasts a year or longer, PHN is a major cause for visits to pain specialists. Treatment with antivirals initiated within 72 hours of onset may reduce severity of the pain and increases the rate of healing of shingles lesions. While there have been few studies, it appears that treatment with antivirals does not prevent PHN, but does decrease its duration.

• FUNGAL INFECTIONS

Tineas

Fungal infections labeled as tineas are usually caused by dermatophytes such as *Trichophyton* and *Microsporum* species. Their medical names are determined by location. They have a common appearance regardless of location. They are sharply marginated, have central clearing, and are reddish-brown in color.

Tinea faciei is located on the face, aka ringworm.

Tinea corporis is located on the trunk and lesions are usually asymmetrical rather than circular (Figure 17.22).

Tinea pedis: Otherwise known as athlete's foot, its presentation differs from those found on the face and trunk. There are three types of lesions: dry moccasin like scale on the soles and sides of the feet, interdigital (between the toes) (Figure 17.23), and the vesicular/bullous form.

FIGURE 17.21 A 14-year-old boy with severe case of herpes zoster in a thoracic distribution. (Used with permission of Richard P. Usatine, MD. From Usatine RP, Smith MA, Mayeux EJ, Jr, Chumley H. *The Color Atlas of Family Medicine*. 2nd ed. McGraw-Hill, Inc; 2013.)

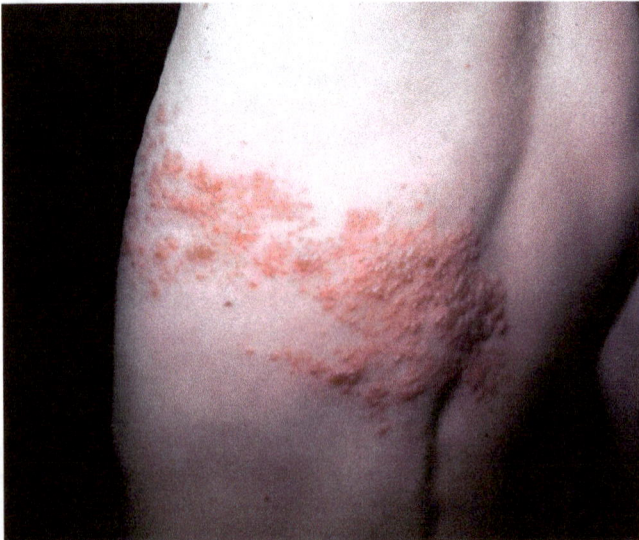

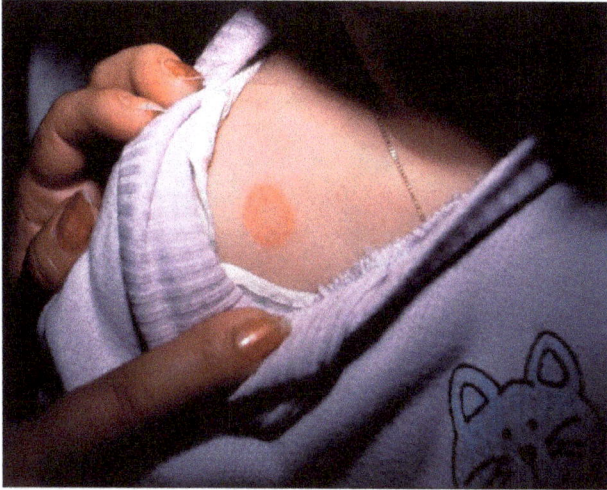

FIGURE 17.22 Tinea corporis on the shoulder of this young girl. This is a very typical annular pattern and the cat on the sweatshirt might be a clue to an infected pet at home spreading a *Microsporum dermatophyte* to its owner. Note the concentric rings with scaling, erythema, and central sparing. (Used with permission of Richard P. Usatine, MD. From Usatine RP, Smith MA, Mayeux EJ, Jr, Chumley H. *The Color Atlas of Family Medicine*. 2nd ed. McGraw-Hill, Inc; 2013.)

Tinea cruris: Also known as jock itch, tinea cruris, located in the groin and genital area, presents like lesions on the face and trunk and patients may contract it via auto-innoculation by pulling on their underwear over tinea pedis (Figure 17.24). Therefore, in order to treat jock itch, antifungals must be applied to the groin *and* the feet to prevent recurrence.

FIGURE 17.23 Tinea pedis seen in the interdigital space between the fourth and fifth digits. This is the most common area to see tinea pedis. (Used with permission of Richard P. Usatine, MD. From Usatine RP, Smith MA, Mayeux EJ, Jr, Chumley H. *The Color Atlas of Family Medicine*. 2nd ed. McGraw-Hill, Inc; 2013.)

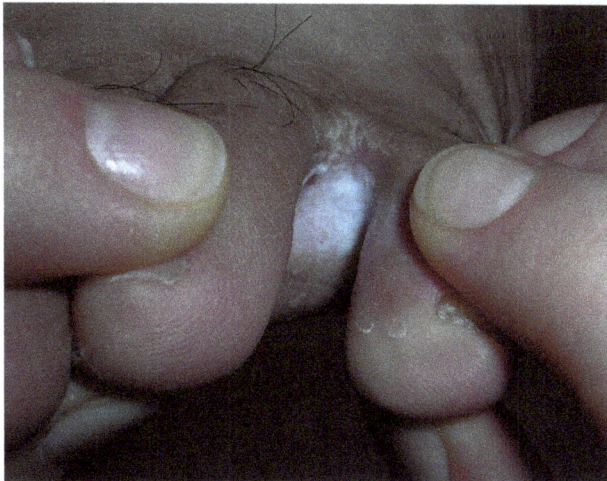

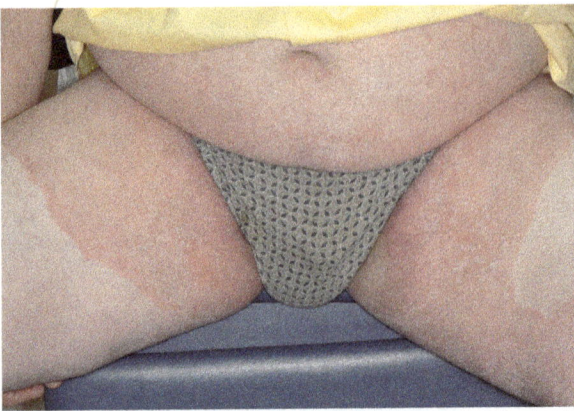

FIGURE 17.24 A 54-year-old man with tinea cruris and corporis for decades despite multiple treatments with oral antifungal medications. His cultures show *T. rubrum* sensitive to all the typical oral antifungal medications, but his tinea never completely clears. He does not have a known immunodeficiency but his immune system appears not to recognize the *T. rubrum* as foreign. (Used with permission of Richard P. Usatine, MD. From Usatine RP, Smith MA, Mayeux EJ, Jr, Chumley H. *The Color Atlas of Family Medicine*. 2nd ed. McGraw-Hill, Inc; 2013.)

Tinea Versicolor

Tinea versicolor is misnamed since it is caused by *Malassezia* species. Many references list it as pityriasis versicolor. While these lesions are a very pale reddish-brown, there is generally no central clearing (Figure 17.25). Sometimes it looks like patches of dry flaky skin on pale complected patients. In patients with darker complexions or suntans, they appear as white patches (Figure 17.26).

Candida

Fungal infections caused by *Candida* species (also known as *Monilia*) are easy to differentiate from other fungal skin infections. Lesions are usually fiery red, may appear

FIGURE 17.25 Large areas of pink tinea versicolor on the shoulder in a cape-like distribution. (Used with permission of Richard P. Usatine, MD. From Usatine RP, Smith MA, Mayeux EJ, Jr, Chumley H. *The Color Atlas of Family Medicine*. 2nd ed. McGraw-Hill, Inc; 2013.)

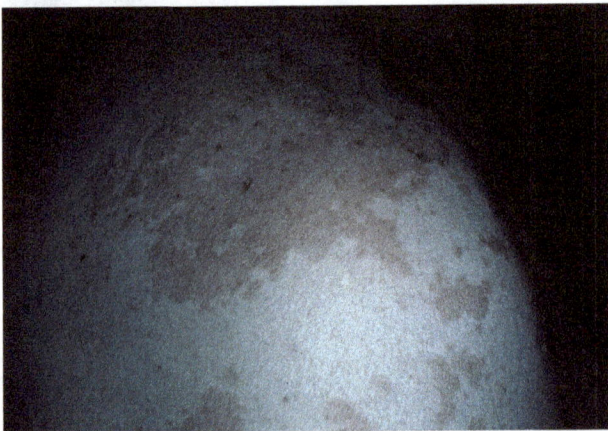

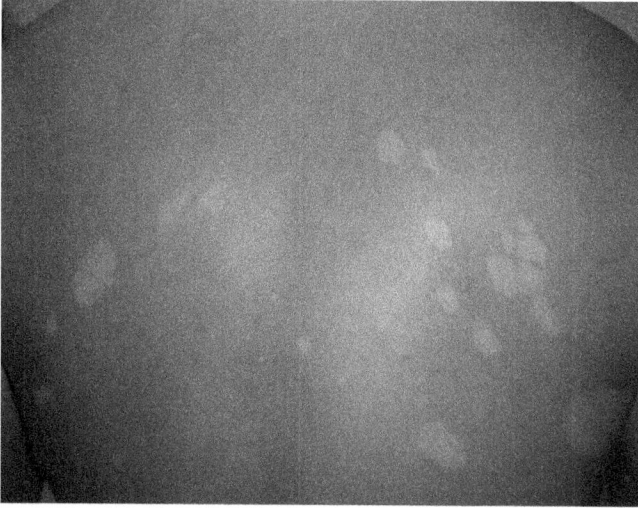

FIGURE 17.26 Patches of hypopigmentation across the back caused by tinea versicolor in a young Latino man. Vitiligo is on the differential diagnosis in this case. A KPH preparation confirmed tinea versicolor. (Used with permission of Richard P. Usatine, MD. From Usatine RP, Smith MA, Mayeux EJ, Jr, Chumley H. *The Color Atlas of Family Medicine.* 2nd ed. McGraw-Hill, Inc; 2013.)

shiny, and are found in moist or intertriginous areas, i.e., under the breasts, genitals, skin folds. In addition, candidal skin infections are not sharply marginated, but they have red, papular "satellite lesions" just outside the main red area (Figure 17.27). In addition, patients who develop candidiasis tend to have compromised immune systems

FIGURE 17.27 Candida inguinal eruption in a 61-year-old man after a course of antibiotics for bronchitis. Note the satellite lesions. (Used with permission of Richard P. Usatine, MD. From Usatine RP, Smith MA, Mayeux EJ, Jr, Chumley H. *The Color Atlas of Family Medicine.* 2nd ed. McGraw-Hill, Inc; 2013.)

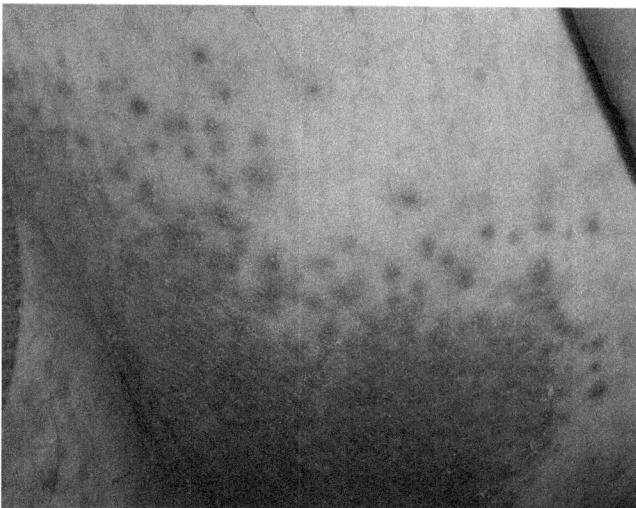

or poorly controlled diabetes mellitus. All patients with candidal skin infections or vaginitis should be questioned and potentially tested for diabetes mellitus if not previously diagnosed, since that may be the initial presenting symptom of their diabetes mellitus.

• DRUG-INDUCED SKIN REACTIONS

Two Important Rules

When asked to evaluate a skin rash in a specific patient for medication etiology, remember two things. First, do not assume that all adverse dermatological reactions occur within 24 to 48 hours of medication administration. If this is a first-time exposure to the medication, the reaction may occur up to 2 weeks after the drug is stopped because it may take the body up to 14 days to fully react immunologically. For example, a patient completes a 7-day regimen of trimethoprim-sulfamethoxazole for a urinary tract infection. Four days later, the symptoms recur, and assuming resistance to the previous regimen, the patient is started on ciprofloxacin. Two days later, the patient develops urticaria. The natural assumption would be that the ciprofloxacin was the causative agent. However, if the initial prescription was the patient's first exposure to a sulfonamide, the skin reaction could be just as easily due to the sulfonamide and not the ciprofloxacin. Second, other infections or autoimmune disorders can also cause these same *drug reactions* and must be *ruled out* before assuming the medication caused the reaction. For example, in a patient presenting with erythema nodosum in Southern Arizona, providers automatically think of valley fever (coccidioidomycosis) as the most likely diagnosis, since it is endemic to the area and erythema nodosum is a very common presentation of that infection. All patients in Southern Arizona will receive a diagnostic workup for coccidioidomycosis if they present with erythema nodosum, regardless of any medication they are taking.

Severe, Potentially Life-Threatening Reactions

There are two sequences of reactions that begin with skin rashes. If patients with that initial dermatological reaction are subsequently given that drug or one in the same pharmacological class, the next reaction may be more severe and even fatal. Patients should be warned never to take that class of medication again for concern over escalation to a more severe reaction in that group and its potentially lethal results. These two types of reactions are discussed in more detail.

IgE-Mediated Reactions

Urticaria Also known as hives, or wheals, urticaria is an IgE-mediated, type 1 immunological reaction. Urticaria presents as multiple pale pink or red raised areas of skin (wheals) that are intensely pruritic (itchy) (Figure 17.28). They may coalesce into larger lesions (Figure 17.29). Individual lesions last only 24 to 36 hours, but as long as the patient is still exposed to the allergen or is untreated, new wheals will continue to appear. Normally antihistamines and in some cases systemic corticosteroids will cause the lesions to stop erupting.

Angioneurotic Edema Also known as angioedema, angioneurotic edema is the second in the sequence of serious IgE-mediated dermatological reactions. Wheals occur in deeper layers of the skin, usually the lips, face, tongue, and eyes, but can affect hands and feet as well (Figure 17.30). Usually nonpruritic, they can coexist with urticaria. Those occurring in the mouth and pharynx can cause local airway obstruction and in more severe cases require tracheostomy and intubation. Rarely the wheals can occur only in the gastrointestinal tract, causing initial manifestations of GI pain/discomfort,

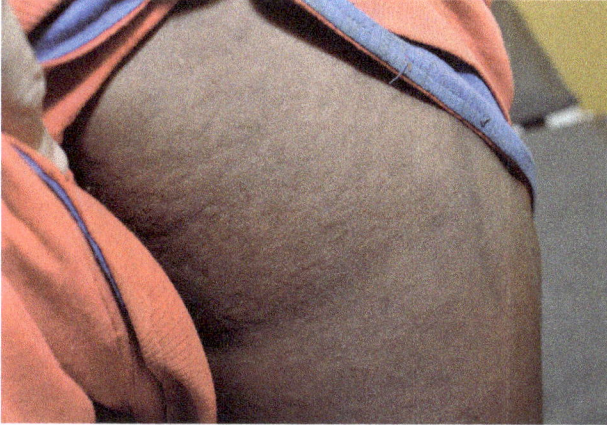

FIGURE 17.28 Urticaria that occurred within an hour after a boy was given ibuprofen to treat a high fever. (Used with permission of Richard P. Usatine, MD. From Usatine RP, Smith MA, Mayeux EJ, Jr, Chumley H. *The Color Atlas of Family Medicine*. 2nd ed. McGraw-Hill, Inc; 2013.)

FIGURE 17.29 Note the confluence of wheals with a well-demarcated border on the arm of the man with acute urticarial due to trimethoprim-sulfamethoxazole. (Used with permission of Richard P. Usatine, MD. From Usatine RP, Smith MA, Mayeux EJ, Jr, Chumley H. *The Color Atlas of Family Medicine*. 2nd ed. McGraw-Hill, Inc; 2013.)

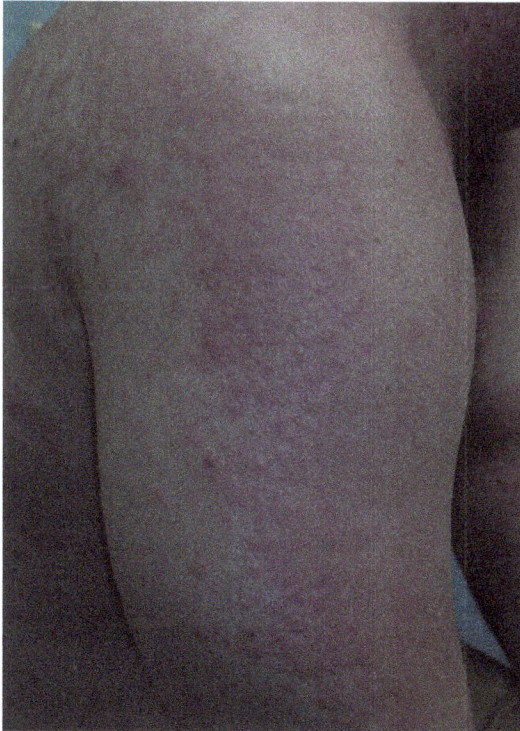

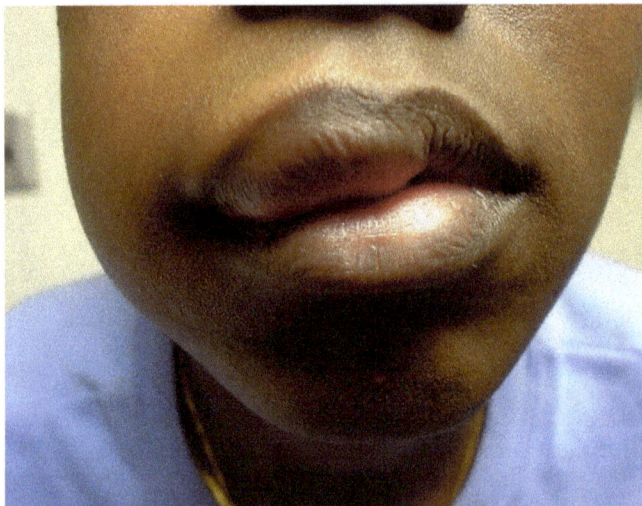

FIGURE 17.30 Young black woman with angioedema after being started on an angiotensin-converting-enzyme (ACE) inhibitor for essential hypertension. (Used with permission of Adrian Casillas, MD.)

nausea and vomiting. Angiotensin converting enzyme inhibitors can cause angioedema. Patients should be warned to go immediately to the emergency room if any unusual swelling in the face occurs.

Anaphylaxis The third and most serious reaction is anaphylaxis, which can be fatal. Therefore, patients with urticaria should be warned about the potentially more severe consequences if exposed to agent or the related agents in the future.

T-Lymphocyte-Mediated Reactions

Erythema Multiforme The term erythema multiforme (EM) indicates that it occurs in multiple forms and is used interchangeably with other stages of this T-lymphocyte-mediated reaction sequence, which makes it somewhat confusing. Patients may present with varying degrees of each reaction, e.g., many patients with toxic epidermal necrolysis syndrome (TENS) will also have oral involvement that is consistent with Stevens-Johnson syndrome.

Classic Erythema Multiforme Also called erythema multiforme minor, or mild to moderate erythema multiforme, it initially presents with a maculopapular/vesicular eruption on the trunk (Figure 17.31) that is usually accompanied by "target lesions" on the hands and forearms (Figure 17.32). This is like urticaria in the IgE-mediated sequence. The presence of target lesions puts the patient at high risk for potentially more severe reactions in the sequence that could result in fatality.

Stevens-Johnson Syndrome Also known as erythema multiforme major, Stevens-Johnson syndrome presents as vesicular and bullous lesions of the mucous membranes including the mouth, eyes, and gastrointestinal tract (Figure 17.33). Like angioedema in the IgE sequence, it can be fatal in some cases.

Toxic Epidermal Necrolysis Also known as TENS (toxic epidermal necrolysis syndrome), it is the last and most dangerous reaction in this sequence. It presents as

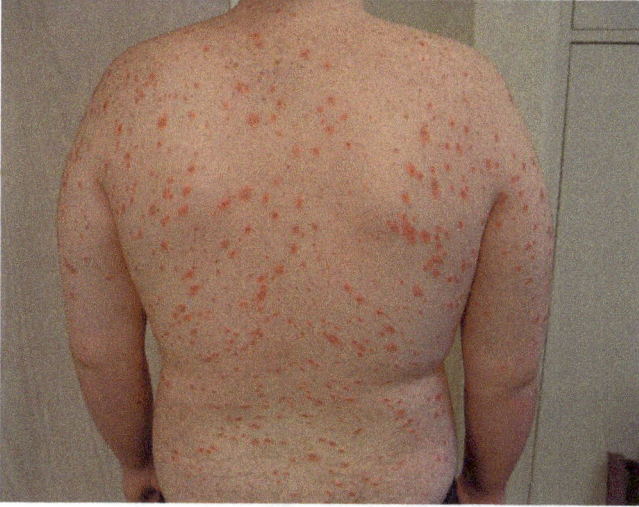

FIGURE 17.31 Target lesions on the back of a 14-year-old boy who received penicillin for pneumonia. (Used with permission of Dan Stulberg, MD.)

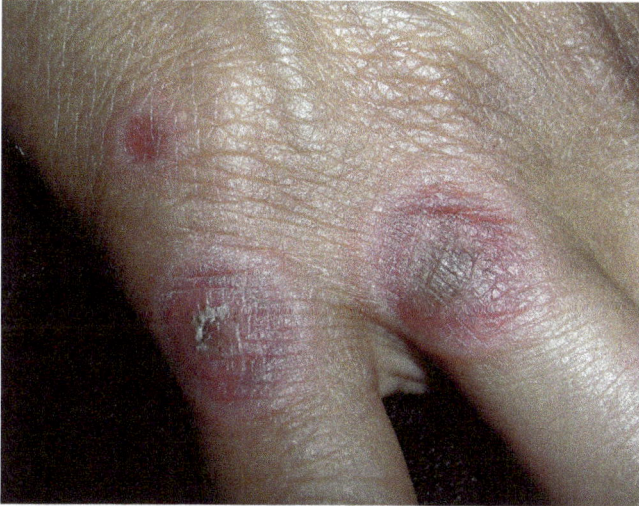

FIGURE 17.32 Erythema multiforme in a 43-year-old woman that recurs every time she breaks out with genital herpes. Target lesions on hand. (Used with permission of Richard P. Usatine, MD. From Usatine RP, Smith MA, Mayeux EJ, Jr, Chumley H. *The Color Atlas of Family Medicine*. 2nd ed. McGraw-Hill, Inc; 2013.)

widespread epidermal necrosis, resembling a massive third-degree burn (Figure 17.34). There is a 20% to 30% mortality despite treatment. Patients are usually treated in a burn unit following treatment protocols used to manage third-degree burns.

Erythema multiforme is like urticaria in that patients with the drug induced form of EM should be warned about the potentially more severe consequences if exposed to that agent or related agents in the future.

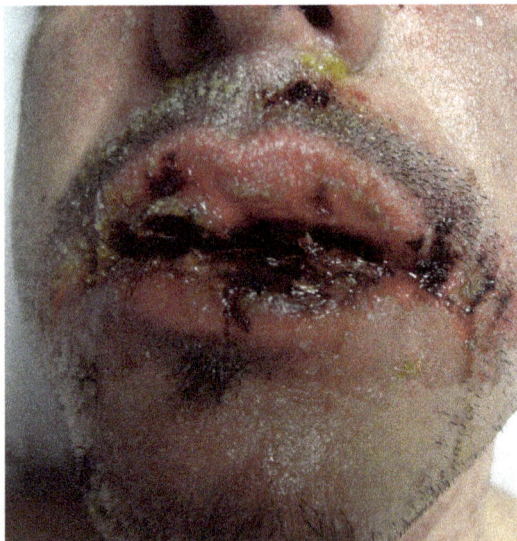

FIGURE 17.33 Stevens-Johnson syndrome that evolved into toxic epidermal necrolysis in a human immunodeficiency virus-positive man with a CDR of 6. He presented to the emergency department with fever and rash on face, eyes, and mouth. Chest x-ray suggested pneumonia, so he was started on azithromycin, ceftriaxone, and trimethoprim-sulfamethoxazole. He developed bulla on skin and a skin biopsy confirmed toxic epidermal necrolysis, possibly secondary to one of the firmed toxic epidermal necrolysis, possibly secondary to one of the antibiotics. He was transferred to a burn unit and given intravenous γ-globulin 1 g/kg for 3 days. The patient survived. Oral lesion. (Used with permission of Robert T. Gilson, MD.)

FIGURE 17.34 Toxic epidermal necrolysis with desquamation of skin on the hand. (Used with permission of the University of Texas Health Sciences Center, Division of Dermatology.)

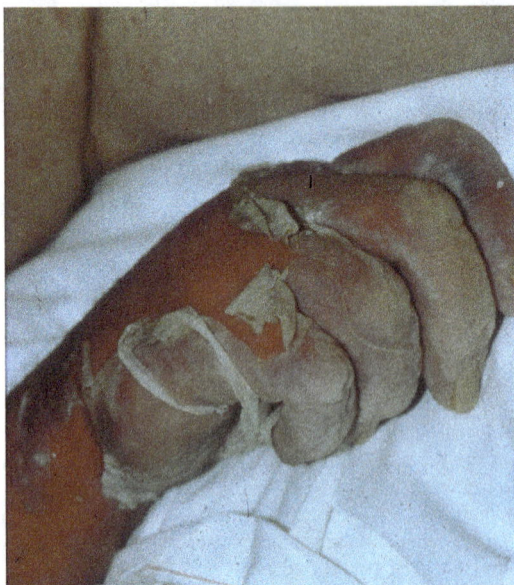

Drug Hypersensitivity Syndrome (DHS) For several decades, DHS was called anticonvulsant hypersensitivity syndrome because when initially described it was most frequently associated with anticonvulsant medication. It is characterized by an initial skin reaction followed by involvement of internal organ systems, including the liver, kidney, central nervous system, and hematopoietic system. Because of the high incidence of eosinophilia, it is also known as drug reaction with eosinophilia and systemic symptoms (DRESS). While it has been reported to be caused by many classes of medications, anticonvulsant drugs, sulfonamides and related drugs are the most frequent causes. DHS presents initially with a fever, followed by a widespread maculo-papular-pustular rash on the trunk, arms, and legs. Eosinophilia occurs in 50% to 90% of cases. Abnormal lymphocytosis is found in 30% of patients and 20% have lymph-adenopathy on physical examination. Headaches occur in 10% to 15% of patients and they can be confused with aseptic meningitis. Internal organ damage occurs last and most patients have elevated liver function tests and/or renal function tests. There is an 8% mortality rate in DHS. Rarely, there are posttreatment autoimmune disorders such as myocarditis, thyroiditis, or pancreatitis, which may manifest itself as type 1 diabetes mellitus.

• MISCELLANEOUS DERMATOLOGICAL DRUG REACIONS

Maculopapular Skin Rashes
These rashes usually occur on the trunk. When pressed, the lesions blanch or lose color. Generally, they are nonimmunological and are not contraindications to future use of the expected causative drug. Examples include measles and the "ampicillin rash."

Erythema Nodosum
Erythema nodosum is easy to diagnose because of its unusual presentation. It presents with red to reddish-brown circular lesions 1 to 2 cm in diameter that only occur from the knees to the feet, usually concentrated on the shins (Figure 17.35). When palpated, they are firm and painful.

Fixed Drug Eruptions
Like erythema nodosum fixed drug eruptions are easy to diagnose because of their unique presentation. Fixed drug reactions occur as red plaques, frequently associated with vesicles. They most frequently occur in the groin, inner thigh, and genitalia. They generally heal in 1 to 3 weeks, many times with hypopigmentation. They are called fixed drug eruptions because reexposure to the same agent causes the lesions to ap-pear on the exact same spot that they occurred initially.

Photosensitivity Reactions
Photosensitivity reactions to chemicals and medications can be divided into two main categories: phototoxic and photoallergic reactions. Phototoxic reactions are nonimmunological reactions manifested by increased susceptibility to sunburn. Phototoxic reactions are by far the most common. While UVB light is the usual cause of sunburn, UVA light is the culprit in drug-induced phototoxic reactions. UVA light reacts with certain medications in the skin, increasing sensitivity to sunburn. It is concentration dependent, so everyone will have the reaction if the drug concentra-tion in the skin is high enough. Lowering the dose will make the reaction less likely to occur. Sunburn sensitivity will occur for as long as there is sufficient concentration of the drug in the skin. Tetracyclines and sulfonamides and related drugs such as di-uretics and sulfonylureas are common causes. The sunburn only occurs in areas that

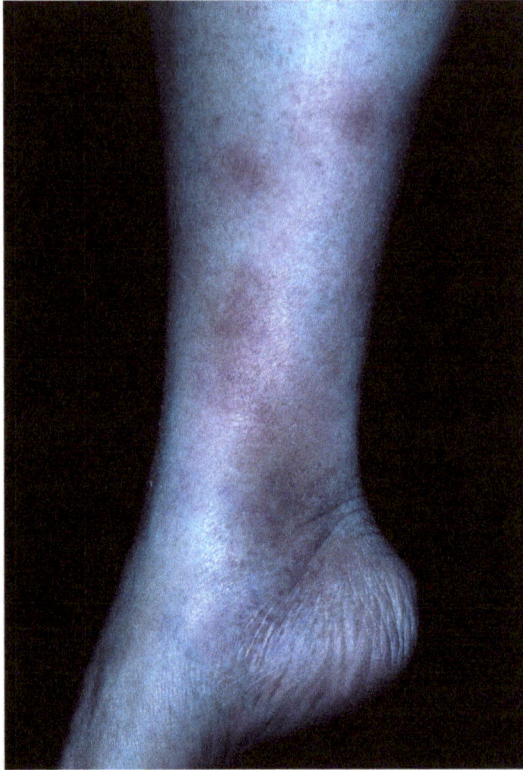

FIGURE 17.35 Erythema nodosum secondary to a group A β-hemolytic *Streptococcus* in a young woman. (Used with permission of Richard P. Usatine, MD. From Usatine RP, Smith MA, Mayeux EJ, Jr, Chumley H. *The Color Atlas of Family Medicine*. 2nd ed. McGraw-Hill, Inc; 2013.)

are exposed to sunlight. Even UVA rays coming through a window and fluorescent lights are enough to cause the reaction.

Photoallergic reactions are uncommon and are immunological in nature, a form of delayed hypersensitivity reaction induced by UVA light in people who have been previously sensitized to the agent. The reaction looks like allergic contact dermatitis and a large percentage of the reactions are due to topical agents and chemicals including those from plants. Mostly, they are limited to sun exposed areas but can spread to nearby areas. While phototoxic reactions end when skin concentrations of the medication fall below interactive levels, photoallergic reactions can persist for extended periods even though the drug is no longer present in the body.

Adverse Reactions to Long-Term Use of High-Potency Fluorinated Topical Corticosteroids

Fluorinated, high-potency topical corticosteroids when used for prolonged periods of time and/or in areas with thin skin, e.g., face and groin, can cause unwanted visible adverse effects. The use of fluorinated topical corticosteroids on the face or in the groin area should only be prescribed by a dermatologist, who is better able to judge the risk of adverse effects versus the potential benefit. Inappropriate use of topical corticosteroids can result in the development of striae, better known as stretch marks and/or atrophy of the skin. Atrophy is an extreme thinning of the skin so that it is tissue paper thin, enabling the easy visualization of arterioles, venules, capillaries, and sometimes nerves.

• KEY REFERENCES

1. de Bruin Weller MS, Rockman H, Knulst AC, Brunijnzeel-Koomen CA. Evaluation of the adult patients with atopic dermatitis. *Clin Exp Allergy.* 2012;43:279-291.
2. Usatine RP, Riojas M. Diagnosis and management of contact dermatitis. *Am Fam Physician.* 2010;82: 249-255.
3. Schwartz JR, Messenger AG, Tosti A, et al. A comprehensive pathophysiology of dandruff and seborrheic dermatitis-towards a more precise definition of scalp health. *Acta Derm Venereol.* 2013;93: 131-137.
4. Gupta AK, Batra R, Bluhm R, Boekhout T, Dawson TL. Skin diseases associated with *Malassezia* species. *J Am Acad Dermatol.* 2004;51:785-798.
5. Keller EC, Tomecki KJ, Chadi Alraies M. Distinguishing cellulitis from its mimics. *Cleve Clin J Med.* 2012;79:547-552.
6. Baldwin HE. Diagnosis and treatment of rosacea: state of the art. *J Drugs Dermatol.* 2012;11:725-730.
7. Varade RS, Burkemper NM. Cutaneous fungal infections in the elderly. *Clin Geriatr Med.* 2013;29: 461-478.
8. Ahmed AM, Pritichard S, Reichenberg J. A review of cutaneuous drug eruptions. *Clin Geriatr Med.* 2013;29:527-545.

CASE 17.1

Helen Autry brings in her 7-year-old son Gene and asks you to take a look at his left arm. You note that there is a red, hot, tender, and swollen area starting at the wrist and ending in his cubital fossa. Helen says it started at his elbow and has spread toward the wrist. There you also note severely excoriated and lichenified skin. The right cubital fossa reveals typical eczematous lesions with mild excoriation and lichenification. Helen and her husband Roy are regular customers in your asthma disease management program. Helen says that she has tried everything to keep him from scratching the itching areas without success. Gene's past medical history is unremarkable except that his patient profile reveals several prescriptions for antihistamine/decongestant combinations for URIs and a single albuterol syrup prescription for a viral chest infection.

a. List the most probable cause for the acute problem *and* the most likely cause for the chronic problems. Explain your rationale.

    _____

    _____

    _____

    _____

    _____

b. List four questions/examinations or lab tests you would ask/conduct/ run to determine the cause of Gene's symptoms. Explain your rationale.

    _____

    _____

    _____

    _____

    _____

One month later, you dispense a 7-day supply of trimethoprim-sulfamethoxazole suspension for Gene's ear infection. About 2 weeks later, Helen calls and is concerned that Gene's skin has just broken out with a red bumpy rash all over his chest, stomach, and back. In addition, on both hands and forearms, there are different lesions that do not itch and look like overlapping pink and red circles. Her son calls them "bull's-eyes." At first, she thought it might be the antibiotic but he has been off that for almost a week! What is Helen most likely describing? What other questions/ examinations/ lab tests could be used to help confirm diagnosis? Explain your rationale.

THREE

Assessment in the Diagnosis and Management of Chronic Diseases and Their Complications

CHAPTER

EIGHTEEN

Essential Hypertension

1. Identify appropriate standards for the diagnosis of hypertension and target blood pressure goals for patients already diagnosed with hypertension.

2. Accurately measure a patient's blood pressure using a sphygmomanometer.

3. Evaluate and identify environmental factors and errors in technique that reduce the accuracy of blood pressure measurements potentially leading to misdiagnosis, over- or undermedication, and poor disease control.

4. Describe the importance of home blood pressure readings in the management of hypertension including patient education on the accuracy and use of home blood pressure devices, and the evaluation of the accuracy of those home measurements.

5. Conduct a comprehensive follow-up visit for a patient with hypertension using appropriate history-taking techniques, physical examination, and laboratory tests. The visit includes assessment of disease control, assessment and support of compliance with lifestyle modifications, and medication regimens, plus evaluate patients for complications from the disease and medication regimen.

Essential hypertension is one of the most common chronic diseases affecting adults. It can occur alone or in combination with comorbidities such as diabetes, dyslipidemia, congestive heart failure, and renal disease.

• ETIOLOGY

Hypertension is a state of persistently elevated blood pressure (BP) due to a wide variety of contributory factors. Excess sodium intake, sodium sensitivity, excessive neurohormonal production, or hypersensitivity (e.g., the renin-angiotensin-aldosterone and sympathetic nervous systems) are well-identified contributory factors. Because of the complexity of the etiology, it is referred to as essential hypertension (EHT) to differentiate it from numerous much less common and in many cases curable, secondary causes such as pheochromocytoma, primary hyperaldosteronism, and coarctation of the aorta. There are also some medications (including OTC and herbal products) that may cause or aggravate BP elevations.

• DIAGNOSIS

It is important to understand the basics of blood pressure readings in order to effectively diagnose and assist patients in managing their hypertension. The top number of the reading refers to the systolic blood pressure and the bottom number refers to diastolic blood pressure. Systolic blood pressure is the amount of pressure exerted when the heart contracts. Diastolic blood pressure refers to the pressure in the arteries when the heart is at rest, passively filling. A diagnosis of hypertension is made in patients under 60 years of age with a blood pressure reading of greater than 140/90 on multiple occasions. New guidelines set greater than 150/90 as the diagnostic cutoff for patients 60 years of age and older. A single reading of a patient's blood pressure above 140/90 and below 180/110 is not diagnostic as blood pressure can be raised during stress, infections, medication use, and exercise, or there are a myriad of errors in technique that can also provide falsely elevated blood pressure readings. However, a single blood pressure measurement >180/110 should be considered diagnostic of hypertension and a referral made so that therapeutic interventions can be initiated immediately.

For most patients, the blood pressure goals are <140/90, even for patients with diabetes mellitus or chronic kidney disease. Accurate measurements of blood pressure are essential to the proper diagnosis and treatment of hypertension. Blood pressure measurements elevated by 5 to 10mm over the diagnostic criteria should be reassessed at different times of the day because many natural factors such as low blood glucose or a full bladder may cause blood pressure to vary throughout the day. In addition, many patients develop "white coat hypertension," blood pressures elevations that only occur in the physician's office and/or in association with a health care provider. To obtain more accurate and meaningful results, blood pressure readings at home should be measured if possible. If a total of at least three readings done at different times of the day and in different settings are all consistently above 140/90, then the diagnosis of hypertension can accurately be made and therapeutic interventions can be initiated. Marked differences in BP readings may be an indication for ambulatory BP monitoring to more accurately assess whether or not the patient has sustained blood pressure values in the hypertension range. An additional consideration in patients with borderline blood pressure levels is to make sure that the cuff size is accurate and that the cuff is centered over the cubital fossa.

• COMPLICATIONS

If not adequately controlled, hypertension can both directly and indirectly lead to complications and possibly death. Uncontrolled hypertension by itself is the leading cause of stroke and congestive heart failure. In addition, it accelerates the rate of atherosclerosis, leading to peripheral artery disease, angina, and myocardial infarction. Finally, by itself, but especially in combination with diabetes mellitus, uncontrolled hypertension can cause renal failure and blindness. It is well established that effective antihypertensive therapy (i.e., attainment of goal blood pressures) can drastically reduce the incidence of these complications. Therefore, the goal of antihypertensive therapy is to prevent these complications by lowering blood pressure to target values.

• BLOOD PRESSURE MEASUREMENT

Unfortunately, due to a variety of factors, many blood pressure readings are inaccurate, causing inappropriate diagnosis and/or inappropriate changes in antihypertensive therapy. Even when taken by skilled medical personnel using proper techniques, blood pressure measurements with a sphygmomanometer on the upper arm with a stethoscope are at best within plus or minus 5 mm of the actual arterial pressure. Using inferior equipment (finger and wrist cuffs), inaccurately calibrated equipment, improper technique, and not addressing potential modifying factors (smoking, caffeine, etc.) can independently or in combination lead to errors of up to plus or minus 30 mm. Table 18.1 lists appropriate blood pressure measurement techniques. Table 18.2 lists common causes for error in measuring blood pressure, which need to be avoided or accounted for to optimize the accuracy of measurement. In addition to technique and other factors that influence blood pressure measuring accuracy, the setting in which the blood pressure is measured can have a significant impact. In patients with hypertension, the vast majority have white coat hypertension. That is, their blood pressure readings are significantly higher in the doctor's office than they are at home or when done by a friend or family member. Therefore, exclusive reliance on office-based readings to guide antihypertensive drug therapy can lead to overmedication and unnecessary adverse effects such as orthostatic hypotension, which can lead to falls and injuries in the elderly. While home blood pressure readings may be preferred, not all home devices are equal in accuracy. There are international standards for validation of a device's accuracy. However, not all brands meet those standards. There are two main sources of information regarding comparative accuracy. Every several years, Consumer Reports magazine compares the accuracy of various manufacturer's devices. The report is available at the web site of the magazine, without a subscription. The other is the dabl Educational Trust web site (http://www.dableducational.com). Only those devices recommended by these two sources are of acceptable accuracy for home monitoring.

• INITIAL VISIT/WORKUP

Once the diagnosis has been confirmed, the initial visit and workup has four primary purposes: (1) assess target organ damage and comorbid diseases; (2) assess lifestyle for potential use of nonpharmacologic therapy; (3) collect baseline laboratory data to prospectively evaluate potential adverse drug reactions due to antihypertensive therapy; and (4) begin the education process for the patient and their social support system.

TABLE 18.1	Blood Pressure Technique

_____ Ensure that patient's bladder has been emptied recently.

_____ Determine when the patient last ate.

_____ Ask when the patient last took medications (antihypertensives and others).

_____ Determine previous BP values by patient's history or from their medical record.

_____ At least 5-minute rest; seated in a chair with a back; feet flat on floor; legs uncrossed.

_____ Locate brachial artery.

_____ Tightly, place cuff on bare skin of upper arm so the middle of the bladder is approximately vertically over the brachial artery (inner aspect of upper arm) and the bottom of the cuff is 1 inch or 2 fingerbreadths above the midline of the cubital fossa.

_____ Make sure the middle of the cuff's width is approximately at the level of the heart (parallel to the middle of the sternum's height)

_____ Find the radial pulse. Inflate cuff until pulse disappears. Note reading and deflate cuff slowly until the pulse reappears, noting the reading (this value approximates the systolic pressure). Fully deflate the cuff and wait at least 60 seconds.

_____ Inflate cuff for an additional 30 mm past (above) the pulse cutoff or 30 mm past what their usual systolic blood pressure readings are. Ensure that the arm is supported on a firm and stable surface with the palm upward.

_____ Place the diaphragm of the stethoscope on the bare skin (not over clothing) of the cubital fossa over the brachial artery so that the entire surface of the diaphragm is evenly in contact with the skin. Avoid pressing so firmly that the brachial artery is compressed.

_____ Release air at slow even rate (mm/heartbeat or 2 to 3 mm/s) until 10 mm past the last sound heard.

_____ Document the BP value (120/78; readings at first and last sounds heard, respectively), the cuff size used, the position of patient (sitting, standing, lying), which arm was used, and the pulse rate and rhythm.

_____ Deflate cuff and wait 1 to 2 minutes before repeating.

Augmentation (for faint first and last sounds)

_____ Raise arm over the patient's head with cuff on, but uninflated; hold for 30 to 60 seconds.

_____ While the arm is still raised, inflate cuff to 50 mm above pulse cutoff or estimated systolic BP.

_____ Make five quick "fists" (clench and unclench) while hand still raised.

_____ Lower the arm, quickly place stethoscope on the cubital fossa.

_____ Release air at a slow, even rate, recording the reading in the usual way, as described above. K1 and K5. Augmentation should double the volume of the Korotkoff sounds.

Home blood pressure monitoring and educating patients on proper BP measurement techniques can begin at this time. A complete medical history and physical examination should be conducted, focusing on the presence or absence of angina, heart failure, stroke, and the metabolic syndrome. Lab tests that should be done include electrolytes, a glycosylated hemoglobin (A1C) for diabetes, a complete fasting lipid panel for dyslipidemia, serum creatinine and urine microalbuminuria for renal damage, and liver function tests that can identify common comorbidities of hypertension and/or serve as baseline values for later evaluation of potential medication adverse effects. A careful history for salt, caffeine, and ethanol intake plus exercise patterns should be done. A smoking history should be obtained. Also, the patient's willingness to undertake modifications to their lifestyle can be assessed. Appropriate weight loss, smoking cessation, an appropriate exercise program, and minimization of salt intake have all been shown to lower blood pressure and may be successfully used individually or in appropriate combinations in patients with blood pressures only slightly above diagnostic cutoffs. All these measures also augment antihypertensive drug therapy for BP control.

TABLE 18.2	Common Errors in Measurement of Blood Pressure

Physiologic/pathophysiologic

a. Nutrition status—	>5 hours postprandial gives 3 to 5 mm false elevation in BP due to norepinephrine release to raise blood glucose
	In the elderly, get drop in BP up to 20 mm 15 to 75 minutes after a meal
b. Bladder status—	Full bladder provides 3 to 5 mm false elevation
c. White coat effect/cuff reactors—	May falsely elevate BP
d. Circadian variability—	Early AM increase due to activation of the reticular activating system

e. Nicotine within 30 minutes/pseudoephedrine within 4 hours/excessive ethanol ingestion within 8 to 10 hours/caffeine ingestion within 2 to 4 hours→false elevation from 3 to 10 mm due to norepinephrine release

f. Cold room temperature/cold hands/cold equipment→3 to 5 mm false elevation

Iatrogenic

a. Inappropriate cuff size—	Width of bladder should cover 40% to 50% of midupper arm
	The length should cover 80% of circumference
	- Too *small* a cuff overestimates BP (falsely high values)
	- Too *large* a cuff underestimates BP (falsely low values)
	Most BP cuffs have white strips that aid in sizing. If the end strip falls between the two measuring strips, the size is OK.
	If end strip falls outside the measuring strips, it is the wrong size—you need to measure
	11 inches (26 cm) or less = small adult size
	11 to 13 inches (27 to 34 cm) = adult size
	13 to 17 inches (35 to 44 cm) = large adult size
	>17 inches (>35 cm) = adult thigh size

IMPORTANT THAT IF THE PATIENT HAS BORDERLINE BP VALUE (SYSTOLIC 140-150 MM/DIASTOLIC 85-100 MM) NEED TO GET THE RIGHT-SIZED BLADDER

b. Instrument problems—	As many as 60% of BP measuring devices are inaccurate
	Calibrate all but mercury manometers every 6 months
	Aneroid needle not at zero—recalibrate
	Aneroid needle moves before deflation begins—leak in system, use another instrument

c. Rounding off (rarely both systolic and diastolic end in zero)

d. Observer bias (tends to let previous BP readings influence subsequent values)

e. Failure to provide 5-minute rest/no talking while measuring *(false elevation of 3 to 5 mm systolic/diastolic BP)*

f. Taking BP without supporting back, or with legs dangling or crossed, e.g., on the examination table *(false elevation of 5 mm systolic/diastolic BP due to isometric exercise for each)*

g. Cubital fossa/cuff not at heart level *(if higher subtract 0.8 mm for every centimeter above heart or if lower add 0.8 mm for every centimeter below heart)*

h. The arm must be supported on the table or by the examiner *(without support false elevation of 3 to 5 mm systolic/diastolic BP)*

i. Cuff not tightly wrapped *(falsely elevated blood pressure)*

j. Inappropriate deflation rate *(too fast diastolic falsely elevated, systolic falsely read lower)(too slow false elevation of diastolic BP)*

k. Diaphragm of the stethoscope applied too firmly *(diastolic reading falsely lowered, or all sounds relatively diminished, and hard to hear accurately, due to compression of the brachial artery)*

• FOLLOW-UP VISITS

At each follow-up visit control of the disease, compliance with medication and life-style changes and any complications related to the drug or disease need to be assessed. Table 18.3 summarizes follow-up parameters and questions to be assessed at each visit.

Control

The target blood pressure for most patients with hypertension is <140/90 regardless of comorbid conditions such as diabetes and chronic renal disease. For patients 60 years of age or older, the new target goal is <150/90. Which blood pressures should be used

TABLE 18.3	Follow-Up Visit Hypertension

CONTROL

S   How have your home blood pressure readings been since last visit?

O   BP, pulse

COMPLIANCE

S   How have things been going with your diet? Exercise?
    What kind of problems have you been having following your diet? Exercise plan?
    What kind of problems have you been having remembering to take your medication?

O   Weight
    Medication refill record

COMPLICATIONS (DISEASE)

S   What other changes or problems have you noticed since your last visit?
    What kind of problems have you noticed during physical activity? **(angina, CHF)**
    What kind of problems have you been having sleeping? **(CHF)**
    Have you had any of the following since your last visit?

Chest pain? **(angina)**	Number of pillows for sleep? **(CHF)**
Shortness of breath? **(CHF, angina)**	Ankle swelling? **(CHF)**
Headache? **(TIA/CVA)**	Dizziness (unsteadiness)? **(TIA/CVA)**
Forgetfulness? **(TIA/CVA)**	Numbness/tingling in extremity? **(TIA/CVA)**
Decreased ability to move extremities? **(TIA/CVA)**	Other unusual symptoms?

O   Observational neurological examination (i.e., watch the patient while interviewing for facial and other movements
    and for coherency of speech and understanding of conversation, and while exiting and entering the examination
    room for ease of mobility and balance **(CVA/TIA)**
    Annual complete history and physical examination including dilated eye examination
    Other physical examinations as indicated by history
    Annual serum creatinine, microalbuminuria **(renal disease),** and if DM, CAD, or metabolic syndrome, A1C and
    lipid profile

COMPLICATIONS (DRUG)

S   How do you feel after standing up from bed or lying on the couch? **(orthostasis)**
    Have you had any of the following since your last visit?

Cough? **(ACEI)**	Swelling face/lips? **(ACEI)**
Last menstrual period? **(ACEI, ARB)**	Ankle swelling? **(CCB, hydralazine, β-blockers, α-blockers)**
Diarrhea? **(aliskiren)**	
Headache? **(CCB, hydralazine, α-blockers)**	Dizziness, especially when you stand up quickly? **(orthostasis)**
Fatigue? **(β-blockers, clonidine)**	
Flushing? **(CCB, hydralazine)**	Muscle weakness? **(diuretics, CCB)**

TABLE 18.3	**Follow-Up Visit Hypertension (*Continued*)**
Dry mouth? **(clonidine)**	Nasal congestion? **(terazosin)**
Swollen, painful breasts? **(spironolactone)**	Problems exercising? **(β-blockers)**
Nocturia, polyuria? **(diuretics)**	Sunburns easily? **(diuretics)**
Joint pain? **(diuretics, hydralazine)**	NSAID use? **(β-blockers, ACEI, ARB, diuretics)**

0 Examinations/laboratory tests to f/u specific symptoms
Orthostasis BP check
Check for pedal edema **(CCB, carvedilol, hydralazine, α-blockers)**
Check pulse for irregularity/bradycardia **(β-blockers, CCB, hydralazine)**
Examine gums for gingival hyperplasia **(CCB)**
Serum creatinine, K^+, Mg^+ **(ACEI, ARB, diuretics)**
Serum uric acid **(diuretics)**

to adjust the patient's drug regimen? Currently, home blood pressures are preferred because of the high incidence of white coat hypertension among patients with hypertension. Using higher office-based blood pressures exclusively introduces the risk of inadvertently overmedicating the patient and inducing orthostatic hypotension.

Patients need to be educated on proper and accurate home blood pressure techniques. At each follow-up visit, remind the patient of the importance of being seated in a supporting chair with feet on the floor for several minutes, arm supported by table at heart level, the proper placement and position of the cuff in relationship to the brachial artery and the level of the heart, in addition to avoiding any modifying factors such as full bladder. Proper documentation of the readings is also important. Patients need to record the blood pressure with pulse rate along with the arm in which it was measured. Their position (sitting, standing, lying) and the time of the day should also be documented. To assess the relative accuracy of home versus office readings, the patient should periodically bring their electronic devices to the office to allow comparison of blood pressure readings with both the office and home devices. Bringing the home device to the office annually or when there seems to be a significant difference between home and office readings can also serve as the periodic review of patient's home technique.

Initially, blood pressures should be taken several times a day. Ideally, this would include readings at home and at work. In elderly patients, at least one reading every day should be taken 30 to 60 minutes after a meal to assess postprandial drops in blood pressures. Most elderly patients with hypertension have a significant postprandial fall in blood pressure, which combined with the antihypertensive therapy may exceed 20 mm. Significant drops in blood pressure can be dangerous, leading to orthostasis or syncope, thus increasing the patient's fall risk and/or precipitating symptoms of other comorbidities such as angina. While the exact cause of this effect is unclear at this time, its frequency and potential severity make it imperative that elderly patients take their blood pressure before eating and 30 to 60 minutes after beginning a meal to ascertain the level of this drop in blood pressure. With these multiple readings, the provider can more accurately adjust the timing and magnitude of any medication or dosage adjustments. It is important to recognize the variations in pharmacodynamic effects of various antihypertensive agents among individual patients. Multiple antihypertensive medications are listed as lasting 12 or 24 hours. However, in some patients the effect may only last 6 to 8 or 16 to 20 hours. This may lead to large gaps of time during which the blood pressure is well above target. In the case of a patient with well-controlled (or lower than desired) blood pressure in the afternoon or evening, but above target values in the morning, the single 24-hour dose can be split into two doses given 12 hours apart. Alternatively, the patient may be given one or more of their 24-hour duration antihypertensives in a single daily dose at bedtime rather than taking all medications in the morning.

One question that frequently arises relates to the safety of blood pressure values well below target values: can blood pressure be lowered too much? While most experts say attempting to achieve blood pressures near normal (120/80) is the ultimate target, others warn of decreased perfusion of vital organs and potential decreased survival. This so called J-curve is controversial. Common sense should direct adjustments in therapeutic regimens. *The overall goal is to lower the blood pressure to below target values without adverse effects such as orthostatic hypotension or drug-specific adverse effects.* Since elevated systolic pressure is probably more damaging, achieving blood pressure levels below the systolic target is probably most important. However, in some patients that may not be attainable without causing troubling side effects. In particular, in elderly patients, the arteries become less flexible (arteriosclerotic), causing the systolic pressure to be more elevated relative to the diastolic pressure. Sometimes this makes it difficult to attain target systolic pressure without lowering diastolic pressure too much. In that situation, have the patients return to measuring their blood pressure several times a day including after meals. Adjusting timing and dosage of existing medicines or changing medicines based on those pressures may enable adequate control. Recent studies in hypertensive patients with type 2 diabetes showed that lowering the target systolic pressure 20 mm (from 140 to 120) failed to further decrease overall cardiovascular mortality, which supports the adage: "*Treat the patient, not the numbers!*"

Another frequently asked question is, "*How fast should the blood pressure be lowered?*" Other than hypertensive emergencies (>200/120), the general rule is to decrease the blood pressure slowly. Lowering blood pressure too quickly, especially with parenteral agents, can precipitate manifestations of ischemia (in the brain, heart, or kidneys). Even adding oral medications too quickly can be counterproductive. First, a minimum amount of time is required for onset and especially maximal effect for each drug at each dosage. Additions made too soon could ultimately result in hypotension. Second, each new drug and dosage increment increases the chances of dose-related side effects. In addition, it takes time for patients to develop routines necessary for optimal adherence with the medication regimen and to learn to accurately measure home blood pressures. In patients with blood pressures >160/100, it is reasonable to initiate therapy with two medications. For patients with readings slightly above target values, a 6-month attempt at one or more lifestyle changes is warranted before initiating drug therapy. Once the blood pressure nears target levels, the emphasis should be on slowly lowering the blood pressure with small adjustments to the therapeutic regimen. Give each new change in therapy a month or more to take effect, since the full effect of many agents is not seen until 6 to 8 weeks after a dosage change or initiation of a new regimen. Once the home blood pressure readings are stabilized at desired levels over several consecutive office visits, all that remains is fine tuning the regimen to maintain its benefits. If pressures climb slightly, check for medication adherence issues or home device accuracy before considering alterations in the regimen. If pressures rise above target levels and all other explanations have been ruled out, have the patient increase the frequency of their testing and return in 30 to 60 days with their home device for an accuracy and technique check. If at that time the pressure remains elevated and no accuracy or technique issues are found, then small changes in the therapeutic regimen may be initiated. Similarly, if blood pressure readings continue to fall, check for orthostasis, recent weight loss, initiation or increase in intensity of exercise or diet programs, changes in levels of activity or stress, changes in hepatic or renal function, and overmedication.

Compliance

Medication refill records can be a source of objective information regarding medication adherence. Since a healthy diet, appropriate weight loss, and exercise all have a positive impact on lowering blood pressure, patients should be encouraged to lower salt intake, exercise regularly, and attain or maintain an ideal body weight in addition to any medication prescribed. At each visit, patients should also be asked about issues or problems with medication adherence and lifestyle changes, providing support, assistance, and positive reinforcement when appropriate.

Complications

At each visit, patients should be questioned regarding symptoms of congestive heart failure, stroke, angina, renal dysfunction, and visual problems. Start with one or more general open-ended questions. If answers are negative, follow up with "Have you had any of the following since your last visit..." listing each potential symptom of a complication in order. Yes answers need to be followed up using the chief complaint history technique. For the first few follow-up visits, make sure you explain the purpose of each of the questions, to educate the patient on things to look for, making sure that if they have any of those symptoms that may signal the onset of complications, they need to be seen immediately.

A complete history and a thorough physical examination are appropriate on an annual basis. The examination should include a dilated ophthalmoscopic examination. Additional annual evaluations include a serum creatinine and microalbuminuria determination to assess renal function, as well as an A1C and a fasting lipid profile in those patients with type 2 diabetes to detect common comorbid conditions. At each visit, an observational neurological examination can be done looking at cranial nerve function during the interview and evaluating motor function as they enter and exit the examination room. If questioning reveals headache or any other potential symptom of a stroke, a thorough neurological examination should be done.

Evaluating complications due to the medication is generally medication specific. Table 18.3 lists major problems with common antihypertensives. For example, for a patient on a thiazide or thiazide-like diuretic questioning about muscle weakness (not cramping) and observing patient's ease getting up out of a chair help detect hypokalemia's early impact on quadriceps muscle weakness. Checking for joint pain will evaluate patients for gout due to elevated uric acid levels depending on the drug therapy. Annual laboratory examinations for electrolytes, fasting glucose and lipids, and uric acid are also warranted. Similarly, with angiotensin-converting-enzyme inhibitors (ACEI) questions about cough and ununusual swelling of the face, mouth, or tongue are warranted. For all patients with blood pressure near or below target, the patient should be evaluated for orthostasis, probing for dizziness or light headedness at each visit and periodically measuring the level of orthostatic changes in blood pressure. This is done by first measuring the blood pressure in the normal manner with the patient seated. Then, while leaving the sphygmomanometer in place, have the patient stand. After properly positioning the cuff at heart level and supporting the patient's arm, retake the blood pressure 30 to 60 seconds after standing. Deflate the cuff, and again repeat the measurement standing, about 1 minute later. A drop in systolic blood pressure of 20 mm or more or a drop in diastolic BP of 10 mm or more at either standing measurement is indicative of orthostasis and warrants adjusting drug therapy to prevent that drop. When checking for orthostasis in elderly patients, make sure to find out when they ate last.

• SUMMARY

The pharmacist, by training, is ideally suited to play a major role in the diagnosis and treatment of hypertension, including patient education and managing patient's medication therapy through prescriptive authority. In addition to knowledge regarding diagnostic criteria and target blood pressure goals, the pharmacist needs to be the expert on the accurate measurement of blood pressure, avoiding the many environmental factors and the multiple potential errors in blood pressure measurement that can eventually lead to poor outcomes. Finally, the pharmacist must be able to fully assess the control of the patient's blood pressure, assess and support adherence to pharmacological and nonpharmacological treatment regimens, and assess the patient for the presence of complications from both the disease and the therapeutic regimen.

• KEY REFERENCES

1. Frohlich ED, Grim C, Labarthe DR, et al. Recommendations for human blood pressure determination by sphygmomanometers. *Circulation.* 1988;77:501A-514A.
2. Perloff D, Grim C, Flack J, et al. Human blood pressure determination by sphygmomanometer *Circulation.* 1993;88:2460-2470.
3. Pickering TG, Hall JE, Appel LJ, et al. Recommendation for blood pressure in humans and experimental animals. Part 1: blood pressure measurement in humans. *Circulation.* 2005;111:697-716.
4. Ogedegbe G, Pickering T. Principles and techniques of blood pressure measurement. *Cardiol Clin.* 2010;28:571-586.
5. Menash GA, Bakris G. Treatment and control of high blood pressure in adults. *Cardiol Clin* 2010;28:609-622.
6. Acelajado MC, Calhoun DA. Resistant hypertension, secondary hypertension and hypertensive crises: diagnostic evaluation and treatment. *Cardiol Clin.* 2010;28:639-654.
7. James PA, Oparil S, Carter BL, et al. Evidenced-based guideline for the management of high blood pressure in adults: report from the panel members appointed to the eighth joint national committee (JNC-8). *JAMA.* 2014;311:507-520.

CASE 18.1

RJ, a 42-year-old male recently diagnosed with mild hypertension, comes to your pharmacy clinic for initiation of antihypertensive therapy. He had four blood pressure readings in the clinic over the last 6 months; all of which were greater than 140/90: 150/100, 150/90, 148/100, and 142/96, all R arm sitting. He also has a strong family history of hypertension on his father's side of the family. Today's reading by the medical aide is 150/90 with a pulse of 92. He had home blood pressure readings twice a day for the last 2 weeks, taken by his wife who is a registered nurse. They range from 120-138/82-88. He had a complete physical examination by his primary care provider 2 weeks ago along with appropriate laboratory tests. All findings and results were normal or unremarkable. What should be your next steps?

CASE 18.2

LK is a 68-year-old female with hypertension previously seen in the pharmacy clinic by a colleague (now on maternity leave) for the last 2 years. Chart review reveals that LK is under good control (120s over 70s) and has been steadily losing weight at the rate of 5 lb per year. She is on chlorthalidone 25 mg q AM, lisinopril 20 mg q AM, and carvedilol 6.25 mg bid. Her home blood pressure readings are excellent over the last 6 months with a slight downward trend in evening and bedtime readings (as low as 100/66). In taking her history, she denies any problems except for occasional dizziness that occurs most frequently after getting up from the dinner table, especially after a big meal (about one to two times/week). The other change is that she has begun to walk 2 miles a day with her new next-door neighbor, with whom she is becoming fast friends. Her sitting blood pressure reading by you today at 11 AM is 110/68 with a pulse of 72. What should you do next?

MS is a 54-year-old male who is regularly seen in your clinic for his hypertension, diabetes, and hyperlipidemia. He has been stable on enalapril 20 mg bid, HCT Z 25 mg q AM, and amlodipine 5 mg q AM for the last 3 years. He is returning today, 2 weeks since his last visit because his systolic blood pressure readings have been consistently over 140 when he awakens in recent weeks. Two weeks ago he was asked to increase the frequency of his blood pressure readings to several times a day, then return today. His blood pressure taken by you today is 144/88 and pulse of 92 with your cuff and 146/90 with his home device. MS typically exhibits white coat hypertension. About 70% of his home readings indicate a systolic pressure between 130 and 140, with the diastolic blood pressure readings typically in the mid- to high 70s. Almost all of the high readings are in the morning before he takes his medication or in the evening before he takes his second enalapril dose. Where do we go from here?

NINETEEN

Dyslipidemia

1. Identify appropriate standards for the diagnosis of dyslipidemia and determine risk and prognosis for developing cardiovascular disease.

2. Use available parameters to measure and monitor target lipid goals for patients under treatment for dyslipidemia.

3. Conduct a comprehensive follow-up visit for a patient with dyslipidemia using appropriate history-taking techniques, physical examination, and laboratory tests. The visit includes assessment of disease control, plus assessment and support of compliance with lifestyle modifications and medication regimens.

4. Evaluate patients for complications from dyslipidemia and the medication regimen.

• INTRODUCTION

In 2011, Centers for Disease Control estimated that 29% of all deaths in the U.S. will be caused by heart and cerebrovascular disease, the vast majority of which are caused by atherosclerotic cardiovascular disease (ASCVD), also known as coronary heart disease (CHD). Atherosclerosis is a process that causes oxidative endothelial damage and inflammation that eventually leads to the formation of cholesterol-laden atheromas or plaque lining the arterial intima. The inflammation ultimately causes the plaque to rupture, which leads to platelet adhesion and aggregation resulting in arterial occlusion. If vessels in the heart and brain are occluded they cause a myocardial infarction or cerebrovascular accidents (strokes or CVA). Since dyslipidemia is a major factor in the atheroscerlotic process, the advent of highly effective cholesterol-lowering medication has become a major tool in preventing atherosclerosis and subsequent heart attacks and strokes. Pharmacists play a key role in monitoring and managing the therapeutic regimens of patients with dyslipidemia.

• TYPES OF LIPIDS

There are three major types of cholesterol found in the bloodstream. They are carried in the blood by lipoproteins, which combine with cholesterol and other fats. LDL cholesterol (low-density lipoprotein or LDL-C) is the cholesterol intimately involved in the formation of arterial plaque and high levels are associated with a greater risk of heart attack and stroke. Since lowering LDL-C blood concentration has been shown to prevent heart attacks and strokes, it is the focus of current lipid-lowering therapy. LDL-C is made by the liver from VLDL cholesterol (very-low-density lipoprotein or VLDL-C), which has the highest concentration of triglycerides. HDL cholesterol (high-density lipoprotein or HDL-C) serves as a scavenger, transporting LDL-C back to the liver for recycling, and maintaining the integrity of the endothelium of the arteries. High levels of HDL-C markedly reduce the incidence of heart attacks and strokes, so increased HDL-C blood levels reduce the risk of cardiovascular disease. Some authors refer to LDL as the "bad" cholesterol and the HDL as the "good" cholesterol. These terms can be very useful in helping patients understand their illness and the importance of treatment goals, i.e., lowering the *bad* cholesterol and raising the *good*. Triglycerides are a fourth type of lipid routinely found in the blood stream. They are important sources for energy, but high levels are associated with the metabolic syndrome and its increased risk for cardiovascular disease and type 2 diabetes mellitus.

• DIAGNOSING DYSLIPIDEMIA AND THE NEED FOR THERAPY

According to the 2002 guidelines (National Cholesterol Education Program Adult Treatment Panel III or NCEP ATP Panel III), diagnosis and the determination of need for therapy were both tied to a risk factor assessment, based in part on LDL-C levels. Normal LDL-C values vary based on risk factors and HDL-C levels. To determine what a normal LDL-C is for an individual, which was also their target LDL-C goal, a series of questions needed to be asked and calculations done (Table 19.1). There are significant controversies surrounding the new, 2013 guidelines and numerous experts have suggested continuing to use the old guidelines for the time being. Therefore, the old criteria and cases to practice calculating older cardiovascular risk and target goals of therapy based on LDL-C are included to enable pharmacists to work with physicians who continue to utilize older guidelines.

TABLE 19.1	Low-Density Lipoprotein (LDL) Goal Calculation (NCEP ATP III)

1. Do you have or have you had a myocardial infarction, heart attack, peripheral artery disease, angina pectoris, abdominal aortic aneurysm, symptomatic caroid artery disease, or diabetes?

   POSITIVE ANSWER TO ANY OF THE ABOVE CORONARY HEART DISEASE (CHD) OR CHD EQUIVALENTS TARGET LDL GOAL **<100 MG/DL**

2. If no CHD or CHD equivalents, conduct risk factor assessment.

   One point for each of the following:

   - Male >45 years old
   - Female >55 years old
   - Family history of premature CHD in parent or sibling (males <55 years old; females <65 years old)
   - Current cigarette smoker (includes those who have quit within 30 days)
   - Hypertension (BP ≥140/90 or on antihypertensive therapy)
   - HDL <40 mg/dL

   SUBTOTAL

   Subtract one risk factor if HDL ≥60 mg/dL

   TOTAL RISK FACTORS

3. Based on the total number of risk factors, calculate target LDL goal

   - **If zero to one total risk factors, Target LDL Goal <160 mg/dL**
   - **If two or total more risk factors, go to Framingham Score Calculation Tool to determine risk of CHD within 10 years (10-year risk)**
     - **If <20% 10-Year Risk, Target LDL Goal <130 mg/dL**
     - **If >20 % 10-Year Risk, Target LDL Goal <100 mg/dL**

From 2002 NCEP 3 Guidelines.

The new, 2013 guidelines eliminate the use of LDL-C target goals! Instead the new guidelines focus on cardiovascular risk, advocating reduction of LDL-C levels by 30% to 50% by choosing the dose and potency of the statin (Table 19.2). The Framingham-based ASCVD risk calculator from NCEP ATP III has been replaced by the new Pooled

TABLE 19.2	2013 ACC/AHA Cholesterol Guidelines

WHO SHOULD BE TREATED WITH A STATIN?

1. Patients with clinical atherosclerotic cardiovascular disease (ASCVD) (high-dose statin, e.g., 80 mg atorvastatin)
2. Patients with LDL 190 mg/dL or higher (high-dose statin)
3. Patients 40 to 75 years of age *with diabetes* without clinical ASCVD and LDL 70 to 189 mg/dL (moderate to high-dose statin)
4. Patients without clinical ASCVD or diabetes, but with LDL 70 to 189 mg/dL, and 7.5% or greater 10-year risk of ASCVD (moderate to high-dose statin, e.g., simvastatin 20 to 40 mg)

If the patient does not fit in one of the above categories, but has 10-year ASCVD risk of 5% to 7.5% with clinical suspicion based on one of the criteria below, the patient may benefit from statin therapy can use the following criteria:

LDL 160 mg/dL or higher or other evidence of genetic dyslipidemia
ASCVD onset in first degree relative males <55: females <65
hs-CRP 2.0 or higher
Ankle to brachial index <0.9
Elevated lifetime risk of ASCVD
Coronary artery calcium scores (CAC) 300 Agatston units or higher or >75 percentile for age, gender, and ethnicity

Data from Stone NJ et al.[15]

Cohort Equations Cardiovascular Risk Calculator found at http://myamericanheart. org/cvriskcalculator. Table 19.2 shows the four categories of patients that will benefit from statin therapy. They include those with clinical ASCVD and those with LDL-C levels higher than 190 mg/dL. In addition, patients with diabetes, without clinical ASCVD, but with LDL-C levels of 70 to 189 mg/dL, plus those *without* diabetes and clinical ASCVD, LDL-C levels 70 to 189 mg/dL, but with a 10-year ASCVD risk of >7.5%, also warrant statin therapy. See Table 19.2 or Key reference 15 for details about the appropriate intensity of statin therapy for each group. Dosage titration of statins to target LDL-C goals has been eliminated. Nonstatin medication use is discouraged.

• OTHER RISK FACTOR MEASUREMENTS

While the focus of the new guidelines is on LDL-C levels, there are other biomarkers that can be used to further assess the risk of developing ASCVD (Table 19.3).

Framingham Study Ratios

The Framingham Study began in 1948 and has traced more than 15,000 patients over their lifetimes to see what risk factors exist for developing cardiovascular diseases of all types. Today, much of the data that we use to set practice standards for most cardiovascular diseases came from the Framingham Study. The study results established ratios of cholesterol values that were definitely linked to markedly increased risk of ASCVD. They found major risks associated with two ratios using HDL-C. If total cholesterol value (TC) divided by the HDL-C (TC/HDL) was >5 or the LDL-C divided by the HDL-C (LDL/HDL) was >3, there was a markedly increased risk of coronary artery disease. These can be useful today in patients with borderline risk profiles to determine whether or not there is significant risk of ASCVD that warrants initiation of cholesterol-lowering therapy. For example, a male patient who is 40, but has hypertension and an HDL-C of 22, a total cholesterol of 239, LDL-C = 150 and smokes, has three risk factors: smoking, low HDL-C, and hypertension. However, he is planning to quit smoking with a quit date next week. He has already begun taking bupropion. If the patient stays quit for 30 days, that would eliminate smoking as a risk factor, giving him

TABLE 19.3	Supplementary Factors Indicating Increased ASCVD Risk
Framingham Ratios	
• TC/HDL-C >5	
• LDL-C/HDL-C >3	
hs–CRP	
• <1.0 mg/L	Low risk
• 1.0 to 3.0 mg/L	Average risk
• >3.0 to 10 mg/L	High risk
• >10 mg/L	Noncardiovascular causes (infection/inflammation)
ApoB/ApoA1 Ratio	
• >0.97 for males	
• >0.86 for females	
Non-HDL Cholesterol	
a. Calculation=TC- HDL-C= non-HDL cholesterol	
b. To determine patient's goal level simply add 30 to their target LDL-C goal.	

just two risk factors under the 2002 guidelines. Assuming his systolic pressure runs between 135 and 145 mm, the Framingham Score Calculation Tool would give him a 10-year risk of heart attack of 12% and an LDL-C target of <130 mg/dL. However, his TC/HDL ratio is well above 5 (10.9) and his LDL/HDL ratio is well above 3 (6.8), indicating major risks for cardiovascular disease. In this case, in addition to quitting smoking, he should be counseled about his risk and advised to increase his exercise and modify his diet to raise his HDL-C above 40 mg/dL and to lower his total and LDL-C cholesterol. The new, 2013 guidelines make no reference to Framingham ratios.

Apolipoprotein B/Apolipoprotein A1 Ratio

Apolipoprotein B is the transporter for LDL-C and binds to the receptors on the cells facilitating deposit. Apolipoprotein A1 plays a similar role for HDL-C. Recent evidence indicates that this ratio is a more accurate marker of risk than the LDL/HDL ratio. An ApoB/ApoA1 ratio of >0.97 for men and >0.86 for women is indicative of increased risk of ASCVD. Additional evidence appears to make it more accurate in subclinical atherosclerosis and may be a better predictor of plaque instability than traditional lipid profiles. Recent studies have shown that a formula to estimate ApoB/ApoA1 ratios, using only HDL and total cholesterol, has excellent correlation with direct measurement in fasting patients. The new, 2013 guidelines make no reference to this ratio.

Non-HDL Cholesterol

Some experts feel that non-HDL cholesterol should be the primary parameter used rather than LDL-C alone since it better predicts the risk of developing ASCVD. One reason is because the LDL-C value is an estimate based on the Friedewald formula using HDL, total cholesterol, and triglycerides and does not include VLDL-C, which is also atherogenic. High triglyceride levels make the estimate much less reliable, hence when testing patients with high triglyceride levels the report may say "unable to calculate" for LDL-C values. The 2002 guidelines accommodated those experts by suggesting the use of non-HDL cholesterol as a secondary goal after current LDL-C goals are met. Target non-HDL-C goals can be calculated by adding 30 mg/dL to each of the three LDL-C levels derived from risk-factor assessment.

C-Reactive Protein High-Sensitivity Assay

Because endothelial inflammation and subsequent plaque rupture are such a major part of the atherosclerotic process, many experts have advocated the use of C-reactive protein high-sensitivity assay (hs-CRP) as an adjunctive marker of ASCVD risk. C-reactive protein is a biomarker of inflammatory activity in the body. Its release from the liver is stimulated by several cytokines including IL-1 and IL-6. CRP stimulates the production of cytokines and chemokines in endothelial cells contributing to the inflammatory endothelial dysfunction that is part of the atherosclerotic process. The American Heart Association and CDC recommend that asymptomatic patients with a 10% to 20% 10-year risk of myocardial infarction hs-CRP be used to further assess CHD risk using the following criteria. An hs-CRP below 1.0 mg/L predicts low risk; an hs-CRP level between 1.0 and 3.0 mg/L indicates average risk, whereas hs-CRP levels above 3.0 mg/L indicate a high risk of CHD. Persistent levels >10 mg/L indicate noncardiovascular causes like an acute infection or inflammation. The JUPITER study showed that rosuvastatin reduced cardiovascular risk by 37% in patients with low/normal cholesterol levels but high hs-CRP levels. Recent studies have shown a genetic variation in hs-CRP levels further adding to the controversy surrounding the accuracy and utility of hs-CRP as a biomarker of cardiovascular disease. The new guidelines use an hs-CRP of 2 mg/L or greater as a potential factor to justify starting statins in patients at very low risk of ASCVD.

• MONITORING/MANAGING DYSLIPIDEMIA

Therapeutic lifestyle changes (low fat diets and exercise) are the mainstay in the treatment of dyslipidemia. However, the majority of patients do not achieve the degree of LDL-C reduction they need from just lifestyle changes. Statins have been shown to markedly reduce the risk from ASCVD. There are two major mechanisms of action that account for this benefit. First, they reduce the synthesis of LDL-C, a major component of atheromatous plaque. Second, they have an anti-inflammatory effect that decreases endothelial reactivity and ultimately reduce the tendency for plaque rupture. Recent studies have shown that adding other cholesterol-lowering agents to statins improves lipid profiles, but has no effect on cardiovascular outcomes. Even though hs-CRP levels are lowered by statins, there is little or no evidence regarding dose-effect relationship for the anti-inflammatory effect. Therefore, cardiovascular risk factors are still used to determine whether or not to start statin therapy.

Monitoring Treatment Efficacy

The lipid profile (total cholesterol, HDL-C, LDL-C, and triglycerides) is the primary measure of therapy effectiveness. From those values, the Framingham ratios (TC/HDL, LDL/HDL) and non-HDL cholesterol levels (TC level minus HDL-C value) can be calculated. ApoB/ApoA1 ratios and hs-CRP must be ordered separately at this time. In patients who choose to try therapeutic lifestyle changes alone as initial therapy, a trial of 6 months is usually appropriate. Lipid profiles are done at baseline and 4 to 12 weeks after initiation of statin therapy and at least annually and up to every 3 months. This 4- to 8-week period allows the statin dose to attain its maximum impact. In the patient attempting therapeutic lifestyle changes alone, repeating the lipid profile every 4 to 8 weeks, over the 6 months, can serve as educational and motivational tools, as well as provide data to the reluctant patient to help them see the need for statin therapy, if appropriate, in the future.

Under the 2002 guidelines, "When do I increase statin doses or add nonstatin medication?", was a frequent concern of providers. Guidelines by definition are *not* absolute requirements, but suggestions based on the best available evidence; therefore, application of common sense is important. As with hypertension, be careful not to "chase numbers." An LDL-C level of 5 mg/dL above the patient's target goal does not mandate an increase in medication dose. As in a patient with hypertension, in an asymptomatic patient near LDL-C target goal, it is perfectly appropriate to wait another 6 months to get another lipid profile. Waiting can serve as motivation for the patient to further improve the intensity of their lifestyle changes. In patients with dyslipidemia, the alternate measurements of risk can assist in the decision regarding potential dose increases. For example, a patient close to target LDL-C goal, but with unfavorable Framingham or ApoB/ApoA1 ratios, and an hs-CRP level >3.0 mg/L would be a more viable candidate for a dose increase. Conversely, in a patient with the same LDL-C levels and favorable alternative parameters, the pharmacist could more comfortably delay a dosage increase. It is not uncommon in a patient with dyslipidemia and type 2 diabetes to have high triglycerides in spite of LDL cholesterol levels below 100 mg/dL. Since excess glucose is the major source of triglycerides, the patient's elevated triglycerides are most likely due to poor control of their diabetes and increasing the statin dose or adding an agent to lower triglycerides, e.g., fibrates would be inappropriate until the patient's A1C is below 7.0. Therefore, in this situation, intensifying therapy for their type 2 diabetes is the treatment of choice to lower the triglyceride level, especially considering that concurrent fibrate therapy markedly increases the risk of musculoskeletal adverse effects of statins, specifically rhabdomyolysis.

Under the new guidelines, if a patient does not meet expected percentage providers are told to check for adherence to statins and lifestyle modifications. There is no provision for increasing statin doses unless the patient moves into a different risk-benefit group, by developing diabetes, having a cardiovascular event, or having their LDL-C levels exceed 190 mg/dL. While all patients taking statins should be monitored for adherence, in patients taking statins other than pitavastatin, atorvastatin, or rosuvastatin, who are apparently not responding to statin therapy with sufficient LDL-C lowering, providers need to verify that the patients are taking their statin after 6 PM in the evening before changing therapy. Many purported cases of ineffectiveness of simvastatin and pravastatin are, in part, due to inappropriate timing of the dose.

• MONITORING FOR COMPLICATIONS OF DYSLIPIDEMIA AND ITS TREATMENT

Disease Complications

Complications of dyslipidemia are those of atherosclerosis: angina pectoris, acute coronary syndrome, peripheral artery disease (intermittent claudication), and stroke (CVA). Therefore, questions about the symptoms of those complications are appropriate at each visit, e.g., chest pain, leg pain when exercising, visual disturbances (Table 19.4). Since dyslipidemia frequently occurs concurrently with hypertension and diabetes, which also cause the same atherosclerotic complications, it is unnecessary to ask questions for each disease, i.e., asking about chest pain once covers common complications for all three comorbid conditions.

Drug Complications

Adverse drug reactions with statins are uncommon. Musculoskeletal disorders and hepatic side effects have been prominent concerns historically. Recently, concerns have been raised regarding statin-induced cognitive adverse effects and a statin-related increased incidence of diabetes.

Musculoskeletal Myalgias occurred in 1.5% to 3.0% of patients in randomized controlled trials of statins. Observational studies have shown a slightly higher incidence, up to 10%. Patients describe symptoms including pain, tenderness, cramping, fatigue, weakness, stiffness, and heaviness. Symptoms are *symmetrical* (occurring in limbs on *both sides* of the body). Muscle symptoms tend to be generalized and proximal (occurring in both upper and lower limbs) and may be worse with exercise. In general, the higher the dose of statin, the more likely muscle symptoms are to occur. Reactions most commonly occur within a month of initiation or dosage increase, but in one study, 15% reported symptom onset after 6 months of therapy. Generally, symptoms resolve within 2 to 8 weeks after discontinuation.

Statins have rarely caused rhabdomyolysis, an acute fulminant, potentially fatal disease of skeletal muscle, involving the destruction of muscle manifested by myoglobinemia, myoglobinuria, brown urine, and eventually renal failure. The annual incidence of statin-induced rhabdomyolysis is 0.0042% (4.2/100,000) with statin monotherapy. Concurrent therapy with fibrates increases the risk of rhabdomyolysis to 200/100,000. Symptoms include diffuse, symmetrical muscle pain and weakness, flu-like symptoms, and low back pain. Creatine kinase (CK) levels are at least 10 times the upper limit of normal, and myoglobin is present in the urine. Published criteria include elevated serum creatinine, but some experts feel that is not necessary for the diagnosis.

The cause of statin muscle side effects is unknown, but has been attributed to effects on coenzyme Q10, selenoproteins, and low cholesterol itself. Multiple studies

TABLE 19.4	Follow-Up Visit Check List for Dyslipidemia

CONTROL

    S   *None since there are no symptoms of poor control other than atherosclerotic complications*

    O   Lipid profile as indicated by level of control (at least annually in stable patients)

COMPLIANCE

    S   *How have things been going with your diet? Exercise?*
        What kind of problems have you been having following your diet? Exercise plan?
        What kind of problems have you been having remembering to take your medication?

    O   Weight
        Medication refill record

COMPLICATIONS (DISEASE)

    S   *What other changes or problems have you noticed since your last visit?*
        What kind of problems have you noticed during physical activity? **(CHF, PAD)**
        What kind of problems have you been having sleeping? **(CHF)**
        Have you had any of the following since your last visit?

Chest pain? **(angina)**	Shortness of breath? **(angina, CHF)**
Headache? **(TIA/CVA)**	Dizziness (unsteadiness)? **(TIA/CVA)**
Forgetfulness? **(TIA/CVA)**	Numbness/tingling in extremity? **(TIA/CVA)**
Ankle swelling? **(CHF)**	Number of pillows for sleep? **(CHF)**
Decreased ability to move extremities? **(TIA/CVA)**	
Leg cramps/pain while exercising? **(PAD)**	
Other unusual symptoms?	

    O   Observational neurological examination (i.e., watch the patient while interviewing for facial and other movements
        and for coherency of speech and understanding of conversation and while exiting and entering examination
        room for ease of mobility and balance) **(CVA/TIA)**
        Annual complete history and physical examination including dilated eye examination
        Other physical examinations as indicated by history
        Electrocardiogram as indicated

COMPLICATIONS (DRUG)

    S   *What other changes or problems have you noticed since your last visit?*
        Have you had any of the following since your last visit?
        Muscle pain or weakness? **(myotoxicity)**
        Fatigue, anorexia, malaise, nausea, vomiting, dark urine? **(hepatotoxicity)**
        Difficulty concentrating or remembering things? **(cognitive effects)**

    O   Examinations/laboratory tests to f/u specific symptoms
        A1C annually
        Creatine kinase, urine myoglobin (as indicated)
        Folstein minimental status examination (as indicated)
        LFTs (as indicated)

have failed to support any individual cause. Patient education should include warnings about symmetrical, diffuse pain, or weakness in the extremities and at each visit patients should be questioned about those symptoms. If a patient complains of musculoskeletal pain/weakness typical of statins, then a careful history should be taken, which includes looking for other medications that may interfere with the metabolism of statins by the liver or other conditions that might increase statin levels (liver or renal disease, depending on the statin). CK serum levels should be drawn.

Thyroid-stimulating-hormone (TSH) levels should also be drawn since hypothyroid disease raises serum cholesterol and CK levels, and may predispose patients to statin myotoxicity. Some authors also suggest 25-OH vitamin D levels because vitamin D deficiency has been associated with statin myotoxicity. Obviously, the presence of clinical and laboratory evidence of rhabdomyolysis requires immediate discontinuation of the statin and treatment. Normal CK levels rule out muscle damage and the decision to discontinue the statin depends on the tolerability of muscle symptoms compared to the level of need for cholesterol reduction. More frequent CK serum levels are indicated to quickly identify any progression of the myotoxicity. Muscle symptoms plus elevated CK levels of less than 10 times the upper limit of normal are more problematic. Guidelines suggest that cautious continuation with frequent clinical and laboratory monitoring can be appropriate. Lower doses or switching to a less lipophilic statin (pravastatin or rosuvastatin) have been suggested, but there are no clinical trials to support their efficacy. Intolerable muscle symptoms, like rhabdomyolysis, require immediate discontinuation. If discontinuation does not resolve muscle symptoms, then a more detailed workup, potentially including muscle biopsy, is indicated.

Hepatotoxicity Hepatotoxicity due to statins has been a controversial issue. Based on reports of increased transaminase levels in early trials, the FDA originally required baseline liver function tests (LFTs), followed by repeat LFTs every 6 months. However, recent evidence has led to uncertainty regarding the need for monitoring with LFTs. First, while there have been cases of acute liver failure thought to be caused by statins they have been confounded by the presence of other hepatotoxic agents. In addition, the rate of purported statin-induced acute hepatic failure is less than that of liver failure due to idiosyncratic causes. Second, nonalcoholic liver disease (NALD) commonly exists in patients with the metabolic syndrome and causes low levels of transaminase elevations. Since dyslipidemia is a major component of the metabolic syndrome, many patients on statins could have elevated LFTs due to the metabolic syndrome, rather than statins, making it problematic to distinguish NALD from the typical statin-induced mild transaminase elevations. Third, several studies have shown that giving statins to patients with mild transaminase elevations, including patients with hepatitis C is safe. In some patients addition of statins actually caused reductions in transaminase levels. Given the additional information, the FDA recently dropped the requirement for both baseline and follow up LFTs for all statins. However, it is appropriate to question patients for potential signs and symptoms of hepatotoxicity at each visit, i.e., fatigue, malaise, anorexia, nausea, vomiting, jaundice, dark urine. Positive responses should be followed up with LFTs.

Diabetes and Cognitive Dysfunction Recent case reports and epidemiologic studies have proposed potential statin-induced cognitive dysfunction and an increased incidence of diabetes in statin users. Several case reports have suggested cognitive dysfunction as an adverse effect of statins. Symptoms include primarily impaired concentration and attention, or long- and short-term memory loss. However, behavioral changes, anxiety, and paranoia have also been reported. Symptom onset ranges from 5 to 270 days and patient recovery time has ranged from a few days to 4 weeks after discontinuing statins. The FDA MedWatch program received 60 case reports of memory loss attributable to statins over a 5-year period. There have been 11 studies looking at cognitive effects of statins as a primary endpoint. Three studies showed improvement in cognitive function; seven showed no difference between patients receiving statins compared to patients receiving placebo. Only one study showed negative effects on some measures of cognitive function. Furthermore, no significant differences in cognitive function were found between patients on statins compared to those on placebo in three studies where cognitive function was a secondary endpoint. The theoretical basis for statin-induced cognitive dysfunction involves the important role of cholesterol in the brain as part of the myelin sheath, but exact mechanisms are unknown. Since statin-induced cognitive impairment is uncommon to rare, patients should be questioned at each visit for changes in concentration, attention, and memory loss. Also in patients exhibiting behavioral changes, the statin should be included in the differential diagnosis of the etiology of the symptoms. If symptoms are thought to be due to a statin, discontinuing the statin for 1 to 3 months appears to be safe, not increasing the risk of cardiovascular events. In patients who have statin-induced cognitive dysfunction, a discussion of risk versus benefit should take place. Various authors and experts have suggested several therapeutic options for patients with likely statin-induced cognitive issues. Most common is switching the patient to a more hydrophilic statin (pravastatin or rosuvastatin), since almost all reports have occurred with more lipophilic statins (simvastatin, atorvastatin). Some experts, who feel that all their patients with cognitive dysfunction had LDL-C levels markedly below 100 mg/dL, have suggested lowering the dose of statin to allow the LDL-C serum level to rise to near the target goal for patients with higher cardiac risk (100 mg/dL). There are no clinical trials to support the efficacy of either of these theoretical options.

In several meta-analyses, researchers noted an increased incidence of diabetes, especially in those patients over 65 who have a history of long-term statin use. The risk ranged from 9% to 13%. While some studies looked at changes in BMI to rule out the metabolic syndrome as a cause of increased diabetes risk, these studies were, at best, hypothesis generating. Given the genetic predisposition of the metabolic syndrome and type 2 diabetes, and the concurrent presence of dyslipidemia in both conditions, it would not be an unexpected finding for the incidence of diabetes to be higher in patients with abnormal cholesterol values. Until better evidence is available, it is appropriate to monitor fasting plasma glucose or A1C levels periodically in all patients on statins.

• KEY REFERENCES

1. Grundy SM, Becker D, Clark LT, et al. Third Report of the National Cholesterol Education Panel (NCEP) Expert Panel: Detection, Evaluation and Treatment of High Blood Cholesterol in Adults (Adult Treatment Panel III): Final Report. *Circulation*. 2002;106:3143-3421.
2. Grundy SM, Cleeman JL, Merz CN, et al. Implications of Recent Clinical Trials for the National Cholesterol Education Programs Adult Treatment Panel III Guidelines. *Circulation*. 2004;110:229-239.
3. Last AR, Ference JD, Falleroni J. Pharmacological treatment of dyslipidemia. *Am Fam Physician*. 2011;85:551-558.
4. Rana JS, Boekholdt SM. Should we change our lipid management strategies to focus on non-high-density lipoprotein cholesterol? *Curr Opin Cardiol*. 2010;26:622-626.
5. Contreras F, Lares M, Castro J, et al. Determination of non-HDL cholesterol in diabetic and hypertensive patients. *Amer J Ther*. 2010;17:337-340.
6. Robinson JG. LDL reduction: how low should we go and is it safe? *Curr Cardiol Rep*. 2008;10:481-487.
7. Sniderman AD, De Graaf J, Couture P. Low-density lipoprotein strategies: target versus maximalist versus population percentile. *Curr Opin Cardiol*. 2012;27:405-411.
8. Battistoni A, Rabattu S, Volpe M. Circulating biomarkers with preventive, diagnostic and prognosic implications in cardiovascular diseases. *Int J Cardiol*. 2012;157:160-168.
9. Sathasivam S. Statin-induced myotoxicity. *Eur J Intern Med*. 2012;23:317-324.
10. Mansi I, Frei CR, Pugh MJ, et al. Statins and musculoskeletal conditions, arthropathies and injuries. *JAMA Intern Med*. 2013;173: 1318-26.
11. Russo MW, Scobey M, Bonkovsky HL. Drug-induced liver injury associated with statins. *Semin Liver Dis*. 2009;29:412-422.
12. Bader T. The myth of statin-induced hepatotoxicity. *Am J Gastroenterol*. 2010;105:978-980.

13. Rojas-Fernandez CH, Cameron JCF. Is statin-associated cognitive impairment clinically relevant? A narrative review and clinical recommendations. *Ann Pharmacother.* 2012;46:549-557.
14. Sampsom UK, MacRae FL, Fazio S. Are statins diabetogenic. *Curr Opin Cardiol.* 2011;26:342-347.
15. Stone NJ, Robinson J, Lichtenstein AH, et al. 2013 ACC/AHA guideline on the treatment of blood cholesterol to reduce atherosclerotic cardiovascular risk in adults: a report of the American College of Cardiology/American Heart Association task force on practice guidelines. [Published online November 12, 2013] Circulation doi:10.1161/01 cir 0000437741.48606.98.
16. Richardson K, Schoen M, French B, et al. Statins and cognitive function: a systematic review. *Ann Intern Med.* 2013;159:688-697.

CASE 19.1

Age:	58
Sex:	Female
Medical Conditions:	Diabetes, BP = 130/80
Family Hx:	Mother died of heart attack at age 47
Smoking Status:	Nonsmoker
Meds:	Glyburide, metformin, HCTZ, lisinopril
Goal LDL: _____	
Results:	TC: 212 LDL: 126 HDL: 42 Trig: 180

What is the LDL-C goal? What would you tell the patient? Explain your rationale.

CASE 19.2

Age:	35
Sex:	Male
Medical Conditions:	None, BP = 130/80
Family Hx:	Unremarkable
Smoking Status:	Just quit ... last cigarette was last weekend
Meds:	None
Goal LDL: _____	

Results: TC: 190   LDL: 145   HDL: 22   Trig: 170

What is the LDL-C goal? What would you tell the patient? Explain your rationale.

CASE 19.3

Age:	75
Sex:	Male
Medical Conditions:	Emphysema
Family Hx:	Mother died of a heart attack at age 80
Smoking Status:	Quit smoking in 1985 (had smoked for 40 years)
Meds:	Albuterol, ipratropium
Goal LDL: _____	
Results:	TC: 185 LDL: 125 HDL: 65 Trig: 165

What is the LDL-C goal? What would you tell the patient? Explain your rationale.

CASE 19.4

Age:	56
Sex:	Female
Medical Conditions:	Allergies, BP = 120/80
Family Hx:	Sister had MI at age 62
Smoking Status:	Nonsmoker
Meds:	Claritin
Goal LDL: _____	
Results:	TC: 225 LDL: 122 HDL: 55 Trig: 230

What is the LDL-C goal? What would you tell the patient? Explain your rationale.

Diabetes Mellitus

1. Identify appropriate standards for the diagnosis of diabetes and determine risk and prognosis for developing complications of poorly controlled diabetes mellitus.

2. Use available parameters to measure and monitor target blood glucose and A1C goals for patients under treatment for diabetes mellitus.

3. Conduct a comprehensive follow-up visit for a patient with diabetes mellitus using appropriate history-taking techniques, physical examination, and laboratory tests. The visit includes assessment of disease control, plus assessment and support of compliance with lifestyle modifications and medication regimens.

4. Evaluate patients for complications from diabetes mellitus and the medication regimen.

• INTRODUCTION

More than 25 million Americans have diabetes mellitus, 90% to 95% of whom have Type 2 diabetes mellitus. The economic burden of diabetes is almost $250 billion annually. Because most patients with Type 2 diabetes have the metabolic syndrome, with concomitant hypertension and hyperlipidemia, the average number of medications per patient ranges from 4.1 to 5.9. Because of the reliance on medication to control diabetes and its comorbid conditions, the pharmacist is a key member of the health care team in the management of patients with diabetes. Not surprisingly, there are numerous studies demonstrating the pharmacist's effectiveness in managing Type 2 diabetes. Therefore, this chapter focuses on the competencies required by pharmacists to assume a primary care role in the treatment of patients with Type 2 diabetes mellitus.

• CLASSIFICATION/ETIOLOGY

There are two main forms of diabetes mellitus (Table 20.1). The first is Type 1 diabetes, also previously known as insulin-dependent diabetes mellitus (IDDM) or juvenile onset diabetes. Type 1 diabetes is an autoimmune disease that results in the destruction of the β cells in the islets of Langerhans in the pancreas. Once 80% to 90% of the β cells are destroyed, severe glucose intolerance develops because of the lack of insulin. With little or no insulin available, patients are unable to use glucose. In response, the body breaks down proteins and fats for energy, frequently resulting in the development of ketoacidosis, which can be fatal. Patients with Type 1 diabetes require insulin injections due to the lack of insulin production to control glucose and prevent ketoacidosis. The exact mechanism for this autoimmune process is unknown, but patients who develop Type 1 diabetes have a genetic predisposition and the β-cell destruction is triggered by either infectious, chemical, or dietary agents. Generally, patients who develop Type 1 diabetes mellitus do so as children or adolescents. In contrast to patients with Type 2 diabetes, who are overweight, patients with Type 1 are usually of normal body shape and weight. In some cases, the destruction is rapid, and the onset is sudden. In others the destruction is slower and may take up to a year to fully develop signs and symptoms.

Type 2 diabetes, also previously known as adult onset or noninsulin dependent (NIDDM), usually occurs in patients over 40 years of age. Patients tend to be obese, and rather than having no insulin tend to be hyperinsulinemic early in the disease

TABLE 20.1	Classification of Diabetes Mellitus

Type 1 Diabetes Mellitus (juvenile or insulin-dependent diabetes mellitus, IDDM)

    Little or no insulin production due to autoimmune destruction of pancreas
    Young age of onset
    Develop ketoacidosis if not tightly controlled
    Slender at diagnosis
    Must be treated with insulin to control glucose and prevent ketoacidosis
    Classic symptoms: polyuria, polyphagia, polydipsia

Type 2 Diabetes Mellitus (adult-onset, noninsulin-dependent diabetes mellitus, NIDDM)

    Hyperinsulinemic/*insulin resistance*
    Decreased insulin effectiveness at the skeletal muscle
    Predisposes to concurrent hyperlipidemia and hypertension (the metabolic syndrome)
    ≥ 40 years of age at onset
    Rarely ketoacidosis even with poor plasma glucose control
    Obese
    Treated with diet/exercise/oral agents, but may require insulin to control glucose
    Asymptomatic or just fatigue as a primary symptom

TABLE 20.2	The Metabolic Syndrome

Metabolic Syndrome consists of insulin resistance, obesity, Type 2 diabetes mellitus, dyslipidemia, and hypertension.

Three or more of the following are needed for the diagnosis of the metabolic syndrome:

1. Abdominal obesity (waist circumference)
   - Men >40 inches
   - Women >35 inches
2. Triglycerides >150 mg/dL
3. HDL cholesterol
   - Men <40 mg/dL
   - Women <50 mg/dL
4. BP >130/85
5. Fasting plasma glucose >100 mg/dL

due to insulin resistance. This prevents insulin from entering cells to provide energy. Because muscles are not getting enough energy, they signal the liver to produce more glucose, causing glycogenolysis and gluconeogenesis. Insulin resistance also contributes to the development of hypertension and dyslipidemia. Therefore, most patients with Type 2 diabetes also have dyslipidemia and hypertension. Those three comorbid diseases along with other factors create the *metabolic syndrome*, which greatly increases the risk of cardiovascular disease (Table 20.2). Because there is some insulin effect, patients with Type 2 diabetes mellitus rarely develop ketoacidosis. Type 2 diabetes can be managed by diet and exercise alone, oral antidiabetic agents, or a combination of both. Eventually many patients will require insulin therapy to optimize control of their plasma glucose.

• DIAGNOSIS

The classical symptoms of diabetes include polyuria (excess/frequent urination), polydipsia (excessive thirst), and polyphagia (excessive hunger). Historically these occur in patients with Type 1 diabetes mellitus, but also can occur in patients with Type 2 diabetes. Polyuria is caused by high-plasma glucose levels exceeding the kidney's threshold to reabsorb glucose. Once the plasma glucose exceeds 160 mg/dL, most patients spill glucose into the urine, creating a hyperosmolar state that causes water to be pulled into the tubules. Most patients notice it as nocturia (frequent urination at night), since they cannot sleep through the night without being awakened by the urge to urinate several times. The higher the plasma glucose levels, the greater the chance of developing dehydration. Excess plasma glucose also creates a hyperosmolar state. Both the polyuria-induced dehydration and the hyperosmolar state stimulate polydipsia (excessive thirst) in an attempt to correct those conditions. Finally, because glucose cannot be effectively utilized, the body is starved for energy so it stimulates polyphagia (excessive eating) in an attempt to correct the glucose/energy deficit.

Symptoms of Type 2 diabetes mellitus are not quite as obvious as in Type 1 diabetes mellitus because they occur more slowly. Fatigue is the most common symptom followed by nocturia. However, patient recognition of nocturia or polyuria may be masked by other conditions associated with aging that also cause more frequent urination, e.g., benign prostatic hypertrophy in males and postbirth trauma conditions such as cystocele or uterine prolapse in postmenopausal women. Frequently, the first sign of diabetes is an episode of vulvovaginal candidiasis (VVC), candidal balanitis, or a cut that easily becomes infected or does not heal normally. Excess glucose in the urine and vaginal fluid predisposes women to developing UTI's or candidiasis and plasma glucose levels above 200 mg/dL impair neutrophil response to any bacterial infection. Therefore, patients over 40 years of age, with VVC or unexpected bacterial infection, should be questioned for symptoms of Type 2 diabetes mellitus and after the infection has been cleared, a fasting plasma glucose should be done. A fasting plasma glucose of >126 mg/dL, a random plasma glucose of ≥ 200 mg/dL, or a A1C (hemoglobin A_{1c}, glycosylated hemoglobin) ≥ 6.5% are all diagnostic of diabetes mellitus. A1C is the percentage of hemoglobin that has glucose attached. Fasting plasma glucose levels of 100 to 125 mg/dL are considered prediabetes, a situation that needs to be addressed by lifestyle changes (weight loss, diet, and exercise). Prediabetes, which is common in patients with the metabolic syndrome, is a warning sign that if the patient continues their present lifestyle they will eventually develop Type 2 diabetes mellitus.

• COMPLICATIONS

There are multiple severe complications in patients with suboptimally controlled diabetes mellitus. Excess levels of plasma glucose directly and indirectly damage blood vessels and nerves, leading to many of the complications. Excess glucose effects on the immune system, coupled with neuropathy and microangiopathy can combine to cause the *diabetic foot*. The important point is that controlling plasma glucose levels prevents or delays the complications of diabetes. Many complications are caused wholly or in part by microangiopathy, the thickening of the basement membrane of tiny blood vessels (precapillary arterioles and capillaries) in all parts of the body. The thickening of blood vessel walls eventually leads to ischemia and cell death. Nephropathy, neuropathy, and retinopathy all have elements of microangiopathy in their etiology. Macroangiopathy refers to the ability of diabetes mellitus to accelerate the rate of atherosclerosis in larger blood vessels, leading to myocardial infarction, stroke, and peripheral artery disease.

In uncontrolled Type 1 diabetes mellitus, the obvious and potentially fatal complication is diabetic ketoacidosis. In patients with Type 2 diabetes, uncontrolled diabetes mellitus can occasionally lead to hyperosmolar non-ketotic coma. Typically plasma glucose levels are well in excess of 1000 mg/dL (but can occur with >600 mg/ dL) and patients present with symptoms of dehydration (polyuria, polydipsia, fever, warm dry skin without sweating). Other symptoms include vision impairment, confusion, hallucinations, weakness, and somnolence. Because less than 20% of patients develop a coma, it is now called hyperosmolar, hyperglycemic, non-ketotic syndrome (HHNS). Typically, it occurs as the result of a combination of poor control and a bacterial infection, which further elevates plasma glucose.

Retinopathy

Diabetic retinopathy is the leading cause of blindness in the United States. Microangiopathy of tiny retinal blood vessels lead to hypoxia of retinal tissue and cellular death and formation of scar tissue. The vessels are also weaker and develop aneurysms, which may rupture, leading to small hemorrhages. The lack of oxygen eventually causes the proliferation of multiple small blood vessels to overcome the hypoxia. Macular edema also occurs. The combination of proliferation of small arterioles and macular edema eventually leads to visual loss. An annual dilated retinal examination by an eye professional is required to detect and monitor retinopathy. Findings of diabetic retinopathy during retinal examination include neovascularization, hard exudates (yellow dots), which are lipid residues of serious leakage from damaged capillaries, soft or cotton wool exudates, which are retinal nerve fiber microinfarcts, and hemorrhages of many shapes and sizes reflecting bleeding in various layers of the retina.

Nephropathy

Diabetes is the leading cause of end-stage renal disease (ESRD) in the United States. Excess blood glucose levels directly cause mesangial expansion, thickening of the basement membrane of the glomerulus, and eventually glomerulosclerosis. Since hypertension by itself causes nephropathy by a different mechanism, patients with Type 2 diabetes are far more likely to develop ESRD. As changes occur in the glomerulus, protein normally retained in the blood stream begins to leak out, causing proteinuria, the earliest sign of decreased renal function. Faced with high blood pressure and high blood glucose levels, renal function progressively decreases. Because of this process, an annual test for microalbuminuria and renal function are required.

Neuropathy

Diabetic neuropathy is the leading cause of nontraumatic amputations in the United States. While the exact cause of diabetic neuropathy is unknown, it appears to be multifactorial. Polyols, glucose by-products, accumulate in peripheral nerves and cause nerve damage. Other advanced glycation end products stimulate the immune system to attack nerves. High glucose levels cause nerves to produce reactive oxygen molecules that are thought to damage neuronal mitochondria. Finally, microangiopathy eventually causes nerve ischemia and death. The result of these processes is progressive loss of sensation usually starting in the feet. In addition to the loss of sensation, some patients will develop lancinating neuropathic pain, which can manifest itself on the bottom of the feet as burning sensations. Starting in the peripheral nerves, diabetic neuropathy can eventually progress to affect the autonomic nervous system where it manifests itself as impotence in males, vaginal dryness in women. Diabetic gastroparesis or paralysis of the gastrointestinal tract eventually develops. Gastroparesis usually occurs in patients who have had peripheral diabetic neuropathy for many years and manifests itself as a feeling of early fullness, belching and bloating, constipation, or diarrhea.

While the pain of diabetic neuropathy can be difficult to treat, the loss of sensation in the feet has far more dangerous consequences, the diabetic foot. When normal patients step on a stone, they sense the discomfort and shift their weight to prevent the stone from breaking the skin. Similarly, pain from tight fitting shoes alerts normal patients to make footwear changes or pad the tight area to prevent blister formation. Patients with diabetic neuropathy cannot feel the stone or the tightness and both may cause significant damage to the skin of the foot. In patients with diabetic neuropathy due to poorly controlled diabetes, microangiopathy to the small blood vessels in the skin is usually well advanced, leaving layers of skin and subdermal tissue with markedly reduced blood flow. The inoculation of bacteria from a stone breaking the skin or a blister rupturing creates a source of infection. Because of the decreased circulation, neutrophils have difficulty reaching the location. In addition, if the plasma glucose is >200 mg/dL, neutrophils respond poorly to chemotactic factors. Finally, because of poor circulation, it can be difficult to get enough antibiotic to the site of infection. Similarly, this microangiopathy can by itself cause ulcerations due to chronic ischemia and deeper ischemia, which eventually leads to gangrene and amputation (Figure 20.1). That is why a comprehensive diabetic foot examination is so important and is required at least annually. The diabetic foot examination checks for peripheral neuropathy with the monofilament examination and vibratory sensation (Table 20.3). Checking for the presence of the dorsalis pedis and posterior tibial pulses evaluates peripheral artery disease (macroangiopathy). Loss of hair on the toes, skin atrophy, delayed capillary fill time, and differences in temperature between feet or between parts of the same foot, all indicate microangiopathy. Care should be taken in evaluating capillary refill time

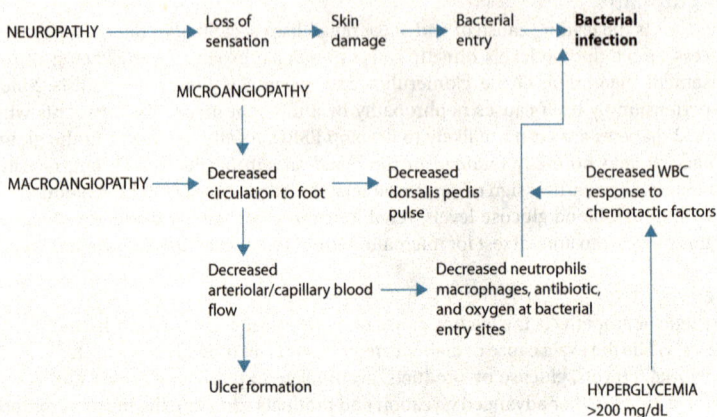

FIGURE 20.1 Pathophysiology of the diabetic foot.

TABLE 20.3	Diabetic Foot Examination

Neuropathy

____sensation (monofilament)
____vibration (128 mHz)
____patellar/Achilles deep tendon reflexes

Microangiopathy

____temperature difference between feet/parts of foot
____skin atrophy
____hair loss on toes
____ulcers/cuts
____color
____capillary refill time (pad of big toe) (<3 seconds)

Macroangiopathy

____leg lift test (raise legs change color/hang over side of exam table and watch complexion turn dusky red)
____palpate dorsalis pedis pulse
____palpate posterior tibial pulse
____edema

Source of trauma/infection

____callouses
____red areas indicating friction
____blisters
____overlapping toes/bunions
____equinus (frozen ankle)

Other

____onychomycosis//tinea pedis

especially in patients with advanced neuropathy. Use of the toe pad on the end of the big toes is the safest. Some references suggest squeezing the toes superiorly to inferiorly, with the thumb on the nail. This is not a good idea since hard pressure may cause a break in the skin from the compressed toenail, setting up a nidus for infection. Finally, looking for potential sources of trauma and infection involves looking for ingrown toenails, blisters, cuts, ulcers, and red areas caused by friction from footwear. Callouses bear special mention. In a patient with peripheral neuropathy, a callous (thick hard skin) is just like a stone. While not breaking the skin, the pressures can cause damage to subcutaneous tissue underneath the callous, which can eventually lead to gangrenous conditions and amputations. Patients are encouraged to inspect their own feet daily for cuts, sores, blisters, and ulcers. A metal camp mirror is very useful for this purpose. Once patients begin to lose sensation in their feet, all foot care needs to be done by a podiatrist. Self-care, even trimming toenails, is not wise. Some experts recommend a brief screening at each provider visit (every 3 to 6 months) since it takes only a few minutes and has been shown to reduce the incidence of amputations.

Macroangiopathy

In addition to microangiopathy's effect on arterioles and capillaries, poorly controlled diabetes accelerates the rate of atherosclerosis by reducing the effectiveness of protective enzymes, while enhancing inflammation among atherosclerotic plaques in larger blood vessels. These deleterious changes increase the incidence of myocardial infarctions, atherosclerotic stroke, and peripheral artery disease. Patients with Type 2 diabetes mellitus also have dyslipidemia and hypertension due to the insulin resistance in the metabolic syndrome, both of which also accelerate atherosclerosis. In establishing target LDL cholesterol levels, diabetes is considered the equivalent of a history of coronary artery disease. Macroangiopathy, through atherosclerosis in larger vessels, combines with microangiopathy to eventually worsen circulatory problems in the extremities.

Infection-Prone

Some textbooks categorize patients with diabetes as immunosuppressed or immunocompromised because they appear to be more susceptible to a wide variety of infections. In reality, under normal circumstances, patients with well-controlled diabetes have similar incidences of bacterial, fungal, and viral infections as do patients without diabetes. However, high blood glucose levels (uncontrolled diabetes mellitus) do increase the risk for fungal and bacterial infections. First excess glucose in urine, sweat, and vaginal fluids predispose patients to urinary tract infections, vulvovaginal candidiasis, candidal balanitis, and soft tissue infections, because the glucose is fuel for microbial growth and has other direct effects to enhance microbial growth. In addition, at plasma glucose levels >200 mg/dL neutrophils and macrophages do not respond as well to chemotactic factors released at the site of bacterial infections, reducing the body's ability to fight infection. However, even patients who normally have excellent control of their blood glucose will be at increased risk during periods surrounding surgery or other trauma due to the release of substances, such as cortisol, that increase blood glucose levels as part of the physiological process to speed the repair of damaged tissue. Similarly, when bacterial infections do occur in patients with excellent control, plasma glucose levels tend to rise because of similar physiological defense and repair processes. In patients who present with a bacterial infection and a mildly elevated plasma glucose level, a fasting plasma glucose should be done several weeks after the infection has cleared to determine if the patient has diabetes or prediabetes.

• INITIAL VISIT

An initial visit for a patient with diabetes has two major components. The first component is to confirm the diagnosis of diabetes mellitus and the metabolic syndrome, the presence of comorbid illness, e.g., dyslipidemia and hypertension, and the absence of

TABLE 20.4	Initial Patient Visit Checklist

CONFIRM DIAGNOSIS

A1C
Fasting plasma glucose
Thyroid panel (TSH, T3, T4)
Fasting lipid panel
BMI
Waist circumference
Blood pressure

PRESENCE OF COMPLICATIONS

Serum creatinine
Microalbuminuria (albumin/creatinine ratio)
Comprehensive diabetic foot examination
Dilated fundoscopic (retinal) examination by optometrist or ophthalmologist
Comprehensive dental examination
Complete cardiovascular history/risk analysis (family history, angina, MI, CVA, PAD, lipid profile, BP)
ECG if indicated
Rule out other potential causes of nocturia (uterine prolapse, cystocele, and benign prostatic hypertrophy)

secondary causes of elevated plasma glucose such as hypothyroidism. The second component is to assess for the presence and severity of complications due to diabetes, hypertension, and dyslipidemia. Initial evaluation will require a complete history and physical examination, with special emphasis on cardiovascular risk factors, peripheral neuropathy, vascular disease, and other potential causes for nocturia such as uterine prolapse or cystocele in females and benign prostatic hypertrophy in males. Because diet and exercise are important components of treatment of Type 2 diabetes, a thorough history of current dietary and exercise habits is an important part of the initial workup. Similarly, a smoking history is needed since smoking accelerates microangiopathy, atherosclerosis (macroangiopathy), and neuropathic complications of diabetes (Table 20.4).

• FOLLOW-UP VISITS

Follow-up visits cover evaluation of control of diabetes mellitus, compliance with the therapeutic regimen, and complications from the disease and the therapeutic regimen (Table 20.5). The general approach to a follow-up visit is to begin with broad open-ended questions to start the dialog about symptoms for each section

TABLE 20.5	Follow-Up Visit Checklist

CONTROL

Subjective

*

How have things been going with your diabetes since your last visit?
What have your home blood glucose readings been? How many times a day do you test?
How many times does the urge to urinate awaken you at night? **(nocturia)**
Skin rash, vaginal rash, or discharge? **(decreased immunological competence due to hyperglycemia)**
How about dizziness, palpitations, mental changes, sweating, hunger? **(hypoglycemia)**

Objective

A1c (HA$_{1c}$, glycosylated hemoglobin) <7% **(measures long-term blood glucose control over the last 3 months blood glucose control)**
Weight

TABLE 20.5	Follow-Up Visit Checklist (*Continued*)

COMPLIANCE

Subjective (Medication)

* *What do you take for your diabetes?*
What kind of problems have you been having remembering to take your medications?
How frequently does it happen? When was the last time it happened?
When did you take your last dose? How much?

Subjective (Exercise)

* *How are you doing with your exercise?*
What kind of exercise do you do? How frequently do you exercise?
What kind of problems have you been having getting your regular exercise done?

Subjective (Diet)

* *How is your diet going?*
What kind of problems have you been having following your diet?
What did you have for dinner last night?

Objective

Weight
Have patients draw up insulin dose if applicable?
Check refill records/do pill count..

COMPLICATIONS

Subjective (Disease)

* *What changes have you noticed since your last visit?*
How have your foot checks been going? How frequently do you check?
CLOSED-ENDED QUESTIONS
Numbness/tingling/pain in your feet? **(neuropathy)**
Chest pain, SOB, DOE, PND? **(angina, CHF)**
Dizziness, memory loss, headache? **(CVA, TIA)**
Visual changes (especially color vision)? **(retinopathy)**
Pedal edema, weight gain, fatigue, nausea, decreased appetite? **(nephropathy)**
Dysuria, frequency? **(UTI, VVC)**
Any sores, cuts, rashes? **(vasculopathy)**

Objective (Disease)

BP
Screening diabetic foot examination including sensory examination with monofilament

ANNUALLY OR AS INDICATED

Complete diabetic foot examination **(checks for macrovascular, microvascular, and neuropathic changes/complications)**
Microalbuminuria (sensitive for greater than 30 mg/L but less than 300 mg/L) (annually if no previous problem). Reported as mg/L or albumin to creatinine ratio (ACR)
BUN/serum creatinine
Dilated ophthalmoscopic examination including visual field
Complete lipid panel

Subjective (Medication)

Hypoglycemia **(sulfonylureas, meglitinides, insulin)**
Nausea, vomiting, diarrhea, heartburn **(metformin, GLP-agonists, gliptins)**
Abdominal pain **(exenatide, gliptins)**
Abnormal taste **(metformin)**

Objective (Medication)

Edema **(glitazones)**
Weight gain **(sulfonylureas, meglinitides, insulin, glitazones)**
Serum amylase/lipase **(GLP-agonists, gliptins)**
Tachypnea **(glitazones, metformin)**

* Initial broad open-ended questions to begin discussion of control, compliance, and complications.

TABLE 20.6	Relationship Between A1C and Estimated Average Glucose Levels
A1C%	**Estimated Average Glucose (95% CI)**
5.0	97 (76 to 120)
6.0	126 (100 to 152)
7.0	154 (123 to 185)
8.0	183 (147 to 217)
9.0	212 (170 to 249)
10.0	240 (193 to 282)
11.0	269 (217 to 314)
12.0	298 (240 to 347)

(control, compliance, complications). Positive responses are followed up with more focused open-ended questions. Similarly, if specific information is not covered in response to broad questions, a focused open-ended question approach is used. Finally, a series of closed-ended questions can be used to double check for the presence of symptoms that may indicate poor control or complications due to the disease or medication regimen.

The A1C is the primary test used to evaluate disease control because it is a measure of average blood glucose over a 3-month period (Table 20.6). In interpreting the A1C, the last month represents half of the value and months 1 and 2 the other half. The target A1C is less than 7%. However, like with hypertension and dyslipidemia there is little difference between an A1C of 6.9 and 7.2 and pharmacists should be slow to add medications for small changes in A1C. Recent studies show that aggressive target values for glucose control, hypertension, and hyperlipidemia do not further reduce morbidity and mortality and in some cases negatively affect overall outcomes. The vast majority of benefit in preventing complications occurs at A1C levels below 8.0% so while achieving target A1C is important, it does not require heroic effort or instant change. Fatigue and nocturia are common symptoms of hyperglycemia that should lessen as A1C levels near target. Urinary tract infections, vulvovaginal candidiasis, candidal balanitis, and candidal rashes may also be symptoms of excess blood glucose. Some experts recommend that in addition to an A1C <7%, fasting or preprandial plasma glucose levels of 70 to 130 mg/dL should be an additional goal. Other experts, based on evidence that high postprandial glucose levels are the most damaging, suggest using 2-hour postprandial plasma glucose levels of less than 140 mg/dL as an additional goal.

While objective monitoring parameters for blood glucose control are well established, and therapy with medication, diet, and exercise consistently lower blood glucose levels, the same cannot be said of weight. Patients with Type 2 diabetes mellitus, who are treated with insulin or sulfonylureas, probably will all gain weight, even though the control of their diabetes improves!! While the exact mechanism is unknown, it can be problematic in that it is thought to potentially increase cardiovascular disease risk. More importantly, it is very frustrating to patients who have been told that the key to diabetes control is to lose weight. This patient frustration can negatively impact regimen adherence and eventually disease control. Metformin, by an unknown mechanism, largely prevents this therapy-induced weight gain, which averages 5 to 10 lb. In general, the higher the A1C, and the more aggressive the blood glucose lowering, the larger the weight gain. Part of the rationale in the new guidelines for using metformin as the initial agent in all patients with Type 2 diabetes mellitus is that if sulfonylureas or insulin must be added for better disease control at a later date, the metformin will prevent or lessen that weight gain. In addition, lowering plasma glucose levels more gradually seems to lessen the weight gain.

While self blood glucose monitoring (SBGM) has been the subject of much discussion in patients with Type 2 diabetes, there are some definite benefits for patients, particularly early in therapy. Two-hour postprandial readings along with a food diary can be used to help educate patients regarding the impact of types and portions of various foods on blood glucose levels. Some recommend the SBGM plus food diary along with nutrition consultation as the only activity for the first 2 weeks in newly diagnosed asymptomatic patients to reinforce the effects of diet on diabetes control. The effect of exercise on blood glucose can be determined by having the patient test blood glucose immediately after exercise and one hour-later. This is particularly important in patients on medications that may cause hypoglycemia. Some patients may choose a basal-bolus insulin regimen, where bolus doses are calculated based on carbohydrate intake and requires testing several times a day. Finally, SBGM has been shown to improve adherence with the therapeutic regimen. Once daily SBGM, with varying times of fasting, preprandial and 2-hour postprandial testing each day, can give the patient and the provider information that may assist in a more accurate adjustment of diet, exercise, and medication, while minimizing the testing burden.

While many of the commonly used medications today rarely cause hypoglycemia, all patients should be educated in the recognition of signs and symptoms of hypoglycemia and its treatment. Symptoms of hypoglycemia include those caused primarily by the body's release of catecholamines in an attempt to raise blood glucose by glycogenolysis. Catecholamines and low blood glucose levels combine to cause behavioral changes ranging from light headedness or agitation to semiconscious or unconscious states (Table 20.7).

In addition to evaluating the control of the patient's diabetes, adherence to all aspects of the therapeutic regimen is evaluated, including diet, exercise, and medications. Finally, each follow-up visit should evaluate the presence and progression of complications due to the disease and drug therapy (Table 20.5). All patients require ophthalmoscopic examination, diabetic foot examination, and microalbuminuria testing annually. A brief diabetic foot examination should be done at each provider

TABLE 20.7	Signs and Symptoms of Hypoglycemia
Sympathomimetic Symptoms	
Shakiness, trembling	
Sweating, chills, clamminess	
Rapid heartbeat/palpitations	
Blurred/impaired vision	
Behavioral Changes	
Nervousness/anxiety	
Anger, stubbornness, sadness	
Irritability/impatience	
Confusion/delirium	
Light headed/dizziness	
Drowsy/sleepy	
Miscellaneous	
Hunger, nausea	
Headaches	
Paresthesias	
Weakness/fatigue	

visit. In between annual examinations, responses to questions at follow-up visits about vision, neuropathy, and other complications will determine the need for more frequent evaluations. Once the first signs of neuropathy, nephropathy, and/or retinopathy are detected, evaluation and follow-up by the appropriate specialist is recommended, in addition to follow-up visits for routine care of diabetes mellitus. Similarly, routine dental care is important since high blood glucose levels increase the incidence of periodontal disease. Finally, most patients with Type 2 diabetes mellitus also have the metabolic syndrome and comorbid diseases of dyslipidemia and hypertension. Many of the questions and tests listed in Table 20.5 for complications of diabetes also apply to hypertension and dyslipidemia. For specific subjective and objective disease and medication monitoring parameters for comorbid disease, see Chapters 18 and 19.

• KEY REFERENCES

1. Anon. Standards of medical care in diabetes-2014. *Diabetes Care*. 2014;37(suppl 1):S14-S80.
2. Anon. Diagnosis and classification of diabetes mellitus. *Diabetes Care*. 2014;37(suppl 1):S81-S90.
3. Haas L, Marynuik M, Beck J, et al. National standards for diabetes self-management education and support. *Diabetes Care*. 2014;37(suppl 1):S144-S153.
4. Boulton AJM, Armstrong DG, Albert SF, et al. Comprehensive foot examination and risk assessment. *Diabetes Care*. 2008;31:1679-1685.
5. Seaquist ER, Anderson J, Childs B, et al. Hypoglycemia and diabetes: a report of a work group of the American Diabetes Association and Endocrine Society. *J Clin Endocrinol Metab*. 2013;98:1845-1859.
6. Blevins T. Control of postprandial glucose levels with insulin in type2 diabetes. *Postgrad Med*. 2011;123:135-147.
7. Russell-Jones D, Kahn R. Insulin associated weight gain in diabetes, causes effects and coping strategies. *Diabetes Obes Metab*. 2007;9:799-812.

CASE 20.1

You are working in the VA refill clinic and Kyle Maloney, a 67-year-old Korean War veteran, comes to the pharmacy to get refills on all his chronic medications for diabetes, cholesterol, and blood pressure. He missed his doctor's appointment this week because they could not get his old 1956 Thunderbird "Betsy" started. He needs enough to last until his next physician visit in 6 weeks. A review of his computerized medical record reveals the following medications and the results of the lab tests he had drawn last week for the missed appointment.

Medications	Lab Test Results	
Metformin	A1C	7.2%
500 mg bid	Microalbuminuria	70 mg/L
	Creat	1.1
Atorvastatin	Tot Chol	232
20 mg q hs	LDL	148
	HDL	46
	TG	126

HCTZ 25 mg q AM
Enalapril 20 mg q AM 10 mg q PM
The clinic nurse vital signs are as follows:

BP: 170/98	Weight: 210 (up 10 lb)	T/P/R: 98.6/80/14

a. Based on this information evaluate the level of control for all three disorders. Explain your rationale.

b. For each of the three diseases list three questions or physical examinations you would conduct to evaluate the level of disease control and/or the presence of disease complications.

Asthma and Chronic Obstructive Pulmonary Disease (COPD)

1. Identify appropriate standards for the diagnosis of asthma and COPD.

2. Use available parameters to measure and monitor target goals for patients being treated for asthma and COPD.

3. Conduct a comprehensive follow-up visit for a patient with asthma or COPD using appropriate history-taking techniques, physical examination, and laboratory tests. The visit includes assessment of disease control, plus assessment and support of compliance with lifestyle modifications and medication regimens.

4. Evaluate patients for complications from asthma, COPD, and the medication regimen used to treat them.

• INTRODUCTION

Roughly 12% of the population of the United States suffers from either asthma or COPD, at an economic cost of over $100 billion annually. COPD is the third leading cause of death in the United States. As with other chronic diseases, pharmacists can play an important role in assisting patients to optimize the benefits from their medication regimen. The pharmacist, either as part of a health care delivery team or in pharmacist-run asthma or COPD disease management programs, has been shown to have a positive clinical and economic benefit on patient outcomes. Since medication is the primary therapeutic modality, pharmacists need to understand the diagnosis, pathophysiology, and treatment of these diseases since patients may attempt self-care of these disorders, require education for proper medication use, or may rely on the pharmacist to help them manage their disease.

• ETIOLOGY/PATHOPHYSIOLOGY/EPIDEMIOLOGY

While both asthma and COPD have major small airway disease components with inflammation and increased airway resistance, they have different etiologies, characteristics, and outcomes (see Table 21.1).

Asthma

Asthma affects patients of all ages. Over 25% of the 25.9 million patients with asthma are children. Asthma is a chronic inflammatory disease of the airways. The inflammation causes airway hyperresponsiveness to various stimuli, leading to bronchospasm, which manifests itself as coughing in the early morning hours, wheezing, breathlessness, and chest tightness. The inflammation also causes airway obstruction that limits airflow that can be reversed with treatment. Long-term untreated disease can lead to airway remodeling that may not be completely reversible. Initially, the pathogenesis was thought to be exclusively due to IgE-mediated reactions involving eosinophils. However, while eosinophilis and IgE are still important elements in the pathogenesis of asthma, over the last several years evidence has shown asthma to be a heterogeneous disease. Different patterns of inflammatory processes that involve multiple cellular mechanisms, result in different disease intensity and varying response to

TABLE 21.1	Differences Between Asthma and COPD	
	Asthma	*COPD*
Bronchospasm	Primary feature	No unless concurrent asthma
Immunology	Eosinophil/IgE mediated	Neutrophil/protease mediated
Cause	Aeroallergens	History of cigarette smoking
Age of onset	Usually childhood/adolescent	Over 40, usually in 50s or 60s
Comorbidities	Allergic rhinitis, atopic dermatitis	Cardiovascular disease, lung cancer, and heart failure
Lung auscultation findings	Expiratory wheezes	Rhonchi, crackles
Symptoms with adequate treatment	Intermittent	Constant and progressively worsen
Changes in lung structure	Some airway remodeling in severe uncontrolled disease	Destruction of alveoli
Reversibility	Yes	Little or none
Acute exacerbations	Yes	Yes
Cough	Usually dry	Productive, if present

guideline-based treatments. Currently, the development of asthma is thought to be due to an interaction among innate immunity, a complex genetic component, and environmental factors, including respiratory syncytial virus, rhinovirus, and airborne allergens. Recent evidence also shows that this process impedes the normal epithelial cell barrier (like atopic dermatitis), which allows antigens to pass into local tissue to create the interaction between the three major pathogenic components. In patients with stable, well-controlled asthma, exacerbations are mostly due to rhinovirus infections. Allergen concentration, suboptimal medication adherence, and other triggering substances or medications are also responsible for exacerbations in poorly controlled asthma.

COPD

While airway inflammation is a major component of COPD, the process is totally different than with asthma. Cigarette smoke and other toxins, e.g., indoor (smoke from burning wood) and outdoor air pollution are the primary causative agents in COPD. These noxious toxins stimulate the release of proteases from neutrophils, which cause alveolar wall destruction (emphysema), mucous hypersecretion (chronic bronchitis), and fibrosis of lung tissue. This process accelerates the normal age-related annual rate of loss of lung function by threefold. Unfortunately, the lung damage is irreversible. Even when exposure to the noxious substance (cigarette smoke) ceases, the accelerated loss of lung function only returns to normal age-related rates of decline. Therefore, in the patient who quits smoking after being diagnosed with COPD, the disease will continue to worsen albeit at a slower, normal rate rather than the accelerated rate induced by smoking. There is a genetic component since only 25% of heavy smokers go on to develop COPD. Historically, COPD occurred primarily in men, because they more frequently smoked than women. Today, with the rise in the number of women who smoke, the incidence of COPD is roughly equally divided between men and women. In addition to losing lung function, exacerbations of COPD are both a clinical and economic burden. Exacerbations of COPD are defined as increased dyspnea for two consecutive days. Triggers for exacerbation include bacterial and viral respiratory tract infections, environmental pollutants, and unknown causes. Some patients have asthma in addition to COPD (asthmatics who smoke) and treatment of these patients involves anti-inflammatory drug therapy used in asthma patients.

• DIAGNOSIS

Spirometry

Spirometry, also known as pulmonary function testing (PFTs), is the major objective measurement of lung function used in the diagnosis of asthma and COPD. Portable instruments are available for office use and procedures have long been standardized. The patient takes a deep breath and blows into the machine as hard and fast as they can for as long as they can. This is repeated several times and if the results are similar, the machine calculates several values. Once initial values are established, two puffs of a short-acting bronchodilator are administered and PFTs are repeated 10 to 20 minutes later. The most important values are the forced expiratory volume during the first second (FEV_1) and the forced vital capacity (FVC), the total amount of air exhaled during the test. Both values vary with gender, age, and height. Both FEV_1 and FVC peak at about 20 to 25 years of age and at approximately 35 years of age begin to slowly decline. The normal annual rate of loss increases with age starting out at 10 to 15 cc/year at 35 and increasing to nearly 60 cc/year by age 70. Changes between the prebronchodilator and postbronchodilator values determine the reversibility and are used to confirm the diagnosis of concurrent asthma.

Asthma

A careful history is required as part of a workup for asthma. Key symptoms include recurrent bouts of wheezing, difficulty breathing, and chest tightness. Some patients' symptoms may manifest themselves primarily as cough during exercise or between 2 and 6 AM, when lung vital capacity is at its lowest due to circadian variation. Identifying situations that precipitate or aggravate symptoms provides important diagnostic clues. Exercise, viral infection, exposure to inhaled allergens, e.g., cat or dog dander, pollen, etc., all can trigger or worsen symptoms. Symptoms that occur or worsen at night, awakening the patient, are common in asthma. Coughing episodes between 2 and 6 AM are almost diagnostic in children. Finally, a personal history of allergic rhinitis or atopic dermatitis is a common finding in patients with asthma, as is a history of asthma, allergic rhinitis, and atopic dermatitis in a direct blood relative. Many patients with asthma also have allergic rhinitis and symptoms of asthma may worsen with exacerbation of allergic rhinitis symptoms. Findings during physical examination can include expiratory wheezing during auscultation of the lungs. However, many times the patients have a normal chest examination. Careful examination of the cubital and popliteal fossa (the hollow of the elbow and knee respectively) for the eczematous rash of atopic dermatitis and an ENT examination for signs of allergic rhinitis (e.g., allergic shiners, nasal crease, Dennie's lines, and pale boggy nasal mucosa, with a thin watery nasal discharge) are important. Lung function needs to be evaluated by spirometry both pre- and postbronchodilator. After baseline values are established, the patient is given two puffs of albuterol by metered dose inhaler (MDI). FEV_1 values should increase by at least 12% 10 to 20 minutes after bronchodilator administration to establish the reversibility of bronchoconstriction that is diagnostic of asthma. Fractional nitric oxide (NO) concentration in exhaled breath (FE_{NO}) is also used as an aid to diagnosis. In classical asthma, sputum eosinophilia and IgE are markers of airway inflammation. Since eosinophils cause the production of NO, the degree of inflammation can be assessed by the amount of NO exhaled. Greater than 50 parts/billion (ppb) (>35 ppb in children) is diagnostic of asthma. However, since the nature of asthma is heterogeneous regarding pathogenesis, some patients will have low NO levels because their asthma is not the predominant type (eosinophilia, plus IgE mediated). However, elevated FE_{NO} levels will predict the likelihood of response to inhaled corticosteroids and can be used for monitoring therapy effectiveness, adjusting doses, confirming medication adherence problems, and identifying suboptimal inhaler technique.

COPD

In patients over 40 years of age, COPD should be suspected with any of the following: history of difficulty breathing (dyspnea) that has tended to worsen over time or worsen with exercise, chronic cough with productive sputum, history of cigarette smoking, or a family history of COPD. However, there are exceptions to the classical pattern listed above. Some patients will not identify difficulty in breathing, but will instead talk about not being able to walk very far without their legs getting tired or heavy. Similarly, a cough may be absent, intermittent or non-productive or be dismissed as an expected consequence of smoking. Patients may have had no exposure to cigarettes, but have regular exposure to wood smoke or industrial or occupational pollutants. Patients need not be current smokers, but usually have a long history of cigarette smoking, which greatly accelerates lung function loss. A history concerning the frequency of possible COPD exacerbations needs to be done. Unfortunately, patients may not recognize them, so questioning should include a history of hospitalizations for respiratory disorders, treatment of lower respiratory disorders with antibiotics, corticosteroids or inhalers, and colds that "go to the chest" and/or "last forever." Physical examination in many cases is normal. In patients with a productive cough, rhonchi or crackles can be heard on auscultation of the lungs. Rhonchi are heard in both inspiration and expiration. They have a low-pitched snoring, gurgling, rattle-like quality. Rhonchi represent secretions/mucous in large airways, and leaving the stethoscope in place and having the patient cough will cause the rhonchi to disappear or drastically change. In addition, breath sounds may be decreased due to destruction of lung tissue and air trapping. In patients with more advanced COPD, the patient will have tachypnea and tachycardia and the pulse oximetry may be less than 92% on room air. In patients with severe and long-standing disease, patients will not be able to speak in complete sentences without taking a breath and may have unusually prominent sternocleidomastoid muscles (in the neck) during each inspiration. Spirometry again establishes airflow limitations and the diagnosis. In COPD, postbronchodilator the FEV_1/FVC is less than 0.70 and the lower the FEV_1, the more severe the COPD. There are standardized questionnaires to measure functional dyspnea severity, such as the Modified Medical Research Council scale (mMRC) and the COPD Assessment Test (CAT). The mMRC uses the degree of breathlessness related to physical activities such as dressing and walking uphill. The CAT uses a 6-point scale and 8 statements regarding the extent of cough, congestion, tightness, breathlessness with exercise, sleep quality, and energy levels. Both are more predictive than FEV_1 alone in predicting mortality.

• CLASSIFICATION

Both asthma and COPD have classification systems based on severity of symptoms and spirometry values that are primarily intended to guide therapy.

Asthma

The asthma classification system distinguishes between intermittent asthma and persistent asthma based on symptoms, nighttime awakenings, interference with normal activity, and the frequency of use of short-acting β-adrenergic inhalers (SABA) and FEV_1 using a peak flowmeter. See the National Asthma Education and Prevention Program's *Expert Panel Report 3 (EPR-3) Guidelines for the Diagnosis and Management of Asthma* for specific details by age. Intermittent asthma is characterized by no more than two episodes of symptoms/week, no more than two episodes/month of nighttime awakenings, SABA use no more than two times/week, no interference with normal activities, and a normal FEV_1 between exacerbations. Persistent asthma is divided into mild, moderate, and severe based on those same parameters. Each level of severity is tied to a specific intensity of treatment.

COPD

The classification system for COPD is international and is composed of three parts: objective airflow limitations, symptoms, and risk of future exacerbations. The first is based on postbronchodilator FEV_1 values with four levels of severity in patients with FEV_1/FVC <0.70, with mild or level one having an FEV_1 greater than or equal to 80% of predicted value, ranging to the fourth level where the FEV_1 is less than 30% of predicted value. Second is a measure of the severity of functional dyspnea using the mMRC or CAT. The third part is the frequency of COPD exacerbations/year. These three parts are combined into an ABCD classification system that is tied to recommended treatment regimens. For specific details, see the Global Initiative for Chronic Obstructive Lung

Disease's (GOLD) *Global Strategy for the Diagnosis, Management and Prevention of Chronic Obstructive Pulmonary Disease: GOLD Executive Summary.*

• COMPLICATIONS

Asthma

Over 3000 people die every year from asthma, and in 7000 additional deaths asthma was a contributing factor. The primary complication of asthma is respiratory failure from acute asthma attacks. The goal of asthma treatment is to prevent these acute attacks by controlling the inflammation with inhaled corticosteroids or drugs that interfere with the effects of leukotrienes and other mediators. Acute asthma attacks due to poorly controlled asthma were the cause of nearly 500,000 hospitalizations and 20 million emergency room visits in 2012. Viral respiratory tract infections are the most common precipitant of an acute asthma attack. Other common causes include exposure to known allergens or triggers of asthma attacks, inadequate use or dose of inhaled corticosteroids, lack of objective monitoring criteria (lack of an asthma action plan). Some patients, especially those with severe asthma, may have a blunted perception of worsening bronchospasm. Peak expiratory flow (PEFR) monitoring with a handheld peak flowmeter, which approximates FEV_1, helps those patients better assess the presence of acute asthma attacks. Most acute asthma attacks respond to standard treatments of intense bronchodilation and hydration. When an acute attack fails to respond to standard therapy, the term status asthmaticus may be used. This is the most difficult form of asthma to treat. Table 21.2 lists subjective and objective parameters that indicate severe acute asthma attacks similar to status asthmaticus.

COPD

The primary cause of death in COPD is respiratory failure either due to chronic deterioration or acute respiratory failure brought on by bacterial or viral pneumonia, which markedly reduces the already severely limited capacity of the lungs. In addition, the years of smoking predisposes patients to cardiovascular disease, e.g., coronary artery disease and stroke. In addition, severe hypoxia poses a risk for fatal

TABLE 21.2	Danger Signs During Acute Asthma Attacks

SUBJECTIVE

Dyspnea at rest
Confusion, obtundation (indication for intubation)
Agitation
Slow or little response to intense bronchodilator treatment

OBJECTIVE

Failure of Asthma Action Plan treatment
Bilateral wheezing on expiration and inhalation
No wheezing in exhausted patients indicates impending respiratory failure
Inability to talk in complete sentences without taking a breath
Use of ancillary respiratory muscles in the neck and chest to assist breathing
Respiratory rate >30/min
Pulse oximetry <90% on room air
Tachycardia >110/ min
Peak expiratory flow rate (PEFR) <50% expected or personal best
Respiratory or mixed acidosis
Partial pressure of O_2 <60 mm Hg

cardiac dysrhythmias. Finally, the smoking markedly increases the risk for lung cancer. Unfortunately, by the time of COPD diagnosis most patients are past middle age and already have symptoms due to the threefold rate of loss of pulmonary function due to the smoking-induced inflammatory process. While the rate of loss of pulmonary function returns to the normal rate after smoking cessation, lung function continues to deteriorate, but at a slower normal rate. Unfortunately, treatment cannot reverse the damage in susceptible people. For people with the most severe disease, Group C and D (GOLD 3 and 4), there are several integrated disease severity indexes that can be used to predict 3-year mortality risk. The first is the BODE index. Parameters of the BODE index include BMI, obstruction of airflow (FEV_1), dyspnea measured via the mMRC, and exercise capacity (6-minute walk test). The second is simpler, the ADO index, where age, dyspnea, and obstruction of airflow (FEV_1) are used.

• INITIAL VISIT

For both asthma and COPD, the initial visit workup consists of several parts. First the diagnosis needs to be confirmed (see "Diagnosis"). Second, the severity of the disease needs to be classified to determine appropriate initial therapy, which entails a history of exacerbations for COPD and aggravating or precipitating factors in asthma. Third, the psychosociological aspects of the disease and support structure for treatment and control of the disease needs to be ascertained, including any potential adherence barriers or issues. Finally, a history and physical examination should be done to ascertain the presence of comorbid conditions that may impact overall health and adjustment of therapy for asthma or COPD, such as cardiovascular disease in COPD or atopic dermatitis and allergic rhinitis in asthma. See Key References 1 and 10 for specific details of initial visit workups.

• FOLLOW-UP VISITS

Like any chronic disease, follow-up visits for asthma and COPD are an important part of optimizing disease control and preventing complications. In asthma, ideally we want to prevent acute attacks and prevent symptoms that may indicate uncontrolled bronchospasm. However, due to the difficulty posed by normal variation of exposure to aeroallergens and other triggers of asthma symptoms, national guidelines recommended a more pragmatic approach to define well-controlled asthma. Five basic parameters are used including frequency of symptoms (cough, chest tightness, etc.), nighttime awakenings, use of rescue inhalers such as albuterol, FEV_1 (PEFR), and limitations on activities caused by asthma. Well-controlled asthma is defined as symptoms no more than 2 days per week, nighttime awakenings no more than two times per month, no limitations of activities due to asthma, use of rescue inhalers no more than 2 days per week, and a peak expiratory flow reading (PEFR) of more than 80% of predicted value or in more severe forms of asthma the patient's personal best (when they are well controlled). Other organizations have tried to simplify that definition by using a "rule of 2s." Asthma is not well controlled if you use a rescue inhaler more than two times a week, have more than two episodes of nighttime symptoms per month, or refill the rescue inhaler more than two times a year. There are self-administered validated instruments that are based on the definition of well controlled that can be used to assist in assessment, including the Asthma Control Test (ACT), the Asthma Control Questionnaire (ACQ), and the Asthma Therapy Assessment Questionnaire (ATAQ). A comprehensive list of subjective and objective data that needs to be collected at each follow-up visit can be found in Table 21.3. Obviously any responses that indicate poor control need to be

TABLE 21.3	Follow-Up Visit Parameters for Asthma

CONTROL

S   HOW HAVE THINGS BEEN GOING WITH YOUR ASTHMA SINCE YOUR LAST VISIT?
Rescue inhaler use
   How many days have you used your rescue inhaler since the last visit?
   How many times every day do you use your rescue inhaler?
   What time of the day do you use your rescue inhaler?
Acute attacks
   How many asthma attacks have you had since your last visit?
   How many visits to the ER/Urgent Care have you had since your last visit?
   What do you think caused each acute attack?
Self-management
   What have your PEFR readings been since your last visit?
   How many times have your PEFR readings been in the yellow or red zone since your last visit?
   What have you done each time?
Medication efficacy
   How is your medication working?
   How well is the self-management plan working to treat your acute attacks?
Trigger exposure
   What kind of changes have there been in your exposure to potential triggers at home and at work?
Closed-ended questions regarding symptoms
   Have you had any of the following since your last visit?

Wheezing?	*Chest tightness?*	*Shortness of breath?*
Coughing?	*Coughing at night?*	*Coughing with exercise?*
Runny/stuffy nose?	*Itching skin/rash?*	*Awaken at night due to cough/dyspnea?*
Decreased ability to do normal activities?		*Heartburn?*
Exposure to animals/dust/pollens/ other triggers?		

O   Auscultate lungs
   Listen for expiratory wheezes
Observe
   Respiratory rate >20/min
   Ability to speak in complete sentences
   Ancillary muscle use during breathing
   Cough rate/type
Measure
   Peak flow/other PFT
   Oxygenation (blood gases or pulse oximetry)
   Change in peak flow after bronchodilator

COMPLIANCE

S   WHAT KIND OF PROBLEMS ARE YOU HAVING REMEMBERING TO TAKE YOUR MEDICATION?
Probe-specific compliance problems
   How often does it happen?
   When was the last time it happened?
   What do you think caused you to miss a dose?
Probe asthma-specific issues
   How are you using your corticosteroid inhaler?
   Does the inhaler make you cough? If so, what do you do about it?
   Confirm spacer use/post-inhalation mouth rinse.
Nonpharmacological interventions
   What things are you doing to reduce your exposure to _____ (patient specific trigger)?
   How are measures to reduce _____ (patient-specific trigger) exposure going?

O   *Check refill rate from patient profile.*
   Have patient demonstrate inhaler/peak flowmeter technique.

TABLE 21.3	Follow-Up Visit Parameters for Asthma (*Continued*)

COMPLICATIONS

S WHAT KIND OF PROBLEMS HAVE YOU BEEN HAVING SINCE YOUR LAST VISIT?
Disease complications
    Productive cough?
    Fever?
Drug-related complications
    Sores in mouth? **difficulty swallowing, hoarseness (inhaled corticosteroids)**
    Trembling? Nervousness? Palpitations? **(β-adrenergic bronchodilators)**

O Disease complications
    Same things as for asthma control, plus
    Take temperature
    Observe sputum characteristics
Drug-related complications
    Tachycardia due to rescue inhaler overuse
    Oral examination for thrush
    Hand tremors upon extension of arms due to rescue inhaler overuse

probed in depth, including when, why, and what, to get specific details that may aid in determining changes in pharmacological or nonpharmacological therapy.

One of the psychological problems in patients with asthma is the anguish of being unable to breath and the sense of no control over symptoms when they occur. Also patients may be unsure what symptoms are an indication of a need for additional care. In the past, these three factors caused visits to the emergency room that did not match the degree of clinical impairment. Eventually asthma action plans were developed and are now required for each patient. The purpose of the asthma action plan is to allow the self-treatment of minor attacks with asthma medication and provide criteria for assessing the severity of the attack, to determine the need for an emergency room visit or call to the physician. The plan is based on PEFR readings. Patients are told to obtain a PEFR upon awakening (because FVC is at its lowest between 2 and 6 AM) and whenever they notice asthma symptoms. Generally, if the PEFR is 80% of predicted/personal best or higher (in the "green zone" or good zone), then nothing additional needs to be done other than continuing to take their long-term control medicine and avoiding triggers. If the readings are in the "yellow zone" (50% to 80% of predicted/personal best), specific directions on using short-acting bronchodilators are indicated. Also, patients are instructed to wait for a certain amount of time to allow the bronchodilator to work, then repeat the PEFR. If the PEFR is back in the green zone (>80%), then nothing else needs to be done. If after treatment the PEFR is still in the yellow zone, patient-specific instructions for the next step are listed, e.g., repeat bronchodilator treatment, go to the emergency room, or call the physician. If any reading is less than 50% of predicted or personal best, it is in the "red zone." The asthma action plan has instructions for patients in the red zone to go to the emergency room immediately. The directions for what to do if the patient has a yellow zone reading is individualized for each patient. Also, the boundaries of PEFR for each zone can be individualized based on the severity of the disease and the sophistication and comfort of the patient with self-care of acute asthma attacks. Self-management of asthma symptoms using an asthma action plan improves disease control and medication adherence. In addition, asthma action plans significantly reduce the frequency of emergency room visits, and markedly enhance the patient's sense of control of their asthma and satisfaction with asthma care.

One thing that should be checked regularly at each routine visit for both asthma and COPD is proper inhaler use. Multiple studies show that more than 90% of patients make at least one error in technique even though they felt they knew how to correctly use their inhalers. Unfortunately, each type of inhaler has its own specific technique. If unsure about proper technique, there are excellent videos available via the Internet. National Jewish Health, world renown for their care of patients with respiratory disease, has an excellent set of instructional videos, for each type of device, posted on You-Tube and available on their web site (http://www.nationaljewish.org/healthinfo/medications/lung-diseases/devices/instructional-videos).

In COPD, the main goal is to relieve dyspnea as much as possible with long-acting bronchodilators and oxygen, and to reduce the numbers of exacerbations. Since smoking is the primary cause of COPD, smoking cessation is the only treatment that will slow the rate of loss of lung function. In nonsmokers, the avoidance of the noxious substances functions like smoking cessation. Questions regarding changes in exercise capacity or ability to do routine activities are a measure of the severity of dyspnea. A comprehensive list of subjective and objective data that needs to be collected at each follow-up visit for COPD can be found in Table 21.4. While not suggested by guidelines, some providers use COPD action plans that are similar in structure, design and purpose to asthma action plans. Signs and symptoms of COPD exacerbations are acute in nature and differ from normal variation and include increased dyspnea, increased sputum volume, worsening tachycardia/tachypnea, and/or increased sputum purulence. In severe forms of both asthma and COPD, hypoxia from the disease can cause several changes in breathing patterns. Signs include an elevated respiratory

TABLE 21.4	Follow-Up Visit Parameters for COPD

CONTROL

S   HOW HAVE THINGS BEEN GOING WITH YOUR COPD SINCE YOUR LAST VISIT?
     Symptoms
         How many days of work have you missed since your last visit?
         What changes have you noticed in your ability to do routine activities or exercise since your last visit?
         What changes in your coughing have occurred since the last visit?
     Exacerbations
         How many COPD exacerbations have you had since your last visit?
         What did you do about it?
         What do you think caused each exacerbation?
     Medication efficacy
         How is your medication working?
     Trigger exposure
         What kind of changes have there been in your exposure to potential triggers at home and at work?
         What is your smoking status?
     Closed-ended questions regarding symptoms
         Have you had any of the following since your last visit?
         Wheezing?   *Chest tightness?*
         Changes in shortness of breath?
         Runny/stuffy nose?

O   Auscultate lungs
         Listen for rhonchi, crackles, decreased breath sounds
     Observe
         Respiratory rate, temperature, pulse
         Ability to speak in complete sentences
         Ancillary muscle use during breathing
         Cough rate/type
     Measure
         Oxygenation (blood gases or pulse oximetry)
         BODE/ADO index depending on severity

TABLE 21.4	Follow-Up Visit Parameters for COPD (*Continued*)

COMPLIANCE

S WHAT KIND OF PROBLEMS ARE YOU HAVING REMEMBERING TO TAKE YOUR MEDICATION?
Probe-specific compliance problems
How often does it happen?
When was the last time it happened?
What do you think caused you to miss a dose?
Nonpharmacological interventions
What kind of problems do you have remembering to do your breathing exercises?
How frequently do you use your oxygen? How long each time?
What kind of problems are you having with your oxygen?

O *Check refill rate from patient profile.*
Have patient demonstrate inhaler/peak flowmeter technique.

COMPLICATIONS

S WHAT KIND OF PROBLEMS HAVE YOU BEEN HAVING SINCE YOUR LAST VISIT?
Disease complications
Productive cough? Change in sputum?
Fever?
Drug-related complications
Sores in mouth? **difficulty swallowing, hoarseness (inhaled corticosteroids)**
Trembling? Nervousness? **(albuterol, salmeterol, formoterol, indacaterol, arformoterol)**
Coughing after inhaler use? **(all)**
Problems urinating? Constipation? Dry mouth? **(tiotropium, ipratropium, aclidinium)**
Palpitations? **(albuterol, salmeterol, formoterol, indacaterol, arformoterol)**

O Disease complications
Same things as for COPD control, plus
Fever?
Observe sputum characteristics (volume/purulence).
Drug-related complications
Tachycardia due to excess bronchodilator use
Oral examination for thrush
Hand tremors upon extension of arms due to excess adrenergic bronchodilator use

rate (>20 breaths/minute), inability to speak in complete sentences without taking a breath, and the contraction of ancillary muscles of respiration in the neck when breathing. In severe COPD, the sternocleidomastoid muscles enlarge due to regular use and in slender patients, protrude even when not taking a breath. Finally, pulse oximetry values less than 91% on room air are abnormally low, but are not uncommon.

• KEY REFERENCES

1. Anon. Expert Panel Report 3 (EPR-3): guidelines for the diagnosis and treatment of asthma summary report 2007. *J Allergy Clin Immunol.* 2007;120:S93-S138.
2. Self TH, Wallace JL, George CM, Howard-Thompson A, Schrock SD. Inhalation therapy: help patients avoid these mistakes. *J Fam Pract.* 2011;60:714-721.
3. Sims MW. Aerosol therapy for obstructive lung diseases. *Chest.* 2011;140:781-788.
4. Dweik RA, Boggs PB, Erzurum SC, et al. An official ATS clinical practice guidline: interpretation of exhaled nitric oxide levels (FE_{NO}) for clinical applications. *Am J Respir Crit Care Med.* 2011;184:602-615.
5. Higgins JC. The "crashing asthmatic." *Am Fam Physician.* 2003;67:997-1004.
6. Liou TG, Kanner RE. Spirometry. *Clin Rev Allergy Immunol.* 2009;37:137-152.
7. Celli BR, Cote CG, Marin JM, et al. The body-mass index, airflow obstruction, dyspnea and exercise capacity index in chronic obstructive pulmonary disease. *N Engl J Med.* 2004;350:1005-1012.

8. Puhan MA, Garcia-Aymerich J, Frey M, et al. Expansion of the prognostic assessment of patients with chronic obstructive pulmonary disease: the updated BODE index and the ADO index. *Lancet.* 2009;374:704-711.

9. Rosenberg SR, Kalhan R. An integrated approach to the medical treatment of chronic obstructive pulmonary disease. *Med Clin North Am.* 2012;96:811-826.

10. Vestbo J, Hurd SS, Agusti AG, et al. Global strategy for the diagnosis, management and prevention of chronic obstructive pulmonary disease: GOLD executive summary. *Am J Respir Crit Care Med.* 2013;187:347-365.

CASE 21.1

Howkani Stopwhesin, a 32-year-old asthmatic, comes to your pharmacy for his third visit in your asthma disease management program. Howkani has a peak flow meter, and an asthma action plan. He is on fluticasone inhaler 110 µg/spray, 3 puffs q AM and albuterol, 2 puffs per action plan up to four times a day.

List four questions you would ask and four objective parameters you would check to evaluate the level of control of Howie's asthma. Explain your rationale.

_____

_____

_____

_____

_____

Heart Failure

1. Conduct a comprehensive follow-up visit for a patient with heart failure using appropriate history-taking techniques, physical examination, and laboratory tests. The visit includes assessment of disease control, assessment and support of compliance with lifestyle modifications and medication regimens, plus evaluate patients for complications from the disease and medication regimen.

• INTRODUCTION

Heart failure (HF), also known as congestive or chronic heart failure, is a significant complication of essential hypertension and atherosclerotic cardiovascular disease. In 2010, more than 6 million people had a diagnosis of heart failure. Pharmacists in a primary care or disease management role routinely assist patients in managing their diabetes, hypertension, and dyslipidemia, all contributing factors to the development of heart failure as a complication of their chronic diseases. Therefore, it is important for pharmacists to understand the clinical course and pathophysiology and to be able to identify signs and symptoms of heart failure.

• ETIOLOGY

President Franklin D. Roosevelt suffered from severe hypertension. During World War II, he developed congestive heart failure as a complication of his uncontrolled hypertension and eventually died of a massive stroke. In his time, hypertension was almost the sole cause of congestive heart failure. However, as we developed drugs to treat hypertension and focused on controlling elevated blood pressure, it became apparent that heart failure had multiple causes. While more than three-fourths of all patients with HF have a history of hypertension, it is now known that heart failure is a complex syndrome where any structural or functional cardiac damage can impair the ability of the ventricles to fill with or eject blood. Heart failure is the result of continual overactivation of the sympathetic nervous system, the renin-angiotensin-aldosterone (RAA) system, as well as the release of other neurohormones, such as B-type natriuretic peptide (BNP), all of which contribute to the pathophysiology of heart failure. The terms preload and afterload are frequently used when discussing heart failure and other cardiovascular diseases. Preload is defined as the amount of blood presented to the heart for pumping. Preload is increased in heart failure. Diuretics, a mainstay of the treatment of heart failure, decrease blood volume presented to the heart for pumping and, therefore, decrease preload. Afterload is defined as the amount of peripheral resistance the heart pumps blood against, i.e. arterial hypertension. Afterload is generally increased in heart failure in the form of hypertension. Many antihypertensives decrease afterload through their effects on reducing peripheral resistance caused by the sympathetic and RAA systems. This combination of increased preload and afterload in heart failure causes a cyclical worsening of heart failure. Both the sympathetic and RAA systems cause remodeling of the ventricles, which eventually leads to left ventricular enlargement, and ventricular wall stiffness and reduced cardiac output.

Patients with heart failure are currently classified as having systolic or diastolic cardiac dysfunction based on left ventricular ejection fraction (LVEF). In both types of heart failure, cardiac output is markedly reduced, resulting in decreased perfusion of peripheral tissues and organs. In patients with heart failure with systolic dysfunction or heart failure with reduced ejection fraction (HFREF), the ejection fraction (EF) is <40% (>60% is normal). This represents a left ventricle that is enlarged and weakened to the extent that it cannot empty the ventricle completely. This most closely corresponds to classic congestive heart failure where uncontrolled hypertension causes the left ventricle to hypertrophy and eventually fail. In patients with diastolic dysfunction or heart failure with preserved ejection fraction (HFPEF), the ejection fraction is between 40% and 55%, which represents a stiff heart that has lost its flexibility and cannot completely fill by stretching, leading to a decreased cardiac output. The major cause of diastolic dysfunction in heart failure is coronary artery disease.

TABLE 22.1	Classification and Treatment of Chronic Heart Failure		
ACC/AHA Stage[a]	NYHA Class[b]	Description	Management
A	Prefailure	No symptoms but risk factors present[c]	Treat obesity, hypertension, diabetes, hyperlipidemia, etc.
B	I	Symptoms with severe exercise	ACEI/ARB, β-blocker, diuretic.
C	II/III	Symptoms with marked (class II) or mild (class III) exercise	Add aldosterone antagonist, digoxin; CRT, hydralazine/nitrate[d].
D	IV	Severe symptoms at rest	Transplant, LVAD.

[a]American College of Cardiology/American Heart Association classification.
[b]New York Heart Association classification.
[c]Risk factors include hypertension, myocardial infarct, diabetes.
[d]For selected populations, eg, African American.
ACEI, angiotensin-converting enzyme inhibitor; ARB, angiotensin receptor blocker; CRT, cardiac resynchronization therapy; LVAD, left ventricular assist device.
(Reproduced with permission from Katzung BG, Masters SB, & Trevor AJ (Eds). Basic & Clinical Pharmacology, 12ed. McGraw-Hill, Inc., 2012. Table 13-3.)

The severity of the heart failure can also be classified. ACC/AHA and New York Heart Association Classification Systems break down severity into four major groups based on activity and symptoms (Table 22.1).

• DIAGNOSIS

Subjective findings in heart failure are classical. In heart failure shortness of breath (SOB) is the attempt of the body to compensate for poor perfusion of peripheral tissue (hypoxia), by increasing the rate and depth of respiration. When it occurs during exertion, e.g., walking up stairs or an incline, it is called dyspnea on exertion (DOE). Paroxysmal nocturnal dyspnea (PND) is awakening 2 to 4 hours after lying down, with shortness of breath or coughing. Sitting up or standing up quickly relieves the symptom. During the day the excess fluid retained from heart failure pools in the lower extremities due to gravity and may manifest itself as ankle edema. When the patient lies down flat, this excess fluid redistributes itself into the intravascular space, markedly increasing preload. The failing heart decompensates and the excess fluid leaks into the lung tissue, causing the respiratory symptoms, a mechanism similar to acute pulmonary edema. By sitting or standing, the excess fluid repools in the lower extremities and the heart which now does not have to pump all the excess fluid is able work better and the fluid in the lungs eventually returns to the intravascular space, reliving the respiratory symptoms. Over time and with repeated episodes, patients begin to realize that they sleep better propped up with several pillows or in a recliner. This sleeping propped up is called orthopnea and is quantified by the number of pillows they use, e.g., two- or three-pillow orthopnea. Orthopnea is relieved in patients admitted for heart failure who are initially placed in a semi-Fowler position by elevating the head of hospital bed 30° to reduce the preload and allow them more restful sleep.

There are multiple objective findings in patients with heart failure. The more severe the heart failure, the more physical signs are seen. Crackles or rales on auscultation can be heard in both lung bases. Lower extremity edema in the ankles and feet (pedal edema) is common as are tachycardia and tachypnea as the body tries to compensate for peripheral tissue hypoxia. Many times the point of maximal impulse (PMI) or apical impulse will be displaced laterally and inferiorly indicating an enlarged heart. Other signs only occur in more severe disease such as internal jugular vein distention (JVD), the hepatojugular reflux (HJR), and an S3 gallop rhythm on cardiac auscultation. Chest x-ray and echocardiogram will show an enlarged heart and fluid in the lungs. An

TABLE 22.2	Framingham Clinical Diagnostic Criteria for Congestive Heart Failure
Major Criteria	**Minor Criteria**
Paroxysmal nocturnal dyspnea (PND) or orthopnea	Ankle edema
Neck vein distension	Nocturnal cough
Crackles/rales	Dyspnea on exertion (DOE)
Cardiomegaly	Hepatomegaly
Acute pulmonary edema	Pleural effusion
S3 gallop	Tachycardia (>120/min)
Hepatojugular reflux	

electrocardiogram may show left ventricular hypertrophy and left axis deviation. Renal function tests (serum creatinine and blood urea nitrogen) may be elevated due to poor kidney perfusion. Likewise venous congestion in the liver can cause elevated serum AST and ALT levels. These lab values return to normal after heart failure is treated and kidney perfusion improves and excessive preload is reduced. There are clinical diagnostic criteria for heart failure. The best known are the Framingham criteria seen in Table 22.2. Definite diagnosis of heart failure requires the presence of two major criteria or one major criterion plus two minor criteria provided other causes have been ruled out. One major new diagnostic test has been added to the array of tests used to confirm heart failure. B-type natriuretic peptide (brain natriuretic peptide or BNP) is released as a response to the degrees of ventricular stretch and ventricular dilation to help the heart compensate by its action to excrete fluid, sodium, and potassium. At levels >100 pg/mL, BNP has a sensitivity of 90% and a specificity of 73%. Levels above 100 pg/mL are diagnostic of heart failure in nonobese patients. BNP levels are particularly useful to rule out heart failure as a cause of dyspnea or to confirm heart failure in patients with marginal criteria for a clinical diagnosis. BNP also has prognostic value. Each 100 pg/mL increase in BNP is associated with a 35% increase in the relative risk of death. Also, in patients discharged from the hospital, a 46% reduction from admissions levels along with a value <300 pg/mL provided significant reductions in morbidity and mortality. NT pro-BNP, the precursor to BNP can also be used but it has different target and diagnostic values.

• MONITORING AT FOLLOW-UP VISITS

Treatment of heart failure is directed at reducing both preload and afterload, primarily through interfering with neurohormonal manifestations. Diuretics, usually loop diuretics, are the initial treatment of choice to remove excess fluid. Next, either an angiotensin-converting-enzyme inhibitor (ACEI) or an angiotensin-receptor blocker (ARB) decreases afterload and ameliorates ventricular remodeling caused by angiotensin. Higher rather than lower doses are preferred. β-Blockers reduce the negative effects of excessive sympathetic activity. The dose of β-blockers must be carefully titrated upward, beginning with low doses to prevent blocking of necessary sympathetic activity and worsening the heart failure. Aldosterone antagonists, such as spironolactone, improve survival and prevent myocardial fibrosis associated with heart failure. These four medications all improve both the morbidity and mortality in systolic dysfunction, but are significantly less effective in diastolic dysfunction where diuretics are the primary therapy. Digoxin, once the mainstay of HF treatment, is now relegated to use as a 5th agent in patients who fail to respond to the 4-drug regimen. The main limitation of this four-drug combination is hypotension, so at each visit careful history for orthostasis and checking for orthostatic hypotension are needed (see Chapter 18). In recent years, the prevalence of diastolic dysfunction has been increasing. Since many patients with diastolic dysfunction may also have some masked systolic dysfunction, new effective strategies are being

TABLE 22.3	Follow-Up Visit for Heart Failure

Control/Compliance/Complications—Disease

Subjective: *How well do you sleep at night? How many times do you wake up from sleeping each night due to cough/dyspnea?* **(PND)**
How many pillows do you sleep on at night? **(orthopnea)**
Tell me about your exercise? What happens when you go out for a walk? Walking up hill? Upstairs? **(SOB, DOE)**
What kind of problems have you had with swelling in your ankles? **(edema, hydralazine)**
What kind of problems do you have remembering to take your medications?
What kind of problems do you have following your low salt diet?
What kind of problems are having with your exercise program?

Objective: Pulse/respiration rates **(tachycardia/tachypnea)**
Check ankles for edema **(fluid retention)**
Weight gain **(fluid retention)**
Auscultation of lungs **(crackles due to pulmonary edema)**
Check PMI/apical impulse **(cardiac enlargement)**
Periodic serum creatinine/BUN **(organ perfusion)**
Serum BNP/NT-proBNP to evaluate therapy efficacy

Complications—Drugs

Subjective: *What happens when you get up quickly from a bed or chair?*
Have you had any of the following since your last visit?

Cough? **(ACEI)**	Swelling is face or lips? **(ACEI)**
Swollen painful breasts? **(spironolactone)**	Muscle weakness? **(diuretics)**
Sunburn? **(diuretics)**	Bright light/yellow green vision? **(digoxin)**
Palpitations? **(digoxin)**	Joint pain? **(diuretics)**

Objective: Blood pressure
Check for orthostatic hypotension
Serum creatinine, Mg^{++}, K^+ **(diuretics, digoxin, ACEI, ARB, spironolactone)**
Serum uric acid **(diuretics)**
Irregular pulse/bradycardia **(digoxin, β-blockers)**
Serum digoxin level if signs or symptoms of digoxin toxicity or worsening HF

employed using BNP levels to determine the level of aggressiveness of therapy in systolic dysfunction, to maximize the benefits of nondiuretic medications have benefit in mixed dysfunction heart failure, and to reduce the incidence of readmissions. The goal of BNP-targeted therapy is to reduce the level to as close to 100 pg/mL as possible without toxicity. See Table 22.3 for a more complete listing of parameters of control, compliance, and complications.

• KEY REFERENCES

1. King M, Kingery J, Casey B. Diagnosis and evaluation of heart failure. *Am Fam Physician.* 2012;85:1161-1168.
2. Chatterjee K. Pathophysiology of systolic and diastolic heart failure. *Med Clin North Am.* 2012;96:891-899.
3. Maestre A, Gil V, Gallego J, et al. Diagnostic accuracy of clinical criteria for identifying systolic and diastolic heart failure: cross-sectional study. *J Eval Clin Pract.* 2009;15:55-61.
4. Motiwala SR, Januzzi JL. The role of natriuretic peptides for guiding management of chronic heart failure. *Clin Pharmacol Ther.* 2013;93:57-67.
5. Rathi S, Deedwania PC. The epidemiology and pathophysiology of heart failure. *Med Clin North Am.* 2012;96:881-890.
6. Campbell RT, Jhund PS, Castagno D, et al. What we have learned about patients with heart failure and preserved ejection fraction from DIG-PEF, CHARM-Preserved and I-Preserve. *J Am Coll Cardiol.* 2012;60:2349-2356.
7. Chowdhury P, Choudhary R, Maisel A. The appropriate use of biomarkers in heart failure. *Med Clin North Am.* 2012;96:901-913.

CASE 22.1

Ralph Malph, a 62-year-old retired Chief Petty Officer who recently moved to your city, presents to your clinic for assistance in controlling his hypertension, type 2 diabetes mellitus, and dyslipidemia. Ralph has had high blood pressure for 15 years and was diagnosed with diabetes and dyslipidemia 8 years ago at the time of his *mild heart attack* (NSTEMI). Both his diabetes and LDL cholesterol are near target goals (A1C = 7.2, LDL = 104). Because of his relocation he has not seen his primary physician in 4 months. His blood pressure has been problematic ever since diagnosis with his readings consistently between 155 and 170/94-104. Today, his first visit to your facility, the intake nurse noted a BP of 178/102. He takes lisinopril 10 mg q AM, chlorthalidone 25 mg q AM, atorvastatin 40 mg q AM and metformin 500 mg bid, but with limited success. He needs refills primarily of his BP medication to last until he sees his new physician at your facility in 3 weeks. Because his records have still not arrived, the intake nurse sends him to you to authorize his refills.

During your interview of Ralph, when you ask him closed-ended questions about potential complications of his chronic diseases. He mentions some difficulty sleeping and some shortness of breath. Further probing reveals he wakes up several times a week about 3 to 4 hours after falling asleep with palpitations and mild breathlessness. Sitting up or going to get a glass of water relieves the problem. He says the episodes are like the dreams he used to have after coming back from Iraq, but without the nightmares, which he has not had in 4 or 5 years. In addition, walking up the slight grade from the mailbox to the house occasionally leaves him winded, which he attributes to old age.

List six additional questions, laboratory tests, or physical examinations you would ask/order or conduct to confirm your suspicion of heart failure.

_____

_____

_____

_____

_____

TWENTY-THREE

Seizure Disorders

LEARNING OBJECTIVE

1. Conduct a comprehensive follow-up visit for a patient with epilepsy using appropriate history-taking techniques, physical examination, and laboratory tests. The visit includes assessment of disease control, assessment and support of adherence with lifestyle modifications and medication regimens, and evaluation for complications from the disease and medication regimen.

• INTRODUCTION

According to most sources, epilepsy is a condition of recurrent, unprovoked seizures caused by an inherent brain abnormality. Seizures occur when the normal chemical and electrical activity of the brain is disturbed, which leads to changes in behavior, function, or attention. These manifestations can include visible abnormal motor activity, loss of consciousness, and/or memory loss, as well as abnormal sensory, psychic, or autonomic symptoms. Focal or generalized, abnormal increased muscular activity due to a seizure is called convulsion. Because many types of epilepsy do not involve convulsions, the term is less often used in the context of epilepsy or seizure disorders.

While all drugs currently used to treat epilepsy are really antiseizure medications, which suppress abnormal electrical and chemical activity in the brain, they are usually called antiepilepsy drugs (AEDs). This is primarily because seizure activity that either consists of a single event and/or has an identifiable reversible cause does not warrant chronic drug therapy.

The pharmacist's role in epilepsy is primarily monitoring the patient's response to drug therapy, preventing adverse effects and assisting with optimal medication adherence.

• ETIOLOGY

Seizures can be triggered by numerous temporary and potentially correctable conditions such as high fever, head trauma, electrolyte disturbances, medications, alcohol withdrawal, vascular malformations, tumor, infection, or stroke. These seizures are considered to be provoked and will not recur once the offending cause is corrected. If seizures occur repeatedly and chronically, and it is not provoked by an identifiable cause, the condition is called epilepsy. Over 3 million people in the United States have epilepsy (0.5% to 1% of the population).

• DIAGNOSIS

While the cause of a seizure disorder and the diagnosis of epilepsy is done primarily by medical personnel and physician specialists, pharmacists need to know the most common causes and how the diagnosis is made. When evaluating a patient for the first time, it is important to obtain a complete and detailed patient history. Ideally, this would include a detailed description from those who have witnessed the patient's seizures. A complete physical examination, including a thorough neurological examination must be performed. In addition to a careful history and examination, selective laboratory screening along with other tests should be performed to look for temporary or reversible causes of the seizure. Therefore, electrolytes, glucose, calcium, magnesium, CBC, renal function, liver function, and toxicology screenings should be determined. A lumbar puncture or spinal tap is performed if the clinical presentation suggests the following: an acute infection that involves the CNS, a history of cancer that is known to metastasize in the brain, or a subarachnoid hemorrhage or stroke. Patients on potentially seizure-inducing medication, e.g., theophylline, should have serum levels measured.

The electroencephalogram (EEG) is used to measure the electrical activity in the brain. If abnormal, it can be helpful in the diagnosis of an epileptic seizure. This test may be able to pinpoint the location in the brain where the seizures start and suggest whether a patient has generalized or partial seizures. Often after a patient's first seizure, the EEG may appear normal. The use of sleep deprivation, hyperventilation, and intermittent photic stimulation is used to increase the brain activity in an attempt to find an abnormal focus via the EEG. However, a normal EEG does not rule out epilepsy after having a seizure.

Finally, if a cause of the patient's seizure is not discovered with the above workup, magnetic resonance imaging (MRI) or in an emergency computerized tomography (CT scan) of the brain should be performed to rule out changes due to the seizure (which may persist for days or weeks), and to identify structural causes of the seizures (infarct or hemorrhage due to a stroke, or mass occupying lesion such as a brain tumor).

• CLASSIFICATION

While there have been several different systems to classify seizures, the most commonly used system is the *simplified international classification of seizures*. The optimal therapeutic plan varies by the specific type of seizure. Each patient's treatment plan should be individualized to the extent possible, based on their specific type of seizure. There are three major categories of seizures: partial seizures (sometimes called focal seizures), generalized seizures, and unclassifiable seizures. *Partial seizures* start in a focal region of the brain (i.e., one side or hemisphere). They can be either simple or complex. *Simple partial seizures do not* cause loss of consciousness or memory, but may involve focal motor activity (jerking of a single limb) and/or sensory abnormalities (visual, auditory, or olfactory). They may also cause abnormal thoughts or perceptions, or even autonomic symptoms such as nausea, flushing, or tingling. *Complex partial seizures do* cause loss of consciousness or memory and have somewhat different presentations. The manifestations are usually repeated motor activities like lip smacking, chewing, swallowing, hand rubbing, walking about without purpose, and/or repeated verbal statements that may be nonsensical word strings. These are termed automatisms. Complex partial seizures were previously called called temporal lobe or psychomotor seizures and patients may still use the terms. Both of these types of partial seizures will remain focal throughout their duration unless they become generalized. However, either type of partial seizure can become secondarily generalized to the entire brain, leading to generalized tonic-clonic seizures, which are referred to as complex partial seizures with secondary generalization. Complex partial seizures comprise about 40% of all adult seizures and simple partial seizures comprise about another 20%.

Primary generalized seizures include absence (previously known as petit mal), tonic-clonic (previously known as grand mal), myoclonic, atonic, and clonic seizures. They originate and spread throughout both hemispheres of the brain. Primary *generalized tonic-clonic* seizures, probably the most familiar to the lay public, comprise about 20% of all adult seizures. They begin with a sudden loss of consciousness and frequently with eyes rolling upward and sometimes with a shout or a cry, due to contraction of respiratory muscles against the closed throat. Then the tonic phase begins, consisting of involuntary strong sustained contraction of the muscles of the extremities, neck, and trunk usually described as stiffening in extension. Patients' facial expressions may appear distorted. This is followed by the clonic phase, which consists of rhythmic types of jerking movements of the extremities. Urinary and/or fecal incontinence may accompany these general tonic-clonic seizures. Also, these are usually followed by upto several hours of drowsiness, known as the post-ictal phase. *Absence seizures*, a less dramatic form of generalized seizures, consist of staring spells. However, they may also include a fluttering of the eyes and/or a nodding of the head. Sometimes, they appear similar to complex partial seizures and the differentiation can require an EEG tracing. These seizures comprise approximately 10% of adult seizures, but a greater percentage in pediatrics. The remainder of generalized seizure types comprises the last 10% of adult seizures.

In addition to this classification of seizure types, there are also various uncommon epilepsy syndromes, e.g., febrile seizures, Lennox-Gastaut syndrome.

• INITIAL VISIT

Once a diagnosis of epilepsy has been confirmed, goals of therapy are to minimize seizure activity and severity, avoid treatment-related side effects, and maintain or improve quality of life. The type of seizure a patient has will determine which medications will be prescribed. Other factors that should be considered when choosing a medication regimen include potential drug-drug, drug-nutrient, and drug-disease interactions, age, gender, individualized goals of therapy, medical history, potential adverse effects, and psychological history. Women represent a special group of patients due to the possibility of anticonvulsants interfering with oral contraceptive efficacy, complicating breast feeding, and potentially causing birth defects. For readers interested in these specific issues, the American Academy of Neurology (AAN) and the American Epilepsy Society have issued three sets of practice guidelines, in 2009, dealing with best practices in women with epilepsy. Roughly two-thirds of patients will respond to drug therapy alone. An additional role for the pharmacist can be to help identify those patients whose seizures are truly resistant to medication and not caused by insufficient dosing or nonadherence. About one-third of patients diagnosed with epilepsy turn out to be resistant to drug therapy and require specialist management.

• FOLLOW-UP VISIT (See Table 23.1)

Control

The extent of the patient's seizure activities since their last visit is the primary measurement of disease control. Ask patients directly using an open-ended question such as, "How many seizures or spells have you had since your last visit?" If the patient did have one or more seizures, there is a need to ask for more details about each episode. Was there a witness who can tell you the details of the seizure? When did it happen? How long did it last? What were they doing before it occurred? Patients may not remember what happened during their episode so it is important to have a witness provide details, wherever possible. In addition, patients should be queried regarding any of the following that may have occurred around or before the time of the seizure: sleep deprivation, ethanol binge, illicit drug use, or a new medication that may lower seizure threshold such as phenothiazines, theophylline, or bupropion. In addition, the pharmacy should be contacted to make sure that the manufacturer of the anticonvulsant has not changed, which could lead to altered serum levels.

One of the problems about relying on subjective information is that the actual numbers of seizures are generally underreported due to lack of patient awareness and/or willful misrepresentation to avoid losing driving privileges. Most states require 3 to 12 months of seizure free status verified in writing by their physician to obtain or renew a driver's license. Sometimes, the patient can injure themselves during a seizure. Observation for potential evidence of trauma such as a cut lip, swollen body part, bruising, limping, or restricted range of movement may require more in-depth questioning and examination to determine if they were caused by a seizure.

Compliance

Adherence to the medication regimen is essential to disease control. Open-ended probes as seen in Table 23.1 can start the discussion. If suboptimal adherence is

TABLE 23.1	Follow-Up Visit Seizure Disorder

CONTROL

S *How many seizures or spells have you had since your last visit?*
Tell me more about the seizure(s).
  When did it happen?
  What were you doing just before it occurred?
  Who witnessed the seizure?
  How long before you were awake and alert after the seizure?
  How did this event compare or differ from previous events?
  What do you think caused this episode?
  Closed-ended questions for potential triggering events
  Alcohol ingestion? Sleeping less than usual? Using street drugs? Taking a new medication?
O If seizure occurs, check with pharmacy to make sure that the manufacturer has not changed
  Observe for injuries (bruises, cuts, etc.)

COMPLIANCE

S *How do you take your medication?*
What kind of problems have you had remembering to take your medication?
What other medications have you taken since your last visit?
O Check pharmacy refill records
  Check serum anticonvulsant levels if appropriate

COMPLICATIONS (DISEASE)

S *How have things been going in your life since your last visit?*
What changes or problems have you noticed since your last visit?
Have you had any of the following since your last visit?

Trouble sleeping?	Changes in mood, behaviors, thoughts, or feelings?
Increased irritability/anger?	Feeling of sadness?

  Lack of interest in normal activities?
  Change in capabilities to work, carry out activities of daily living?
  Thoughts of suicide?
O Administer Neurological Disorders Depression Inventory for Epilepsy (NDDI-E) at baseline, periodically or based on
    findings during visit.
  Directed examination/evaluation of site of potential injury due to seizure.

COMPLICATIONS (DRUG)

S *What kind of changes or problems have you noticed since your last visit?*
Have you had any of the following since your last visit?

Nausea, vomiting, anorexia? **(all)**	Changes in vision? **(all)**
Trouble speaking? **(all)**	Dizziness? **(all)**
Trouble with learning/memory? **(all)**	Drowsiness? **(all)**
Confusion? **(all)**	Lethargy/fatigue? **(all)**
Balance/movement problems? **(all)**	Tremor? **(all)**

  Fever, infection? **(CBZ, LMTG, LEV, FEL, OX, PHTN, VAL)**
  Fatigue, easy bleeding/bruisability? **(same as above)**
  Fever, dark urine, malaise, yellow eyes? **(FEL,VAL, PHTN)**
  Skin rash? **(all)**
  Blistering of skin around mouth, lips, eyes, nose? **(CBZ, LMTG)**
  Pains in bones/muscle (not joints)? **(CBZ, PB, PRIM, PHTN, VAL)**
  Increased weight? **(VAL, GABA, TIAG, LMTG, PRE)**
  Swelling in ankles? **(GABA, PRE, TOP, VAL)**
  Confusion, muscle weakness/spasm? **(CBZ, OX)**
  Severe back pain? **(TOP)**

(Continued)

TABLE 23.1	Follow-Up Visit Seizure Disorder (*Continued*)
O	Screening neurological examination, primarily testing cerebellar and cognitive functions **(all)**
	Visual acuity examination **(all)**
	CBC with differential **(CBZ, LMTG, LEV, FEL, OX, PHTN)**[a]
	Liver function tests **(all)**[b]
	Serum creatinine, urinalysis **(all)**[b]
	Temperature **(all)**[b]
	Vitamin D levels, bone scan **(CBZ, PB, PRIM, PHTN, VAL)**[c]
	Check for edema, weight **(GABA, PRE, TIAG, TOP, VAL)**
	Serum electrolytes **(CBZ, OX)**[d]
	Renal ultrasound **(TOP)**[e]

Abbreviations: CBZ, carbamazepine; FEL, felbamate; GABA, gabapentin; LEV, levetiracetam; LMTG, lamotrigine; OX, oxcarbazepine; PB, phenobarbital; PHTN, phenytoin; PRIM, primidone; TIAG, tiagabine; TOP, topiramate; VAL, valproate.
[a]Baseline and periodically to detect anemia, granulocytopenia, aplastic anemia, and in all patients with skin rash.
[b]Baseline and in all patients with skin rash or symptoms of liver disease.
[c]In all patients complaining of nonjoint or muscle pain.
[d]In all patients with confusion or other signs of hyponatremia.
[e]In all patients complaining of severe back pain.

suspected as a cause for inadequate seizure control, pharmacy refill records can be checked and reliable serum drug levels can be measured. Suboptimal adherence is common among patients with epilepsy because of potentially complex regimens, frequent annoying adverse effects, and the nature of the disease. In particular, patients with well-controlled epilepsy are known to take "medication holidays" to demonstrate they are not controlled by medication or that they do not really need it. These holidays may start out as just a dose or two, but may expand to longer periods. This is complicated by the fact that in many seizure disorders, there are periods where no electrical discharges that cause seizures are generated. If the holiday coincides with a period of seizure inactivity, then the holiday can last for weeks or months until a seizure recurs.

Complications of the Disease

In addition to seizures, the major complications are psychosocial in nature. Many patients struggle with a loss of independence and can become depressed. Some epileptic patients are unemployed regardless of their college education. Due to increased risk from injury, many patients have activity restrictions, which can make them feel isolated and alone. Many patients develop poor self-esteem when they have problems getting insurance or keeping a suitable job. Family and friends can also struggle to adapt to a person with epilepsy. For providers, patients, and families who want to gain insight into these issues, the Brainstorm series of books by Steven Schachter offer insight into the feelings of patients with epilepsy and those of their family and friends.

Depression is a common complication of epilepsy. Over half of all patients with uncontrolled epilepsy are depressed and the risk of suicide is several times higher than in patients without seizures. In 2008, the FDA issued "black box warnings" based on their analysis of clinical trials of a higher suicide rate in patients on all anticonvulsant medications compared to placebo. The mechanism relating epilepsy and anticonvulsants to depression and suicide is unknown. It may be epilepsy, medications, or a combination of both. Regardless of the cause, providers must be diligent in screening for depression at each visit. Asking general questions about their life, work, or family as appropriate can provide clues to negative changes in their life. Observing for changes in mood and affect plus asking direct open-ended questions regarding symptoms of depression or thoughts of suicide should be done at each visit. A more objective measure specifically designed for patients with epilepsy, the Neurological Disorders Depression Inventory for Epilepsy (NDDI-E), should be administered at baseline during the initial visit and thereafter, either periodically or as indicated by findings during subsequent visits. Patients, suspected of having depression, need to be referred to a qualified mental health provider.

Complications of Drugs

Most antiepileptic drugs are metabolized in the liver and many are CYP 450 inducers or inhibitors. Given the nature and properties of antiepileptic drugs (AEDs), there is a high risk for significant drug-drug interactions involving not only other AEDs, but many medications for comorbid conditions as well. The pharmacist's role is to analyze all the patient's medications, even those for comorbid conditions for potential significant interactions. In addition, the pharmacist should educate the patient to ask about potential interactions before starting any other medications. This is all in addition to routine education about their disease and proper use of their individual medications.

Many AEDs share adverse effects as a class. Most cause some incidence of gastric upset, anorexia, nausea, or vomiting. These can be minimized by starting with a low dose and titrating upward slowly. All can cause disruptions and adverse effects related to the central nervous system (CNS) including visual disturbances, drowsiness, fatigue, lethargy, trouble with memory and learning, confusion, or tremor. Probing for these symptoms should be done at each visit along with administration of the Folstein mini-mental status examination (MMSE) as indicated. Seizure medications can impair cerebellar function (movement and balance). This effect is evaluated with the portion of a neurological examination that tests for cerebellar function (gait, balance, and nystagmus). These CNS signs and symptoms are more frequent when initiating therapy and when increasing dosages or adding additional anticonvulsants or other medication with CNS depressant properties. In addition, cerebellar or cognitive impairment may be an indication of excess medication serum levels. Fortunately, most decrease with time. Problems with cognition can be common and very troublesome, but patient perceptions of cognition problems can be based primarily on mood rather than actual performance and the persistence of complaints should prompt a more thorough investigation for signs and symptoms of depression.

Many AEDs have been implicated in drug hypersensitivity syndrome, also known as anticonvulsant hypersensitivity syndrome, or DRESS (drug reaction with eosinophilia and systemic symptoms). It occurs more frequently with the older AEDs. It has been estimated to occur in one of every 10,000 patients. Since it is associated with an 8% mortality rate, it is important to ask during every visit about skin rashes. Drug hypersensitivity syndrome (DHS) includes not only a widespread maculopapular-papular rash on the trunk, arms, and legs but systemic signs as well. DHS usually presents with a high fever followed by the rash. Systemic effects include eosinophilia in 50% to 90% of the cases. Thirty percent have abnormal lymphocytosis and 20% have lymphadenopathy. Eventually, the liver and/or kidneys become involved as indicated by elevated AST or ALT levels and/or proteinuria, or elevated serum creatinine, respectively.

Individual AEDs are associated with a variety of adverse drugs reactions including granulocytopenia, aplastic anemia, Stevens-Johnson syndrome, drug-induced hepatitis, and hyperammonemia. Therefore, it is important to monitor specific medications via liver function tests, complete blood counts, basic metabolic panels, and ammonia levels to look for possible adverse effects of drug therapy (Table 23.1).

• SUMMARY

The pharmacist's role in epilepsy is primarily monitoring and adjusting drug therapy to prevent seizures, minimize adverse effects, and optimize quality of life. Using careful history taking and focused physical assessment, the pharmacist applies their knowledge of the presentation of various types of seizures, the unwanted effects for each anticonvulsant, and their medication adherence support skills to assist the patient in optimizing therapy.

• KEY REFERENCES

1. Elger CE, Schmidt D. Modern management of epilepsy: a practical approach. *Epilepsy Behav.* 2008;12:501-539.
2. French JA, Pedley TA. Initial management of epilepsy. *N Engl J Med.* 2008;359:166-176.
3. Schachter SC. Seizure disorders. *Med Clin North Am.* 2009;93:343-351.
4. Leeman BA, Cole AJ. Advancements in the treatment of epilepsy. *Annu Rev Med.* 2008;59:503-523.
5. Landmark CJ, Johannssen SI. Pharmacological management of epilepsy. *Drugs.* 2008;68:1925-1939.
6. Raspall-Chaure M, Neville BG, Scott RC. The medical management of epilepsy in children. *Lancet Neurol.* 2008;7:57-69.
7. Stein MA, Kanner AM. Management of newly diagnosed epilepsy: a practical guide to monotherapy. *Drugs.* 2009;69:199-222.
8. Stephen LJ, Brodie MJ. Selection of antiepileptic drugs in adults. *Neurol Clin.* 2009;27:967-992.
9. Schacter SC. *Brainstorms: Epilepsy in Our Words. Personal Accounts of Living with Seizures.* New York: Raven Press; 1993.
10. Schacter SC. *The Brainstorms Companion: Epilepsy in Our View.* New York: Raven Press; 1995.
11. Saiz-Diaz RA, Sancho J, Serratosa J. Antiepileptic drug interactions. *Neurologist.* 2008;14:S55-S65.

CASE 23.1

JT, a 23-year-old male graduate student with a 3-year history of complex partial seizures with occasional secondary generalization, presents to your pharmacy disease management clinic for adjustment of his antiseizure regimen. Initially controlled on valproate, a 25-kg weight gain over 28 months prompted a change to lamotrigine. Lamotrigine was slowly titrated upward over several months. A week ago, just as he reached a maintenance dose of 200 mg bid, he developed erythema multiforme and was hospitalized temporarily because it appeared as if it was progressing to Stevens-Johnson syndrome. The drug was discontinued and high-dose corticosteroids started. No mucous membrane lesions developed and he was discharged 9 days ago on carbamazepine 100 mg bid. The neurologist recommended a slow upward titration to approximately 8 to 10/mg/kg or a serum level of about 8 μg/mL. Carbamazepine serum level drawn yesterday was 1.1 μg/mL (target range 5 to 12 mcg/ml).

a. List six questions you would ask/laboratory tests you would order or physical examinations you would perform to evaluate the efficacy and potential adverse effects of carbamazepine in JT?

_____

_____

_____

_____

_____

b. During the visit, JT revealed that he had had no generalized seizures. However, his mother thought he might have had a brief spell 2 days after leaving the hospital consisting of just some walking around in a daze. He feels it was the carbamazepine that made him "spaced out." JT says that spaced out feeling has gotten better the last 2 days. JT's cerebellar examination as well as a complete neurological screening examination were normal. Discuss the impact of your findings and your plan.

_____

_____

_____

_____

_____

FOUR

Assessment of Potential Drug-Related Problems

TWENTY-FOUR

Liver and Renal Disease

1. Interpret the findings for potential drug-induced liver damage and the presence or absence of other common hepatic disorders given the results of liver function tests.

2. Differentiate between acute hepatocellular, obstructive, and the two types of chronic liver dysfunction using liver function tests.

3. Differentiate drug-induced liver disease from other causes of liver pathology, using knowledge of liver function tests and other signs and symptoms.

4. Interpret the findings for potential drug-induced renal damage, complications from chronic diseases such as hypertension and diabetes mellitus and the presence or absence of other common renal disorders given the results of renal function tests.

• INTRODUCTION

Pharmacists in a variety of patient care practice environments are routinely required to evaluate patient's liver function tests (LFTs) and renal function tests (RFTs) to differentiate between adverse medication effects and other causes of hepatic and renal dysfunction. The purpose of this chapter is to teach pharmacists how to evaluate patients for damage to the liver and the kidney, including those caused by complications of chronic disease, adverse drug effects, and other diseases of the liver and kidney. Pharmacists also interpret LFTs and RFTs to monitor patients taking medications with potential hepatotoxic or nephrotoxic adverse effects. Pharmacists also interpret certain RFTs to assist in the dosing of medications that are primarily excreted by the kidney.

• LIVER FUNCTION TESTS

The term liver function tests is a misnomer, because unlike renal function tests that measure both damage to and the effectiveness of the kidney, LFTs only measure damage to various structures in the liver and gallbladder. While RFTs can be used to determine the dose of medications primarily cleared from the body via the kidney, LFTs, since they measure only damage and not function, cannot be used to determine doses of medications metabolized in the liver (Table 24.1).

Aminotransferases

Aspartate aminotransferase (AST) and alanine aminotransferase (ALT) are synthesized primarily in hepatocytes. Upon the destruction of hepatocytes these enzymes are released into the blood stream, causing serum levels to rise. The presence of elevated levels of AST and ALT in the serum usually indicate of hepatocellular damage. However, there are several issues that need to be considered when interpreting elevated levels of AST and ALT. The first issue concerns normal values. Most laboratory tests have a normal bell-shaped distribution in a given population; therefore, assessment of normal is more reliable. AST and ALT levels have a skewed distribution characterized by a long tail at the high end of the scale. This means that 2.5% of patients' purported "abnormal" levels are actually normal for them. This skewing is more pronounced in nonwhite males. Therefore, slight elevations of aminotransferases (less than 1.5 times the upper limit of normal) may not indicate liver disease. The second issue involves the lack of relative specificity of these enzymes to the liver. AST is widely distributed throughout skeletal and cardiac muscle as well as the liver. Prior to the advent of serum troponin

TABLE 24.1	Laboratory Tests Used to Evaluate Liver Function	
Lab Test	*Normal Range*	*Sources Other Than Liver*
AST (aspartate aminotransferase)	<35 units/L	Cardiac and skeletal muscle ++++
ALT (alanine aminotransferase)	<35 units/L	Skeletal muscle ++
GGTP (γ-glutamyl transpeptidase)	1 to 94 units/L	
ALKALINE PHOSPHATASE	30 to 120 units/L	Bone
TOTAL BILIRUBIN	0.3 to 1.0 mg/dL	From heme breakdown
DIRECT BILIRUBIN (Conjugated)		
TOTAL PROTEIN	6.0 to 8.3 g/dL	
ALBUMIN	3.5 to 5.5 g/dL	
A/G RATIO (albumin/globulin ratio)	>1	Total protein minus albumin = globulin
INR (based on Prothrombin time)	0.9 to 1.1 (1)	

levels, elevated AST levels were used to diagnose acute myocardial infarction. In addition, vigorous exercise or muscle trauma can cause marked elevations in serum AST levels. While ALT is far more specific to hepatocytes, it is found in other tissues and may occasionally be the source of spurious elevations of ALT.

Alkaline Phosphatase

Alkaline phosphatase (AP or alk phos) is a group of iso-enzymes that cleave inorganic phosphate from organophosphates primarily in the bone and microvilli of the canaliculi lining the intrahepatic bile ducts. In LFTs, elevated levels of AP indicate obstruction of the biliary system. In extrahepatic obstruction such as gallstones, the AP may rise more slowly than other LFTs. Isolated elevations of AP can also occur normally in pregnancy (placental source), growing children, and in bone disorders, such as Paget's disease.

Serum Proteins

The liver is responsible for protein synthesis. Therefore, in chronic liver disease such as cirrhosis, synthesis of protein is eventually impaired and serum levels fall. Because *albumin*, one of the major indicators of chronic hepatocellular damage, has a half-life of 20 days in the body, it is unaffected by brief periods of acute or mild hepatocellular damage. Serum *globulin* measures α- and β-globulins, which are synthesized in the liver, plus γ-globulins, which are synthesized by plasma cells and lymphocytes. *Prothrombin*, a clotting agent with a half-life of 60 hours, is more sensitive to liver damage. Prothrombin levels are approximated with the prothrombin time, which measures the time for a blood sample to clot when tissue clotting factors are added to the sample and combine with prothrombin to make the blood clot. Because of variations in the strength of different manufacturers' tissue factors, an international normalized ratio (INR) is used to express prothrombin activity (and levels) instead of the prothrombin time. The normal INR is 1. As prothrombin activity decreases the INR value rises. Because a decrease of 80% in prothrombin levels is required for the INR to start to rise, it makes an excellent indicator of chronic hepatocellular damage along with a decrease in serum albumin. Another manipulation of serum protein levels, the *albumin to globulin ratio (A/G ratio)*, can be an even more sensitive indicator of chronic hepatocellular damage. Normally the A/G ratio is greater than 1. As chronic liver damage increases over time, the production of albumin falls along with that of α- and β-globulins. Simultaneously, the liver damage decreases the liver's ability to process antigens, which causes an increase in the synthesis of γ-globulins outside the damaged liver, which maintains a normal or elevated serum globulin level. If not given on the lab test report, the globulin can be calculated by subtracting the albumin serum level from the total protein serum level. An *A/G ratio* of less than 1 indicates significant, permanent destruction of a large number of hepatocytes as found in cirrhosis.

Other Common Biomarkers of Liver Damage

The γ-*glutamyl transpeptidase (GGTP)* and *serum bilirubin* levels can be used as adjuncts in the diagnosis of types of liver diseases. While specific to the liver, the GGTP is not routinely included in LFT panels because it is too sensitive and is frequently elevated in the absence of liver disease. Medications that cause CYP450 enzyme induction markedly raise GGTP levels. However, GGTP should be done in a case of isolated elevation of AP to confirm its liver origin, since both AP and GGTP are elevated in obstructive liver disease.

Since the advent of AST, ALT, and AP enzyme tests, the utility of serum bilirubin levels has markedly decreased, but can still be used to confirm results from other tests. Bilirubin is a by-product of hemoglobin catabolism and is transported to the liver, where it is quickly conjugated via hepatic glucuronidation and sulfation and is immediately excreted via the bile duct into the intestine. Roughly 10% of serum bilirubin is conjugated (also known as direct bilirubin). The remaining 90% is unconjugated (also known as indirect bilirubin). Ratios of direct and indirect bilirubin were used historically to attempt to differentiate between hepatocellular and obstructive liver disease, but were too unreliable. When total bilirubin levels near 3 mg/dL, check the conjunctiva, frenulum of the tongue, and nail beds for the yellow discoloration of jaundice. In addition, hemolysis can cause marked elevation of total bilirubin and is accompanied by a normochromic, normocytic anemia and a reticulocytosis on the complete blood count.

• INTERPRETING LIVER FUNCTION TESTS

The etiology and type of liver disorder or disease cannot be diagnosed by laboratory test alone. The combination of LFTs with the clinical picture, via a careful history and physical examination are essential to accurate diagnosis. There are four major types of liver damage: acute hepatocellular, severe chronic hepatocellular (cirrhosis), obstructive (cholestatic), and mild chronic hepatocellular (hepatitis C). All four types can be caused by medication and other pathological conditions of the liver. The pharmacist is frequently asked to try to differentiate between drug-induced liver disease and that caused by traditional etiologies. To be effective in this role, the pharmacist needs to know the type of liver injury each drug causes, matching the LFTs and the clinical picture to specific drugs. For example, phenothiazines cause cholestatic liver disease. In a patient on a phenothiazine, a cholestatic pattern would be seen, i.e., AP levels at least three to five times the upper limit of normal with mild elevations of AST and ALT. If the patient's values showed AST and ALT levels >1000 units/dL and a normal AP, then the phenothiazine could be ruled out as a cause of the patient's liver injury. Similarly, the pharmacist must be familiar with the LFTs and clinical presentation patterns of other common causes of liver injury and disease. Unfortunately, many times the exact etiology may elude accurate identification because of the limitations inherent in the available laboratory tests, or patient history and physical findings. In those cases, the suspected offending medication can be discontinued and the patient monitored for resolution of subjective and objective parameters, which can sometimes help confirm a drug-induced cause.

Acute Hepatocellular Damage

Regardless of the cause, acute hepatocellular damage presents with markedly elevated (>300 units/dL) AST and ALT levels as the primary laboratory test abnormality. Mild elevations of AP and unconjugated (indirect) bilirubin can also occur. Isoniazid, acetaminophen, allopurinol, valproic acid, and kava kava are examples of drugs/herbs that cause classical acute hepatocellular damage. These drugs are also said to cause drug-induced hepatitis since the symptoms, physical findings, and LFT patterns mimic viral hepatitis. Typically, other LFTs are normal or only mildly elevated. These medications have all been reported to cause liver failure and death if the drug is not discontinued. Patients may also present with symptoms associated with acute viral hepatitis, including fatigue, malaise, mild fever, anorexia, and nausea. Other than jaundice, physical examination is usually normal. Occasionally, patients will experience mild hepatic tenderness on palpation or percussion. To differentiate from other etiologies, patients should be questioned about herbal and nonprescription medication use, recent travel, transfusions, unprotected sexual intercourse, or tattoos. Given the routine immunization for hepatitis, blood tests for *active* hepatitis A, B, and C should be done, i.e., anti-hepatitis A IgM for hepatitis A, both anti-hepatitis B surface antigen and anti-hepatitis B core antigen IgM for hepatitis B, and HCV-RNA for hepatitis C. Laboratories may list these as a Hepatitis Panel on their order forms.

Cholestatic or Obstructive Damage

Regardless of the cause, cholestatic liver disease presents with markedly elevated serum AP levels, at least three and usually more than five times the upper limit of normal, plus a mild elevation of AST/ALT (<300 units/dL). Anabolic steroids, estrogens, phenothiazines, cyclosporine, and erythromycin are examples of drugs that cause a classical cholestatic pattern of liver injury (also known as cholestatic jaundice or drug-induced cholestasis) (Table 24.2). Drugs that cause cholestasis affect canaliculi of the intrahepatic bile ducts. Patients may present with symptoms that mimic gallbladder disease which includes cramping right upper quadrant (RUQ) abdominal pain or may be relatively asymptomatic. Physical examination may reveal a positive Murphy sign (pain during inspiration while palpating just under the right rib cage) or RUQ tenderness on palpation. Serum conjugated bilirubin (direct) is usually increased (>20%) if the swelling in the canaliculi obstructs the bile ducts, because the hepatocytes are mostly undamaged and continue to efficiently conjugate bilirubin. To differentiate drug-induced cholestasis from other etiologies, patients should be questioned about a personal or family history of gallbladder disease since Native Americans and Hispanic populations have a high incidence of gallbladder disease, relative to other ethnic populations. In addition, the patient should be questioned about recent fractures, medications that may cause osteomalacia, or recent growth spurts in adolescents, all of which cause isolated elevations of AP values. Abdominal examination should include inspection for scars typical of cholecystectomy. Abdominal ultrasound can reveal gallstones, obstructive masses of the gallbladder, or head of the pancreas if present. A GGTP level should be ordered to confirm the liver as the source of AP since it too is concentrated in the bile canaliculi. A normal GGTP indicates a further workup for bone disorders such as osteomalacia and Paget's disease.

Some references refer to "mixed" drug-induced liver disease, where all three enzymes are elevated (AST/ALT/AP). Of interest is that viral hepatitis, particularly hepatitis A, can present with what appears to be a cholestatic pattern early in the course of the disease before changing to a pattern typical of acute hepatocellular injury. Whether or not medications, which cause liver injury, also present with that pattern is unknown. However, a careful review of cases labeled as mixed reveal a variety of criteria about lab test values. For example, some cases used any AP elevation to label it mixed, while some used 1.5 to 2 times the upper limit of normal. Some cases looked for other organs as the source of the excess AP and some ignored the possibility of an alternate source.

TABLE 24.2	Lab Findings in Common Liver Diseases				
Lab Test	Acute Hepatocellular	Obstructive (Cholestatic)	Cirrhosis	Chronic Mild Hepatocellular	Hemolytic Anemia
AST	**>300**	<300	Variable	<100	Normal
ALT	**>300**	<300	Variable	<100	Normal
ALKALINE PHOSPHATASE	<3 × Increase	**> 3 to 5 × Increase**	<3 × Increase	<3 × Increase	Normal
TOTAL BILIRUBIN	Variable Increase	Up to 30 mg/dL	Variable Increase	Normal	**>6 mg/dL**
DIRECT BILIRUBIN	Variable	>50% to 80%	Variable	Normal	<20%
TOTAL PROTEIN	Normal	Normal	**Decrease**	Normal	Normal
ALBUMIN	Normal	Normal	**Decrease**	Normal	Normal
A/G RATIO	>1	>1	**<1**	>1	>1
PROTHROMBIN TIME (INR)	Normal	Normal	**Increase**	Normal	normal

Similar variations and issues also occurred in criteria for AST and ALT. Application of the criteria used in this chapter for acute hepatocellular and cholestasis to the purported mixed cases greatly clarifies the true nature of the liver injury, sorting all but a few into the four categories of hepatic injury.

Chronic Hepatocellular Damage (Cirrhosis)

The hallmark of cirrhosis or severe chronic liver disease is the decrease in capacity to synthesize proteins by the liver. Albumin and prothrombin are two primary proteins whose synthesis becomes impaired as fatty metamorphosis and fibrosis of the liver permanently decreases hepatic function. Albumin is measured via the serum albumin and the A/G ratio, while prothrombin levels are measured via the INR. In cirrhosis, serum albumin levels fall and the A/G ratio falls below 1. Simultaneously, the INR rises above 1.0. The changes in laboratory values show that the patient's hepatocytes and hepatic sinusoids are being replaced by fibrous material, which eventually leads to the classic signs and symptoms of cirrhosis. The fibrosis eventually leads to decreased blood flow from the portal vein through the fibrous liver into the hepatic vein, leading to portal hypertension. Low albumin levels decrease plasma oncotic pressure. Portal hypertension and low albumin serum levels trigger a series of steps including activation of the renin-angiotensin system that causes hyperaldosteronism and increased intravascular volume. The increased intravascular volume, portal hypertension, and low albumin combine to push fluid into the abdominal cavity, creating an enlarged and distended abdomen, known as *ascites* (Figure 24.1). Worsening portal hypertension causes splenomegaly, and varices in the splanchnic bed, primarily in the walls of the esophagus

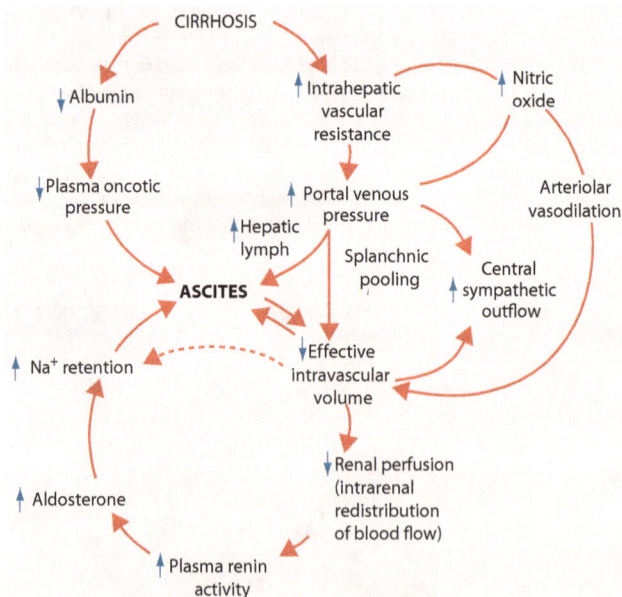

FIGURE 24.1 Factors involved in the development of ascites. (From Chung RT, Podolsky DK. Cirrhosis and its complications. In: Kasper DL, Braunwald E, Fauci AS, et al., eds. *Harrison's Principles of Internal Medicine*. 16th ed. New York, NY: McGraw-Hill; 2005:1858-1869, with permission. Copyright © McGraw-Hill Education LLC.)

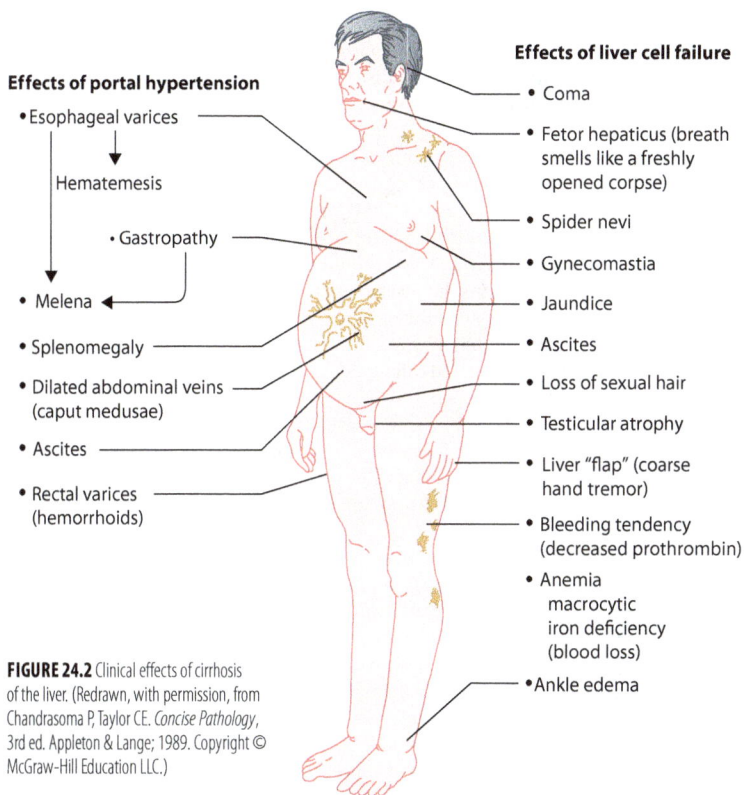

FIGURE 24.2 Clinical effects of cirrhosis of the liver. (Redrawn, with permission, from Chandrasoma P, Taylor CE. *Concise Pathology*, 3rd ed. Appleton & Lange; 1989. Copyright © McGraw-Hill Education LLC.)

Effects of portal hypertension

• Esophageal varices
  ↓
  Hematemesis
    • Gastropathy
  ↓
• Melena ←
• Splenomegaly
• Dilated abdominal veins (caput medusae)
• Ascites
• Rectal varices (hemorrhoids)

Effects of liver cell failure

• Coma
• Fetor hepaticus (breath smells like a freshly opened corpse)
• Spider nevi
• Gynecomastia
• Jaundice
• Ascites
• Loss of sexual hair
• Testicular atrophy
• Liver "flap" (coarse hand tremor)
• Bleeding tendency (decreased prothrombin)
• Anemia macrocytic iron deficiency (blood loss)
• Ankle edema

(*esophageal varices*) and rectum (*hemorrhoids*). Physical examination reveals palmar erythema, spider angiomata (*spider nevi*) on the trunk, gynecomastia, testicular atrophy, hepatomegaly (a firm, hard enlarged liver), splenomegaly, and ascites with fluid wave. Serum bilirubin levels are increased and the patient appears jaundiced, AST and ALT levels are usually normal to or only modestly elevated. As the fibrosis worsens and liver function falls, the liver's capacity to convert amino acids to urea falls and the serum blood urea nitrogen (BUN) falls below normal. A low BUN is a particularly ominous sign, indicating near total liver failure and an inability to metabolize toxins and medications. Eventually, esophageal varices may rupture, leading to significant upper gastrointestinal bleeding. Along with a low BUN, terminal patients develop hepatic encephalopathy and hepatorenal syndrome when the kidneys fail (Figure 24.2).

Chronic/Recurrent Mild Hepatocellular Damage

Currently, one of the more perplexing situations to evaluate is the asymptomatic patient with a single abnormal finding or periodically recurring mildly elevated AST and ALT (<100 units/dL).

First, is this the patient's normal value? The issue is already clouded by the skewing of the distribution, discussed earlier. In addition, the inherent limitations of the accuracy of the testing process further widens the range of actual "normal" values compared to listed normal ranges. Second, has the patient recently ingested more than normal levels of ethanol or is abusing ethanol and has the early stages of cirrhosis? Third, does the patient have chronic hepatitis B or C? Fourth, is it due to the statin the patient is taking? Finally, is it due to nonalcoholic liver disease because the patient has the metabolic syndrome? All of these are possible answers, which makes assessment more complex.

Nonalcoholic fatty liver disease (NAFLD) is one of the major causes of chronic or recurrent mild hepatocellular damage. NAFLD comprises two major variants. Simple steatosis, which is benign, comprises the majority of patients with NAFLD, whereas nonalcoholic steatohepatitis (NASH) is associated with significant inflammation and eventually leads to cirrhosis. The estimated incidence of NAFLD is 20% to 50%. Fortunately, the incidence of NASH is only 3% to 5%. NAFLD is associated with the metabolic syndrome and insulin resistance. Type 2 diabetes is a major risk factor for developing NASH. At this time, the only way to distinguish between the types of NAFLD is a liver biopsy and that may not be accurate in early stages of the disease. While there are some computerized calculations based on a combination of physical factors and laboratory tests, they are still being studied for accuracy and clinical utility. Similarly, hepatic elastography, which measures steatosis via liver tissue elasticity using computerized ultrasonography, can determine the extent of the disease but cannot distinguish between NAFLD variants. Generally, NASH should be suspected when ALT and AST levels exceed 100 units/dL but do not reach acute hepatocellular levels (>300 units/dL).

Recently, the US Preventive Services Task Force (USPSTF) recommended that all adults born between 1945 and 1965 get screened for hepatitis C, since 75% of the nearly 4 million people in the United States with hepatitis C were "baby boomers." Hepatitis C is the leading cause of death from liver disease in the United States. Most patients (80%), regardless of the severity of symptoms of acute hepatitis C, go on to develop chronic hepatitis C, which can manifest itself in intermittent or chronic mild elevations in ALT and AST. Interestingly, up to one-third of patients with chronic hepatitis C have normal LFTs. If untreated, it may eventually cause cirrhosis and all its complications. Similarly, hepatitis B can become a chronic disease. The risk of developing chronic hepatitis B depends on the age of the initial infection. Twenty-five to fifty percent of children who become infected and 6% to 10% of children whose initial infection occurs after age 5 go on to develop chronic hepatitis B. If untreated, it too eventually leads to cirrhosis and its complications. Therefore, patients with mild chronic or intermittent mild elevations should be tested for hepatitis B and C. In chronic hepatitis C, anti-HCV antibodies, measured by either enzyme immunoassay (EIA) or radioimmunoblot assay (RIBA) will be positive. Due to the potential number of false positives with the EIA method, most experts recommend the HCV-RNA, which directly measures viral products through polymerase chain reaction (PCR) assay. In chronic hepatitis B, the hepatitis B surface antigen (HBsAg) is the primary screening test. If the HBsAg is positive, a panel of other hepatitis B antigens and antibodies is ordered to determine the specific stage of the infection (acute versus resolving versus chronic).

The role of ethanol ingestion as a cause of mild chronic or intermittent AST or ALT elevations is unclear. While guidelines suggest up to two alcoholic beverages a day is beneficial, the implication is that higher levels of intake will lead to hepatocellular damage and elevated ALT and AST values. Unfortunately, there is a great deal of variability among individuals regarding a dose-response relationship between ethanol ingestion and elevation of AST and ALT values. In some cases, patients who have ingested excessive amounts of ethanol for several days before LFTs are drawn have normal AST and ALT levels. In others, beneficial intake results in mildly elevated AST and ALT values. Patients should be questioned carefully regarding recent ethanol use. If ethanol is a suspected cause, have the patient discontinue ethanol intake for 4 to 6 weeks to allow the hepatocytes to recover, then repeat LFTs. Whatever the results of the follow-up LFTs, the significant numbers of patients with NAFLD and chronic hepatitis B/C make attribution of test results to ethanol problematic. Similarly, the above factors and the co-occurrence of dyslipidemia with the metabolic syndrome or type 2 diabetes led the FDA to recently remove the requirements for baseline and follow up LFTs in statin users. See Chapter 19 for further discussion of the hepatotoxicity of statins.

• SERUM RENAL FUNCTION TESTS

In order to interpret serum tests of renal function accurately, understanding the general pathophysiology of nephron loss is important. In slow onset or chronic renal disease when nephrons are damaged, the remaining nephrons increase their filtration rates. This "hyperfiltration phenomenon" allows the kidneys to lose up to 50% of their function before changes are seen on common markers in the blood, e.g., serum creatinine. Therefore, serum levels of markers of renal function such as creatinine, BUN, and cystatin C are relatively insensitive to the early stages of renal damage, but are more accurate in monitoring the progression of chronic renal failure.

Serum Creatinine

Creatinine is a metabolic breakdown product of creatine, a substance found in muscle cells. Creatine exists as creatine phosphate, which is the primary source of phosphorous used in the regeneration of adenosine triphosphate (ATP) to transform chemical energy into muscle action. Creatinine is produced in muscle as a breakdown product of creatine and in healthy patients the production and excretion of creatinine are equal, which makes the serum creatinine a good marker of kidney function. While the normal value is listed at 0.7 to 1.5 mg/dL, a variety of issues can impact "normal" levels. The first is the assay method used. In 2003, results varied up to 41% between the various assays used. A decade later, the maximal variance is less than 15%. Differences in muscle mass will change the levels of creatinine. Women, who have less muscle mass than men, will have lower values for serum creatinine. African-Americans tend to have more muscle mass than other ethnicities and thus have higher creatinine serum levels. Therefore, an African-American male body builder may have a serum creatinine of 1.8 mg/dL that is actually normal for him, while a 75-year-old thin frail female with a serum creatinine of 1.0 mg/dL may have significant renal impairment, all due to differences in muscle mass. In addition, about 15% of creatinine found in urine is secreted through the tubules and drugs such as trimethoprim and cimetidine, which block that secretion, can falsely elevate serum creatinine levels. Finally, serum creatinine is slow to change in acute renal disease and may take several days to accurately reflect changes in actual renal function. In spite of these variances, serum creatinine is used to estimate the creatinine clearance and the glomerular filtration rate to monitor the progression of chronic renal disease.

Blood Urea Nitrogen

The BUN was the first serum test used to measure renal function. It actually measures the levels of *serum* urea, a breakdown product of amino acid metabolism by the liver via the arginine-ornithine cycle. The BUN has both advantages and disadvantages, in estimating renal function compared to the serum creatinine. Its major advantage is that a large percentage is reabsorbed at the same rate as sodium, chloride, and water and is sensitive to urine flow; therefore, it responds more quickly to acute change in glomerular filtration such as volume depletion and decreases in renal blood flow due to hypotension, blood loss, dehydration, or congestive heart failure (CHF). Its major disadvantage is that the serum levels of urea vary with the amount of protein intake. Therefore, patients on high protein diets, such as Atkins, or on hyperalimentation will have an elevated BUN, but a normal serum creatinine. Similarly, patients with a significant upper gastrointestinal bleed will have an elevated BUN and normal serum creatinine due to the excess protein absorbed from digested red blood cells and other serum proteins. Severe liver damage (cirrhosis), drastically slows the body's capacity to metabolize amino acids to urea and leads to falsely lowered BUN levels. In patients with cirrhosis, a BUN level below the lower limit of normal can be a sign of end-stage liver disease.

To adjust for the other causes of elevated BUN, the *BUN/serum creatinine ratio* is used. If both values are in the normal range the ratio does not help. The normal ratio is between 10 and 20 to 1. Any value greater than 20 indicates the BUN is elevated due to poor perfusion (pre-renal azotemia), or large protein intake rather than any inherent damage or disease in the kidney.

Estimated Glomerular Filtration rate

Measuring the glomerular filtration rate (GFR) is difficult and cumbersome. An intravenous injection of exogenous substances such as inulin, or I-iothalamate intravenously, then collection of blood and urine samples must be done at specific times. Therefore, they are relegated primarily to research use. Clinically, we used to measure creatinine clearance, which required an accurate 24-hour urine collection and a serum creatinine. The major source of error was failure to collect all the urine. Today GFR is estimated using parameters for age, weight, gender, race, body surface area, and serum creatinine levels, depending on the method used. There is some controversy regarding whether to use actual, ideal or lean body weight. These methods are generally equivalent to a creatinine clearance estimate of GFR and only require a serum creatinine (Table 24.3). There are three methods to measure estimated glomerular filtration rates (eGFRs) that are commonly used. The Cockcroft-Gault equation uses age, weight, and serum creatinine, an adjustment factor for females in a simple mathematical formula. The modified diet in renal disease equation (MDRD) uses a complex formula involving serum creatinine and age with adjustments for both females and African-Americans and is based on a study using I-iothalamate GFR measurements. Finally, there is the chronic kidney disease epidemiology collaborative equation (CKD-EPI), which uses a complex formula involving gender, serum creatinine, and age. Most recently, a formula was developed substituting cystatin C for creatinine and one combining creatinine and cystatin C. Cystatin C is a protease inhibitor produced at steady state in all nucleated cells. It is filtered at the glomerulus, but is neither reabsorbed like urea nor secreted by tubules like creatinine. It is a newer test with less experience but is theoretically more accurate. While these three methods provide similar results, the

TABLE 24.3	Formulas for Calculating Estimated Glomerular Filtration Rates (eGFRs)

Cockcroft-Gault

$$CrCl = (140 - age) \times \frac{IBW}{Scr \times 72} \times 0.85 \text{ (if female)}$$

MDRD (modified diet in renal disease four criteria with standardized serum creatinine)

$eGFR = 175 \times SCr^{-1.154} \times age^{-0.203} \times 0.742 \text{ (if female)} \times 1.1212 \text{ (if African American)}$

CKD-EPI (for males with serum creatinine <0.9 mg/dL)

$eGFR = 141 \times SCr/0.9^{-0.411} \times 0.993^{age} \times 1.159 \text{ (if African American)}$

standardization of creatinine assays has impacted estimates using older methodology such as Cockcroft-Gault. Since 2008, the standardized serum creatinine values are slightly lower than unstandardized values previously used. Because of these changes, today the Cockcroft-Gault equation, which was based on unstandardized serum creatinine values, tends to slightly overestimate the creatinine clearance. However, most of the pharmacokinetic drug dosing protocols for patients with impaired renal function use the Cockcroft-Gault methodology. Until protocols are developed for drug dosing using the MDRD and CKD-EPI, the older methodology should still be utilized recognizing that Cockcroft-Gault slightly overestimates creatinine clearance. Remember that pharmacokinetic dosing based on any renal parameter has always been an approximation requiring adjustments based on clinical judgment and other objective measures, rather than absolute calculation. Finally, for patients with normal or near-normal renal function, most laboratories do not report actual eGFR (calculated using the MDRD), but use eGFR >60 cc/min. Actual calculated eGFRs are only reported for eGFRs <60 cc/min, since that is the agreed upon definition of mildly to moderately decreased renal function.

• URINE RENAL FUNCTION TESTS

One of the disadvantages of serum RFTs is their relative lack of sensitivity to early and small changes in renal function. Urinalysis, on the other hand, is an accurate method to detect early and small changes in renal function. Protein and formed elements in the urine are the primary tools used to indicate early changes in renal function.

Urine Protein/Albumin

The glomerulus is normally impermeable to large protein molecules, such as albumin. Low molecular weight globulins, which are small enough to pass the glomerulus, are mostly reabsorbed in the tubules, so protein levels in the urine are normally very low (<100 mg/24 hours). Protein excretion from the kidneys can be measured in three ways, a 24-hour urine collection, an estimated 24-hour excretion using a 4-hour collection, and by urine test strip in a random sample. Random sample urine test strips for protein can be read without additional equipment, but only detect excretion rates of >300 mg/24 hours. Clinical proteinuria (albumin and globulins) is defined as >500 mg/day. Care is needed in evaluating individual random urine dipstick readings, because exercise, running, fever, infection, and trauma (e.g., dirt bike riding, football) all cause transient increases in urinary protein and albumin excretion. A single 1+ test strip reading should result in questioning about activities known to facilitate excretion. If an identifiable cause cannot be found, then the dipstick should be repeated later. Repeated 1+ protein test strip readings warrant a further workup for impaired renal function. Since albumin in the urine is a more sensitive indicator, it is relied on for early detection of renal damage in conditions known to have renal complications such as hypertension and diabetes mellitus. Albuminuria is measured in two primary ways: the urinary albumin excretion rate (AER), which uses a 4-hour urine collection to estimate 24-hour excretion and the urinary albumin to creatinine ratio (ACR), which uses a single random sample. Macroalbuminuria is defined as excretion rates of >300 mg/g/24 hours, while microalbuminuria is defined as excretion rates of 30 to 299 mg/24 hours. Because of its increased sensitivity, tests for smaller amounts of albumin (microalbuminuria) is preferred. Whenever urine is collected over a 4- or 24-hour period, accuracy due to missed urine collections can be a problem. Therefore, it is probably best to routinely use random urine samples. Random tests for microalbuminuria that measure ACR also use test strips, but require a special analyzer to accurately measure the sample. Because the ACR uses creatinine, it tends to under-estimate albumin excretion in males, due to their larger muscle mass.

Formed Elements

In addition to the presence of albumin in the urine, formed elements such as casts, red blood cells (RBCs), white blood cells (WBCs), and insoluble crystals can indicate kidney damage. Formed elements are seen with microscopic analysis of urine samples.

Hematuria A few RBCs can be found during microscopic urinalysis in patients without intrinsic renal damage. As with proteinuria and albuminuria, exercise, fever, and trauma can result in a few RBCs in the urine. However, even >2 to 3 RBCs/hpf in several samples can indicate renal damage. Significant hematuria may cause the urine to turn orange or pink depending on the number of RBCs. Similarly, urine residue containing RBCs may result in small red to dark reddish-brown stains on underwear. Also in women of childbearing age, RBCs from menstrual blood can be carried into the urine, usually accompanied by epithelial cells. Persistent hematuria requires further workup to rule out more serious problems such as neoplasm, infection, renal calculus, or trauma.

Pyuria WBCs in the urine are usually indicative of infection or inflammation in the urinary tract, occurring commonly in urinary tract infections. Pyuria is defined as >10 WBCs/hpf.

Casts Casts are cylindrical masses of glycoprotein formed in the tubules. The presence of casts in the urine is called cylindruria. Hyaline casts are common and carry no pathological significance. As casts form, they can surround RBCs, WBCs, and epithelial cells. The presence of WBC casts usually indicates infection or inflammation. RBC casts indicate significant damage to the kidney as do epithelial casts.

• MISCELLANEOUS DIAGNOSTIC TESTS

Medical imaging studies including ultrasound, CT scans, and MRI are used to detect masses and structural abnormalities. In addition, other substances found in the urine may indicate other systemic diseases, i.e., ketones in the urine may indicate diabetic ketoacidosis; bilirubin and its metabolites may indicate liver or biliary abnormalities.

• CAUSES OF ABNORMAL RENAL FUNCTION TESTS

When faced with lab test results that indicate potential renal damage, one must consider the problem to be potentially located anywhere in the urinary tract or it can be caused by other organ systems in the body. Decreased renal perfusion due to dehydration or CHF can cause temporary elevations in serum markers such as serum creatinine, BUN. Once hydrated or when CHF is treated, renal perfusion returns to normal along with the values of serum RFTS. Bleeding into the upper gastrointestinal tract can cause elevations in BUN levels and the BUN/creatinine ratio. Severe liver disease can cause abnormally low BUN values. Within the urinary tract, laboratory test abnormalities can be indicative of damage to the kidney itself, i.e., glomerulus, tubules, or interstitial tissue. Damage to these parts of the urinary tract can be caused by neoplasm, infection, autoimmune disease, and numerous medications and will result in abnormal serum and urine tests. In addition, problems with the ureters, bladder, and in males the prostate gland can result in abnormalities in both serum and urinary markers of renal function, but may require imaging to determine the location of damage. By themselves, RFTs usually cannot determine whether the renal injury is acute or chronic. Generally, that determination requires additional history, the clinical course of the event, and at times also requires other studies to determine the exact cause.

• KEY REFERENCES

1. Winger J, Michelfelder A. Diagnostic approach to the patient with jaundice. *Prim Care.* 2011;38:469-482.
2. Johnston DE. Special considerations in interpreting liver function tests. *Am Fam Physician.* 1999;59: 2223-2230.
3. Thapa BR, Walia A. Liver function tests and their interpretation. *Indian J Pediat.* 2007;74:663-671.
4. Carey E, Carey WD. Non-invasive tests for liver disease, fibrosis and cirrhosis: is the liver biopsy obsolete? *Cleve Clin J Med.* 2010;77:519-527.
5. Lee WM. Drug-induced hepatotoxicity. *N Engl J Med.* 2003;349:474-485.
6. Navarro VJ, Senior JR. Drug-related hepatotoxicity. *N Engl J Med.* 2006;354:731-739.
7. Aboud G, Kaplowitz N. Drug-induced liver injury. *Drug Saf.* 2007;30:277-294.
8. Corsini A, Ganey P, Ju C, et al. Current challenges and controversies in drug-induced hepatic injury. *Drug Saf.* 2012;35:1099-1117.
9. Giboney PT. Mildly elevated liver transaminase levels in the asymptomatic patient. *Am Fam Physician.* 2005;71:1105-1110.
10. Vernon G, Baranova A, Younossi ZM. Systematic review: the epidemiology and natural history of non-alcoholic fatty liver disease and non-alcoholic steatohepatitis in adults. *Aliment Pharmacol Ther.* 2011;34:274-285.
11. Barsic N, Lerotic I, Smircic-Duvnjak L, et al. Overview and developments in non-invasive diagnosis of nonalcoholic fatty liver disease. *World J Gastroenterol.* 2012;18:3945-3954.
12. Ghany MG, Strader DB, Thomas, DL, Seef LB. Diagnosis, management, and treatment of hepatitis C. *Hepatology.* 2009;49:1335-1374.
13. Weinbaum CM, Williams I, Mast EE, et al. Recommendations for identification and public health management of persons with chronic hepatitis B virus infection. *Morb Mortal Wkly Recomm Rep.* 2008;57(RR08):1-20.
14. Killeen AA, Ashwood ER, Ventura CB, Styer P. Recent trends in performance and current state of creatinine assays. *Arch Pathol Lab Med.* 2013;137:496-502.
15. Van Pottelbergh G, Van Heden L, Mathei C, Degryse J. Methods to evaluate renal function in elderly patients: a systematic literature review. *Age Ageing.* 2010;39:542-548.
16. Koyner JL. Assessment and diagnosis of renal dysfunction in the ICU. *Chest.* 2012;141:1584-1594.
17. Tesch GH. Review: serum and urine biomarkers in kidney disease: a pathophysiological perspective. *Nephrology.* 2010;15:609-616.
18. Shipak MG, Matsushita K, Arnlov J, et al. Cytostatin C versus creatinine in determining risk based on kidney function. *N Engl J Med.* 2013;369:932-943.
19. Stevens PE, Levin A. Evaluation and management of chronic kidney disease: synopsis of the kidney disease: improving global outcomes 2012 clinical practice guideline. *Ann Intern Med.* 2013;158:825-830.
20. Younes N, Cleary PA, Steffes MW, et al. Comparison of urinary albumin-creatinine ratio and albumin excretion rate in the diabetes control and complications trial/epidemiology of diabetes interventions and complications study. *Clin J Am Soc Nephrol.* 2010;5:1235-1242.
21. Rostoker G, Andrivet P, Pham I, Griuncelli M, Adnot S. Accuracy and limitations of equations for predicting glomerular filtration rate during follow-up of patients with non-diabetic nephropathies. *BMC Nephrol.* 2009;10:16-26.
22. Richardson M. Precision vs approximation: the trade off in assessing kidney function and drug dosing. *Pharmacotherapy.* 2010;30:758-761.
23. Nyman HA, Dowling TC, Hudson JQ, et al. Comparative evaluation of the Cockcrot-Gault equation and the modification of diet in renal disease study equation for drug dosing: an opinion of the nephrology practice and research network of the American College of Clinical Pharmacy. *Pharmacotherapy.* 2011;31:1130-1144.
24. Dowling TC, Matzke GR, Murphy JE, Burckart GJ. Evaluation of renal drug dosing, prescribing information and clinical pharmacist approaches. *Pharmacotherapy.* 2010;30:776-786.
25. Dowling TC, Wang R, Ferucci L, Sorkin JD. Glomerular filtration rate equations overestimate creatinine clearance in older individuals enrolled in the Baltimore longitutdinal study on aging: impact on renal drug dosing. *Pharmacotherapy.* 2013;33:912-921.

CASE 24.1
INTERPRETING LIVER AND RENAL FUNCTION TESTS

Total Protein 8.2 g/L
Albumin 5.0 g/L
ALT 600 units/L
AST 390 units/L
Alk Phos 54 units/L
INR 1.0
Bilirubin 4.0 mg/dL

CASE 24.2
INTERPRETING LIVER AND RENAL FUNCTION TESTS

Total Protein 5.6 g/L
Albumin 2.7 g/L
ALT 60 units/L
AST 39 unit/L
Alk Phos 104 units/L
INR 2.0
Bilirubin 4.0 mg/dL
BUN 2 mg/dL
Serum Creatinine 1.0 mg/dL
eGFR >60 mL/min

INTERPRETING LIVER AND RENAL FUNCTION TESTS

Total Protein 8.1 g/L
Albumin 5.0 g/L
ALT 200 units/L
AST 194 units/L
Alk Phos 640 units/L
INR 1.0
Bilirubin 4.0 mg/dL
Direct Bilirubin 2.4 mg/dL
BUN 45 mg/dL
Serum Creatinine 3.0 mg/dL
eGFR 38 mL/min
Urine Albumin/Creatinine 2000 mg/g

CASE 24.4
INTERPRETING LIVER RENAL FUNCTION TESTS

Total Protein 8.2 g/L
Albumin 5.0 g/L
ALT 65 units/L
AST 52 units/L
Alk Phos 94 units/L
INR 1.0
Bilirubin 0.9 mg/dL
BUN 11 mg/dL
Serum Creatinine 0.8 mg/dL

CASE 24.5
INTERPRETING LIVER FUNCTION TESTS

Total Protein 6.1 g/L
Albumin 3.0 g/L
ALT 650 units/L
AST 520 units/L
Alk Phos 94 units/L
INR 2.5
Bilirubin 3.0 mg/dL
BUN 64 mg/dL
eGFR >60
Serum Creatinine 1.0 mg/dL

CASE 24.6
LIVER DISEASE

Harvey Wallbanger, a rotund 68-year-old Native American war veteran, who supplements his veteran's pension by bartending at the Arizona Inn, presents to clinic complaining of a weeklong history of fatigue, malaise, and nausea without vomiting. He came in because he noticed his urine had gotten dark brown. Harvey's only health problems are severe osteoarthritis of both knees and hips for which he takes 4 to 6 g/day of tylenol and the recent onset of hemorrhoids for which he was given Anusol HC about 6 weeks ago. His only other pertinent medical history is a recent trip to rural Costa Rica as chaperone for a group of teens who were part of a church-sponsored community help program, where he lived with local people.

a. List two probable causes for his problem. Explain your rationale.

_____

_____

_____

_____

_____

b. List four questions you would ask or examinations you would perform to help confirm your diagnosis. Explain your rationale.

_____

_____

_____

_____

_____

c. Below are results of lab tests ordered. What is your assessment of Harvey's complaints? Explain your rationale

Total Bilirubin	10 mg/dL	Total Protein	5.2 g/L	Alk Phos	102 units/L
AST units/L	310	Albumin	2.5 g/L	BUN	12 mg/dL
ALT units/L	540	INR	2.0	Serum Creatinine	0.8 mg/dL

_____

_____

_____

_____

_____

CHAPTER

TWENTY-FIVE

Anemia, Bleeding, and Infection

LEARNING OBJECTIVES

1. Interpret the findings for anemia and its causes, the presence or absence of bacterial infections, and evidence of adverse hematological effects of medication given the results of a complete blood count.

2. Evaluate for evidence of bleeding due to overanticoagulation when monitoring patients on anticoagulants.

3. Use knowledge of the complete blood count and other signs and symptoms to monitor the response to treatment for anemias and infections.

• INTRODUCTION

The purpose of this chapter is to teach pharmacists how to evaluate patients for anemia, bacterial infection, bleeding, and adverse hematological drug effects. Management of anticoagulant therapy, including adjustment of doses, as well as medications that cause various hematological disorders, can be readily found in pharmacotherapy textbooks and other resources. Therefore, these topics are not covered in this chapter. Pharmacists in a variety of patient care practice environments are routinely required to evaluate patients' complete blood counts to evaluate for potential adverse medication effects and response to treatment. Pharmacists working in anticoagulation clinics routinely monitor for evidence of bleeding due to overanticoagulation. Pharmacists also monitor responses of treatments for various anemias and infections. Finally, pharmacists are also asked to evaluate for the presence of drug-induced adverse effects to the hematologic system.

• INTERPRETING THE COMPLETE BLOOD COUNT

This review is not intended to be a comprehensive listing of all possible abnormalities, but focuses on the common hematological abnormalities that are typically seen by pharmacists in dealing with adult patients. The complete blood count (CBC) consists of three major components: red cells (RBC), white cells (WBC), and platelets. When evaluating the results of a CBC, consideration should be given to gender, ethnicity, and normal variation. Up to 5% of the population, without any disease, will routinely have values that are outside the "normal" values. In addition, different references cite small differences in normal values. Therefore, this review will use a common sense approach to CBC interpretation and easy to remember normal and abnormal values.

Red Cells

When looking at the red cell portion of the CBC, the first thing is to determine whether or not the patient is anemic. Anemia is defined as a decreased red cell mass, manifested as below normal levels of hematocrit (HCT) and red cell count (RBC). *Hematocrit* is the percentage of blood volume that comprises red blood cells. Values differ in adults by gender due to a combination of the erythropoietic effect of higher levels of testosterone in males, and regular blood loss due to menses in females. Normal values are 42% to 50% in males and 36% to 45% in females. Hemoglobin (HGB) is the oxygen carrying moiety within erythrocytes (RBC). Anemias are characterized by amounts of hemoglobin <13.5 g/dL in males or 12.0 g/dL in females. The *red cell count (RBC)* is done by instrument and normal values range from 4.5 to 5.9×10^6 in males and 4.1 to 5.1×10^6 in females. The normal values may be slightly higher for patients with chronic hypoxia such as patients with COPD, those living at high altitude or who are heavy

TABLE 25.1	Signs and Symptoms of Significant Anemia (Caused by Hypoxia or Hypovolemia)
Fatigue, weakness, malaise, decreased exercise tolerance	
Headache	
Tachycardia	
Tachypnea	
Orthostatic hypotension	
Dizziness	
Pale conjunctiva, nail bed, frenulum of tongue	
Shortness of breath	
Dyspnea on exertion	
Exacerbation of cardiac disease (angina, CHF)	

TABLE 25.2	Classification of Anemias	
Color	Cell Size	Causes
NORMOCHROMIC	NORMOCYTIC	Acute blood loss
Normal red cell color due to normal	Normal size red blood cells	Hemolytic anemia
amount of oxygenated hemoglobin	MCV 80 to 100	Chronic renal failure
in each red blood cell		Anemia of chronic disease (inflammation, infection, cancer)
NORMOCHROMIC	MACROCYTIC	Folic acid deficiency
	Large red blood cells	Vitamin B$_{12}$ deficiency
	MCV >100	
HYPOCHROMIC	MICROCYTIC	Iron deficiency
Pale red blood cells due to low	Small red blood cells	Chronic blood loss
levels of oxygenated hemoglobin in	MCV <80	Pyridoxine deficiency
each red blood cell		

smokers. Patients with anemia may have symptoms that are caused by physiological responses to poor oxygenation of the tissues, due to the lowered oxygen-carrying capacity of the blood (Table 25.1).

If the patient is anemic, the next step is to determine the type of anemia. There are three main types of anemia defined by the color and size of the red blood cell (Table 25.2). Cell size and color are determined by the *red cell indices*, which are mathematical manipulations of RBC, HCT, and hemoglobin (HGB) values. *Mean corpuscular volume* (*MCV*) is used to determine average red blood cell size. The MCV is calculated by dividing 10 times the HCT by the RBC count. Normal values are 80 to 100. Patients with a low HCT and a normal MCV are said to have a normocytic or normal red cell anemia. Patients with a low HCT and an MCV of less than 80 have a microcytic or small red cell anemia. Finally, patients with a low HCT and an MCV >100 have a macrocytic or large red cell anemia. The *mean corpuscular hemoglobin* (*MCH*) is the hemoglobin value × 10 divided by the RBC count. The *mean corpuscular hemoglobin content* (*MCHC*) is the hemoglobin × 100 divided by the HCT. Anemias with normal values for MCH or MCHC are termed normochromic anemias, because the amount of oxygenated hemoglobin that gives blood its red color is normal, while anemias with low MCH/MCHC levels are called hypochromic anemias due to lower levels of oxygenated hemoglobin, which results in less intense red color of blood.

There are multiple causes of the three types of anemia. *Normochromic, normocytic anemias* have normal cell size and color and are caused by either destruction or sudden loss of red cells such as hemolytic anemia, acute blood loss, or by disorders of erythropoietin production/efficacy, usually classified as anemias of chronic disease. Causes of anemias of chronic diseases include chronic infections (HIV, hepatitis B/C, bacterial endocarditis, or osteomyelitis), autoimmune diseases (rheumatoid arthritis, Crohn disease, systemic lupus erythematosus), lymphomas, and chronic liver or renal disease. *Hypochromic, microcytic anemias* are primarily caused by iron deficiency due to poor nutrition or chronic blood loss. Finally, *normochromic, macrocytic anemias* are caused by vitamin B$_{12}$ or folate deficiencies.

There are several important parameters that assist in the diagnosis or in monitoring the response to therapy. The first is the *red blood cell distribution widths* (*RDW*), which is a measurement of the variation in red blood cell size in the sample and is calculated by instrument. The normal value is 11% to 15%. It is high in anemias caused by iron, folate, and B$_{12}$ deficiencies, and is primarily used in distinguishing iron deficiency anemias from other common causes of microcytosis such as thalassemia. Two terms are often associated with abnormal RDW. *Anisocytosis* means that on microscopic examination of blood there are a variety of red blood cell sizes on the peripheral smear (also measured by instrument) and is present in anemias due to iron, folate, and B_{12} deficiencies. *Poikilocytosis* means that there are a variety of shapes of red blood cells and is typically found in macrocytic anemias and in sickle cell anemia. The second important value is the *reticulocyte count*. Reticulocytes are immature red blood cells and the normal value is 0.5% to 2.5%. In patients with anemias due to iron, folate, and B_{12} deficiencies, using very small amounts of the deficient vitamin or mineral for 5 to 7 days will cause the reticulocyte percentage to go to double digits. Before the days of accurate serum levels of folate, B_{12}, and iron, giving very small amounts and getting a marked response was used diagnostically (Castle test to distinguish folate from B_{12} deficiency). Failure to respond with double digit *reticulocytosis* indicates that there is some other cause for the anemia than the vitamin or mineral deficiency. Today, the reticulocyte count is used primarily to monitor the efficacy of replacement therapy. The reticulocyte count can also be reported as the *reticulocyte index (RI) or corrected reticulocyte count*, which is more accurate, since it adjusts the reticulocyte percentage by multiplying it by the actual HCT divided by 45.

Other Helpful Tests to Evaluate Anemias

Iron deficiency anemia is the most common form of anemia. Among nutritional causes, poor dietary intake and pregnancy (which increases demand for iron) are common causes. Chronic blood loss is also a common cause. Above average, monthly menstrual blood loss and upper gastrointestinal bleeding are the most common etiologies. All red blood cell parameters are below normal except for RDW, which many times is elevated. In addition, a serum ferritin level of less than $10\,\mu g/mL$, is the most accurate indication of iron deficiency, reflecting severely depleted iron stores. While not routinely used in the diagnosis, serum transferrin levels (<30%) and serum iron levels (<$50\,\mu g/mL$) will be decreased. Total iron-binding capacity may be increased (>$250\,\mu g/mL$) in an attempt to capture more iron as it is absorbed into the blood stream from the gastrointestinal tract.

    Macrocytic anemias due to vitamin B_{12} or folic acid deficiencies, may have reduced or normal hemoglobin levels even though their MCV is >100. Generally, low B_{12} and folate blood levels are found depending on the specific deficiency. However, serum folate levels vary based on folate intake; therefore, RBC folate levels are a more accurate indication of folate status. Serum folate levels <$5\,\mu g/L$ and RBC folate levels <$166\,\mu g/L$ are diagnostic of folate deficiency. Similarly, about 5% of patients with B_{12} deficiency will have a normal or near normal serum B_{12} level due to the presence of other B_{12}-like substances. Therefore, in most patients with B_{12} levels in the low normal range, serum methylmalonic acid (MMA) and homocysteine levels will be drawn. In B_{12} deficiency, both will be elevated. They can also be used to confirm folate deficiency since the MMA level will be normal with an elevated homocysteine level. Both macrocytic anemias will have megaloblasts (large immature red cells). Because of that finding, B_{12} and folate deficiency anemias are sometimes referred to as megaloblastic anemias. In both deficiencies, hypersegmented neutrophils (>6 nucleated segments) are often present. In addition to an increased RDW and anisocytosis, macrocytic anemias may also present with poikilocytosis.

    Most macrocytic anemias are caused either by low intake of folate or B_{12}, or by diseases that cause malabsorption of nutrients (including B_{12} and folic acid) from the intestine, e.g., tropical sprue, pernicious anemia. Pernicious anemia is a classical malabsorption syndrome that causes B_{12} deficiency. The absorption of B_{12} requires an active process that involves both gastric acid and a protein called intrinsic factor, which are both produced by the parietal cells of the gastric lining. An autoimmune process attacks and destroys the parietal cells, leading to low B_{12} levels along with achlorhydria and a lack of intrinsic factor that leads to a macrocytic anemia. In addition, B_{12} deficiencies, like pernicious anemia, have other nonhematological complications including irreversible peripheral neuropathy, cognitive decline, and cardiac muscle damage, leading to congestive heart failure. Therefore, it is critical to accurately obtain a specific cause for a macrocytic anemia, since giving folic acid supplements to a patient with a B_{12} deficiency may partially correct or "mask" the anemia, but allow the neurological and cardiovascular damage to progress. That is why the amount of folate in over-the-counter vitamins is limited to 400 µg, to prevent the masking of pernicious anemia or B_{12} deficiency. Another cause of macrocytic anemia of interest to pharmacists is prescription medications. Traditional anticonvulsants such as phenytoin and carbamazepine, through induction of CYP450 enzymes, and methotrexate by direct antagonism can cause folate deficiencies. Chronic use of proton pump inhibitors, such as omeprazole and the diabetic medication metformin, have been reported to cause B_{12} deficiencies.

White Cells

There are five major types of white blood cells. Neutrophils, also known as segmented neutrophils (segs) or polymorphonuclear cells (PMNs or polys), are the primary defense against bacterial infections since they ingest and digest foreign proteins. Immature neutrophils are called bands or stabs and are normally not in circulation. Lymphocytes are the primary defense against viruses, fungi, mycobacterium, and malignant neoplasms. Lymphocytes are also involved in producing antibodies to a variety of viruses and bacteria, which subsequently provide immunity against those organisms. Monocytes are in circulation only 16 to 36 hours before they transform into tissue macrophages, which are active for months to years. They are the garbage collectors, ingesting foreign proteins, old red cells, plasma lipids, and plasma proteins. Macrophages are also an important component of both cell-mediated and antibody-mediated immune processes. Eosinophils are associated with IgE-mediated immune processes such as asthma, allergic rhinitis, atopic dermatitis, and urticaria, as well as with parasitic infections. The function of basophils is not clearly known, but they are thought to participate in both immediate and delayed hypersensitivity reactions. All precursors of white cells are produced in the bone marrow. PMNs continue to differentiate in the bone marrow, while lymphocytes differentiate in lymphatic tissue. Granulocytes (neutrophils, basophils, and eosinophils) have a short duration of existence in serum, ranging from 1 to 5 days. On the other hand, lymphocytes persist in serum for almost 90 days.

The white blood count consists of a *total white blood cell count (WBC)* and when the total white count is outside of normal the laboratory will automatically do a *differential white count*, which consists of measuring the percentages of each of the five types plus bands or stabs. Some facilities require a specific request for a differential count if the total white count is normal. However, most current automated instruments will automatically do a differential white blood cell count. Unfortunately, each process has its own normal range, which leads to a variety of normal values. For example, references for the lower limit of normal for the total white cell count can range from 4000 to 5000 cells/microliter (µL), and the upper normal levels range from 10,000 to 11,500 cells/µL. For the examples and exercises, 5000 to 10,000 cells/µL will be considered normal. Some conditions require an absolute cell count of each type for diagnostic purposes. To calculate the absolute count of a particular cell type multiply the percentage (as a decimal value) by the total white blood cell count. For a total white cell

TABLE 25.3	Normal White Blood Cell Counts
Total White Blood Cell Count	5000 to 10,000 cells/μL
Differential White Count	
Neutrophils **(PMNs, segs)**	35% to 75%
Immature neutrophils **(bands, stabs)**	0% to 5%
	<1500 absolute cell count = neutropenia
Lymphocytes	30% to 45%
Monocytes	1% to 4%
Basophils	0% to 1%
Eosinophils	0% to 3%
	>600 Absolute cell count = eosinophilia
	Leukopenia ≤ 5000 cells/μL
	Leukocytosis ≥ 10,000 cells/μL

count of 8500 cells/μL and 4% eosinophils (0.04), the absolute count of eosinophils is 340. Unfortunately, reference values may also vary for several absolute counts. For example, the definition of eosinophilia (above normal numbers of eosinophils) ranges from 350 to 600 cells/μL. For the examples and exercises in this chapter, >600 cells/μL will be used to determine the presence of eosinophilia. In practice, most results from commercial laboratories list normal values for their procedures or tests. Abnormal values are indicated by an additional symbol, an H for higher than normal values, and L for lower than normal levels. See Table 25.3 for normal values and definitions. Also somewhat confusing is the relationship between the percentages of each cell type in the differential count and the absolute cell count. For example, during bacterial infections, the absolute neutrophil count substantially increases, while other cell type counts remain constant. In the differential count, the percent of neutrophils will rise dramatically, along with the absolute neutrophil count, while the percent of the other cell types, particularly the lymphocytes, will fall to below normal levels even though the absolute cell count is unchanged.

Using the WBC Count to Confirm the Diagnosis of Bacterial Infections and Monitor Treatment Efficacy

Bacterial infections induce an elevated total white count (*leukocytosis*) with a predominance of neutrophils. When neutrophils are released from the bone marrow, most end up adhering to the endothelial walls of the blood vessels, and normally the CBC measures only those neutrophils *not* adhering to the endothelium. When a bacterial infection occurs, the original responding neutrophils attack the bacteria, causing a release of chemotactic factors that cause the neutrophils adhering to the vascular endothelium to be liberated into the blood and travel to the site of infection. Those same chemotactic factors stimulate the bone marrow to release stored mature neutrophils. In a bacterial infection, these two factors cause the total white blood cell count to rise above 10,000 cells/μL and the combined percentage of mature and immature neutrophils to exceed 80% of the total white blood cell count. If a bacterial infection is severe or long standing, the marrow releases immature neutrophils into the blood stream to help battle the infection. Historically, this is called a *left shift*. A left shift is present when the total WBC count indicates bacterial infection (>10,000 WBC + >80% of WBC are PMNs, stabs, or bands) plus the percentage of immature neutrophils (bands/stabs) rise to double digits (≥10%). The total WBC count and differential can also be used to monitor the efficacy of antibiotic therapy and the resolution of the bacterial infection. As the neutrophils, with the aid of an antibiotic, successfully fight the bacterial infection, the total WBC count, absolute neutrophil count, and percentage of neutrophils will return toward normal, along with the percentages of the other cell types in the differential white blood cell count.

Other Causes of Leukocytosis

When the total WBC count rises above 12,000 cells/µL, and there is no evidence of bacterial infection, consideration must be given to the possibility of leukemias and lymphomas. The specific diagnosis requires a peripheral blood smear examined under the microscope and several other specific tests that are beyond the scope of this textbook.

Drug Induced Decreases in Red and White Blood Cells

Many medications have adverse effects on the bone marrow. Obviously, most cytotoxic cancer chemotherapy, which interferes with all rapidly growing cells, also negatively impacts the production of white blood cells in the bone marrow. Other medications have the same impact, but through different mechanisms ranging from pharmacological side effects to hypersensitivity or idiosyncratic reactions. Pharmacists need to monitor patients on medications with potential bone marrow adverse effects to prevent infectious complications. Granulocytes (neutrophils, basophils, and eosinophils) are the most susceptible to the toxic drug effects due to their short half-lives in the blood compared to lymphocytes and macrophages, which have much longer half-lives in tissue and blood. Eventually, they too will be impacted by continuous exposure to a bone marrow toxin. Since neutrophils are so important to defend against bacterial infections, we focus on their absolute counts. *Neutropenia* is defined as an absolute count of less than 1500 cells/µL. Once the levels drop below 500 cells/µL, normal bacterial flora in the oral cavity, gastrointestinal tract, and other parts of the body can cause serious infections. *Granulocytopenia* is a below normal number of neutrophils, basophils, and eosinophils. *Agranulocytosis* indicates granulocytopenia, plus the lack of production of granulocytes in the marrow and requires a bone marrow biopsy for diagnosis. Agranulocytosis carries a much more ominous prognosis than granulocytopenia, so care must be exerted not to use the terms interchangeably. Similarly, *pancytopenia* indicates below normal numbers of red blood cells, white blood cells, and platelets in the blood, whereas *aplastic anemia* refers to a pancytopenia, plus the lack of bone marrow production of all three formed elements in the blood and requires a bone marrow biopsy for diagnosis. With medications that cause decreases in the number of granulocytes, the absolute counts of the granulocytes will fall, along with their percentages of the total white cell count. The absolute counts of lymphocyte and monocytes, because of their longer half-life in serum, will remain unchanged, but the percentages will markedly increase due to the decrease in the absolute number of granulocytes.

Platelet Count

The final formed element of blood made by the bone marrow, platelets, is important to the blood clotting process, especially in arteries. In atherosclerotic cardiovascular disease (strokes and myocardial infarctions), platelet aggregation starts the infarction process. We use drugs like aspirin that interfere with platelet aggregation to prevent or reduce the risk of those events. These platelet inhibitors can also cause abnormal bleeding. While normal values can vary by lab, 150,000 to 400,000/µL is a representative normal range. Values below normal (*thrombocytopenia*) increase the risk of bleeding and values above normal (*thrombocytosis*) tend to increase the risk of clotting. In addition to the numbers of platelets, there are also tests of platelets' ability to aggregate. Most tests are primarily used for research purposes. While the mechanism of action of aspirin is known, there are no practical methods for measuring its effect on platelet aggregation. However, for antiplatelet medications that primarily impact P2Y12, there are now reliable "point-of-service" tests that show promise in helping gauge effectiveness and adjusting doses of clopidogrel, prasugrel, and ticagrelor.

• MONITORING ANTICOAGULATED PATIENTS FOR BLEEDING

Anticoagulants are used to prevent pulmonary embolisms, myocardial infarctions, strokes, deep vein thrombosis, and venous thromboembolism. While monitoring patients on anticoagulants, the pharmacist checks for signs and symptoms of blood clots (stroke, pulmonary embolism) to evaluate the efficacy of the anticoagulant. In addition, some agents have specific tests and procedures that help pharmacists measure optimal anticoagulation and adjust doses. Finally, anticoagulants can also cause bleeding if given in higher doses or to patients with enhanced sensitivity to their effects. Therefore, it is important that pharmacists understand how to evaluate patients for bleeding, the major adverse effect of these medications.

The easiest way to conduct an interview for potential symptoms of bleeding is a modified review of systems (ROS) process (Table 25.4). If lab values indicate overanticoagulation, then a complete ROS should be done. If anticoagulation parameters are normal, then an individualized, but briefer version based on previous patient experiences and education is indicated. During the first few follow-up visits after initiation of anticoagulation therapy, a complete ROS should be done since it also serves as an educational process to teach patients what to look for as symptoms of bleeding

TABLE 25.4	Evaluating Hemorrhagic Complications of Anticoagulants

HEAD AND NECK

    Nose bleeds
    Bleeding gums after brushing
    Visual or conjunctival changes
    Headache
        Intracranial bleed
        CVA
        Hypoxia

SKIN

    Subepidermal bleeding
        Elderly
        Other medication
    Easy bruisability
    Excessive bleeding from cuts and scrapes

GASTROINTESTINAL

    History of peptic ulcer disease
    Ulcerogenic drug use
    Heartburn
    Retroperitoneal bleed
    Hematemesis
    Melena
    Hematochezia

GENITOURINARY

    Hematuria
    Excessive menses or vaginal bleeding

MISCELLANEOUS

    Hemarthrosis
    Hemoptysis

complications. What the pharmacist focuses on are changes or new symptoms that might indicate potential bleeding complications.

Head and Neck

One of the most common signs of bleeding is bleeding of the gums during and after brushing the teeth. Also bleeding from the nose can also be an indication of excessive anticoagulation. Visual changes and decreased visual acuity may indicate a hyphema (bleeding into the anterior chamber of the eye). Subconjunctival hemorrhages can also occur more readily in anticoagulated patients. Both of these are usually associated with trauma to the surrounding area or violent movement of the head, e.g., during sneezing. New onset headaches can indicate a hemorrhagic cerebrovascular accident, an intracranial or subdural bleed, or hypoxia in a severely anemic patient and warrant a neurological examination. Finally, check for paleness in the conjunctiva, frenulum of the tongue, and lips as a sign of significant anemia.

Skin

Another common site for detecting bleeding due to excessive anticoagulation is the skin. Excessive bleeding from cuts, e.g., shaving in males, may indicate overanticoagulation. Similarly, new onset of easy bruisability (bruising due to nominal trauma) or large deep bruises from minimal trauma may be an indication of overanticoagulation. Finally, bleeding just under the skin may warrant further investigation. Many times, it may be hard to distinguish the cause of subepidermal bleeding, especially in elderly patients, in whom it can occur naturally because of increased fragility of small arteries and veins due to aging. Similar effects can be caused by newly added medications, such as angiotensin-converting-enzyme inhibitors or nonsteroidal anti-inflammatory medications, which have mild anticoagulant effects of their own. Like the conjunctiva and tongue, the nail beds can be checked for loss of color, which represents significant anemia.

Gastrointestinal Tract

In patients with a history of peptic ulcer disease or on medications that may be ulcerogenic (corticosteroids, NSAIDs), checking for signs and symptoms of bleeding from the gastrointestinal (GI) tract is important. Symptoms such as heartburn and very dark stool may be an indication of upper GI tract bleeding. Large quantities of upper GI bleeding may cause melena (black tarry stools) or hematemesis in the form of bright red blood or coffee-ground vomitus. Pharmacists should be vigilant, especially in older patients, for a retroperitoneal bleed, which may start out as fullness or bloating, and eventually lead to more severe abdominal discomfort and pain. Finally, hematochezia or rectal bleeding of bright red blood can arise from the sigmoid colon or rectum or anal fissures, in patient with hemorrhoids, can be due to excessive anticoagulation.

Genitourinary (GU) Tract

Hematuria can be a sign of bleeding due to excessive anticoagulation in both genders. Microscopic amounts of hematuria cannot be detected by noting any change in color of the urine. However, small amounts of bleeding may present as pink, red, or red-brown stains on underwear or toilet paper. Gross hematuria may change the urine to colors ranging from pink to reddish brown depending on the amount of blood and the concentration of bilirubin by-products (urobilin) that cause urine to be yellow. In menstruating females, increased volumes and/or duration of menses can be an indicator of excess anticoagulation.

Miscellaneous

Trauma to joints, in addition to visible hematomas (bruises), may also cause hemarthrosis (bleeding into the joint) in anticoagulated patients. Knees and elbows are the most commonly affected. Pain, swelling, warmth, stiffness, and/or reduced range of motion are signs of bleeding into the joint space. In patients with COPD, hemoptysis can occur.

• KEY REFERENCES

1. Tefferi A, Hanson CA, Inwards DJ. How to interpret and pursue an abnormal complete blood count in adults. *Mayo Clin Proc.* 2005;80:923-936.
2. Kaferle K, Strzoda CE. Evaluation of macrocytosis. *Am Fam Physician.* 2009;79:203-208.
3. Bryan LJ, Zakai NA. Why is my patient anemic? *Hematol Oncol Clin North Am.* 2012;26:205-230.
4. Pang WW, Schrier SL. Anemia in the elderly. *Curr Opin Hematol.* 2012;19:133-140.
5. Cerny J, Rosmarin AG. Why does my patient have leukocytosis? *Hematol Oncol Clin North Am.* 2012;26: 303-319.
6. Reagan JL, Castillo JJ. Why is my patient neutropenic? *Hematol Oncol Clin North Am.* 2012;26:253-266.
7. Bhatt V, Saleem A. Review: drug-induced neutropenia—pathophysiology, clinical features and management. *Ann Clin Lab Sci.* 2004;34:132-137.
8. Carey PJ. Drug-induced myelosupression, diagnosis and management. *Drug Saf.* 2003;26:691-706.
9. Wong EY, Rose MG. Why does my patient have thrombocytopenia? *Hematol Oncol Clin North Am.* 2012;26:231-252.

CASE 25.1

CJ is a 27- year-old female who presents with the primary complaint of fatigue. Other pertinent medical history includes long-standing menorrhagia and perennial allergic rhinitis. Interpret the CBC and relevant lab tests.

_____

_____

_____

_____

_____

HCT	27%	TOTAL WBC	7200
HGB	8	PMN	60%
MCV	75	BANDS	–0–
MCH	23	LYMPH	25%
MCHC	30	MONOS	4%
RETIC	0.3%	BASO	2%
		EOS	9%
Platelets	400,000		
Ferritin	6 ng/mL		

CASE 25.2

AB is a 66-year-old male, who has been on phenytoin and phenobarbital for 50 years for a seizure disorder, presents because his wife thinks he does not look well. When asked, he admits to fatigue and tiring easily. Interpret the CBC and relevant lab tests.

HCT	28%	TOTAL WBC	5400
HGB	12.4	PMN	50%
MCV	119	BAND	0%
MCH	28	LYMPHS	44%
MCHC	34	MONOS	4%
RETIC	0.4%	BASO	–0–
		EOS	2%
Platelets	150,000	Hypersegmented PMNs	

Anisocytosis and poikilocytosis

B_{12} and folate serum levels are both normal. So a Castle test is ordered.
After 5 days of 1 μg IM of folic acid/day, reticulocyte count = 17%

CASE 25.3

KJ is a 53-year-old female with a 25-year history of rheumatoid arthritis, who was admitted June 1 with a 6-day history of severe cough and fever. The patient was diagnosed with bacterial pneumonia, based on bilateral consolidated infiltrates in both lower lobes, and antibiotics were started the same day. Interpret the CBC and relevant lab tests.

			June 1	June 8
HCT	32%	TOTAL WBC	12,400	9800
HGB	12	PMN	68%	58%
MCV	88	BANDS	17%	3%
MCH	32	LYMPHS	13%	31%
MCHC	34	MONO	2%	3%
RETIC	0.8%	BASO	0%	1%
		EOS	0%	4%

Ferritin = 100 ng/ml,   folate/B_{12} = wnl

_____

_____

_____

_____

_____

Answer Keys

CASE 3.1
ANSWER KEY

I	Appendectomy	1967
A	Hypertension	1993
TP	Sore throat	4/4/94
A	Obesity	1990
I	Positive PPD	1981 (INH prophylaxis completed 2/82)
TP	Ankle sprain	2/10/99
I	Open reduction	L Humerus FX 7/79
TP	Cellulitis L hand	9/89
A	Congestive heart failure—mild	6/99
TP	Constipation	5/55
TP	Diaper rash (monilial)	7/50
A	Childhood immunizations completed	7/54
A	Penicillin allergy (hives)	10/60
I	Elevated liver function tests	5/91
I	Headache, vascular	1990
A	Diabetes mellitus	1999
A	Proteinuria	7/2003

PROBLEM LIST

Date of Onset/Number.		Active Problems	Inactive/Resolved Problems	Date Resolved
	00	HEALTH MAINTENANCE		
1954		Immunizations complete		
1960	1	PENICILLIN ALLERGY		
		Hives		
1967	2		APPENDECTOMY	10/67
7/79	3		OPEN REDUCTION L HUMEROUS FX	1980
1981	4		Positive PPD	
			INH prophylaxis completed	2/82
1990	5	OBESITY		
1990	6	VASCULAR HEADACHE		
1993	7	HYPERTENSION		
NAME	Barnaby Jones			
DOB	6/18/49			
SS/REG#				

PROBLEM LIST

Date of Onset/Number.		Active Problems	Inactive/Resolved Problems	Date Resolved
1999	8	DIABETES MELLITUS		
2003		Proteinuria		
1999	9	CONGESTIVE HEART FAILURE		
NAME	Barnaby Jones			
DOB	6/18/49			
SS/REG#				

CASE 3.2
ANSWER KEY

TP Runny nose/bad cold

S- Patient presents with 7 to 10 days of runny nose, and dull frontal headache, only partially relieved by ibuprofen. Has had this happen in the past usually in fall and spring. Pain is localized just below the eyes and now his upper teeth have begun to ache. Also complains of bloodshot eyes, and occasional sneezing. Denies fever or purulent nasal discharge. Denies previous MD visit for this problem, other health problems (thyroid/DM/BP, cardiac, glaucoma), other medications, or breathing difficulties.

O- TPR 99/84/15 BP 124/78

Patient has marked allergic shiners bilaterally.

Sounds mildly congested, crumpled Kleenex in R hand

Eyes markedly injected bilaterally without discharge

ENT- negative for transillumination, palpation/percussion of maxillary sinuses but has pale boggy turbinates

A- Allergic rhinitis and conjunctivitis

P- Stop diphenhydramine LA, start chlorpheniramine 8 mg 1 bid for remainder of spring

If no relief of nasal/eye problems to MD

If symptoms worsen, fever or purulent discharge to MD/ ER

Warned patient re drowsiness, dry mouth

Joe Pharmacist Pharm D #10777

CASE 3.3
ANSWER KEY

3 BP

S-   Patient here for routine f/u visit. No problems since last visit other than some dry mouth, which started about 2 days after clonidine started, but has gotten better since then. Home BPs range 130-160/88-95. Denies dizziness or other problems. Will be going on vacation for 5 weeks, requests additional refill to last until next appointment. Working real hard to lose weight and cut back on sodium intake.

O-   BP   148/88 LA sitting

       140/86 RA sitting

       Weight down 6 lbs since last visit—162 today

       No edema

       SMAC-12 wnl

A-   BP under better control since starting clonidine

P.   Continue clonidine 2 mg bid

       Continue chlorthalidone 25 mg qAM

       RTC 2 months

       Monitor dry mouth

       Continue home BP bid

       Call pharmacy for extra refill

Joe Pharmacist Pharm D #10777

CASE 7.1
ANSWER KEY

SM, a regular customer at your store, comes in to pick up her mother's prescription. As she pays for the prescription, she asks: "Is there anything better than Actifed for this cold I've got? I'm tired of being stuffed up. It's been six days!"

a. Based on the information above, what are three likely causes for SM's symptoms? Explain your rationale.

> *Allergic rhinitis* → *lasted 6 days*
> *Viral URI* → *lasted 6 days*
> *Super virus* → *lasted 6 days*
> *Bacterial sinusitis* → *probably not as likely due to short time period but could be a complication of allergic rhinitis*
> *Vasomotor rhinitis* → *lasted 6 days*

b. List 10 questions you would ask, physical examinations you would conduct, or lab tests you would order to identify the etiology of SM's symptoms.

> *Describe the nasal discharge at 3 pm*
> > *Clear, watery* → *allergic rhinitis, vasomotor rhinitis*
> > *Clear, mucoid* → *viral URI, supervirus*
> > *Opaque, mucoid* → *viral URI, supervirus*
> > *Green tinged, mucoid* → *viral URI, supervirus*
> > *Purulent, dark yellow, brown, bloody* → *bacterial sinusitis*
> *Fever* → *URI, bacterial sinusitis, supervirus*
> *Itchy watery eyes* → *allergic rhinitis*
> *Cough?* → *viral URI, supervirus*
> *Hx of maxillary tooth pain* → *bacterial sinusitis*
> *Others have it?* → *viral URI, supervirus*
> *Personal/family hx of atopic dermatitis, asthma, allergic rhinitis* → *allergic rhinitis*
> *Has it gotten better then worse?* → *bacterial sinusitis*
> *Pain worse when bends over?* → *bacterial sinusitis*
> *Facial tenderness/fullness?* → *bacterial sinusitis*
> *Pain on palpation/percussion of maxillary or frontal sinuses* → *bacterial sinusitis*
> *Bad tasting/smelling mucous* → *bacterial sinusitis*
> *No light dispersion on transillumination of maxillary sinuses* → *bacterial sinusitis*
> *Nasal examination* → *pale boggy turbinates* → *allergic rhinitis*
> *Nasal examination* → *normal appearance in color* → *viral URI, vasomotor rhinitis, bacterial sinusitis*
> *Allergic shiners, nasal crease, or Dennie lines?* → *allergic rhinitis*
> *CBC* → *>710,000 WBC; >80% PMU* → *bacterial sinusitis*

Iloff Medkem, a first-year pharmacy student, has the "2014Crud," which began 8 days ago with fever, rhinorrhea, facial fullness, myalgias, and arthralgia. After 5 days he began to feel better. However, his rhinorrhea returned 2 days ago as a mucoid discharge. Today he presents with pain under both eyes and the discharge has markedly changed.

a.   List three questions you would ask to clarify his problem.

History is typical of classical bacterial sinusitis

How has the discharge changed? → *purulent, dark yellow, or brown at 3 pm*
Foul tasting/smelling discharge
Pain worse when bends over
Maxillary tooth pain
Fever

b.   List three physical examinations you would perform to clarify the diagnosis.

Palpate/percuss maxillary/frontal sinuses → *pain* → *bacterial sinusitis*
No light dispersion on transillumination of maxillary sinuses → *bacterial sinusitis*
Have patient blow nose into tissue → *purulent, dark yellow, brown discharge* → *bacterial sinusitis*
Take temperature → *fever* → *bacterial sinusitis*
Palpate maxillary teeth → *pain* → *bacterial sinusitis*

c.   What is the most likely diagnoses if the questions and examinations you listed above are positive?

Classical history and physical findings in bacterial sinusitis

CASE 7.3
ANSWER KEY

Howican Paddle presents to the pharmacy with a 3-day history of right ear discomfort with decreased hearing. This morning he woke up with a small yellow stain on his pillow.

a. What are the two most likely causes of his symptoms? Explain your rationale.

Ruptured TM 2° acute otitis media (AOM)
Otitis externa (OE)
Chronic suppurative otitis media (CSOM)

b. List two questions you would ask to help identify the cause. Explain your rationale.

Did the ear pain go away?   Yes ⟶ *AOM with ruptured TM*
                                                    No ⟶ *Otitis externa (OE)*
History of recurrent ear problems? ⟶ Yes ⟶ *CSOM*
Hx of swimming or picking in ears? ⟶ Yes ⟶ *OE*
Does it hurt when you lay on the ear? ⟶ Yes ⟶ *OE*
Hx of recent URI or allergic rhinitis ⟶ Yes ⟶ *AOM*

c. For each of the diagnoses listed in question a above, list expected findings on ear examination.

AOM
     Red TM, loss of landmarks, pinpoint perforation in TM
     Decreased hearing
     No pain on pinna pull/tragus pressure

OE
     Pain on pinna pull/tragus pressure
     Swollen red external ear canal, colorful growths in external canal
     TM wnl (if visualized)
     Hearing varies depending on the degree of obstruction of the external canal

CSOM
     Large central perforation of TM
     Significant hearing loss

CASE 7.4
ANSWER KEY

FF, a 33-year-old fourth-grade teacher asks what would be good for this bad sore throat he has had for the last 48 hours.

List 10 questions/physical examinations/lab tests you would want to ask, conduct or order to confirm your assessment.

Rapid Antigen Detection Test (RADT) ⁻⁺→ *streptococcal pharyngitis*

Throat culture ⁻⁺→ *for Group A β-hemolytic strep* → *streptococcal pharyngitis*

Positive Monospot test ⁻⁺→ *mononucleosis*

Sudden onset ⁻⁺→ *streptococcal pharyngitis*

Gradual onset ⁻⁺→ *post-nasal drip 2° to allergic rhinitis/URI or mononucleosis*

Nausea and vomiting ⁻⁺→ *streptococcal pharyngitis*

Pain severe lasting all day ⁻⁺→ *streptococcal pharyngitis, mononucleosis, HFMD*

Pain in AM only ⁻⁺→ *post-nasal drip 2° to allergic rhinitis/URI*

Duration longer than 72 hours ⁻⁺→ *viral pharyngitis, post-nasal drip, mononucleosis, HFMD*

Fatigue and /or jaundice ⁻⁺→ *mononucleosis*

Runny stuffy nose ⁻⁺→ *allergic rhinitis, viral URI*

Cough ⁻⁺→ *allergic rhinitis, viral URI*

Tonsils swollen ⁻⁺→ *mononucleosis, streptococcal pharyngitis, viral pharyngitis*

Red posterior pharynx/tonsils ⁻⁺→ *mononucleosis, streptococcal pharyngitis*

Pus on tonsils/posterior pharynx ⁻⁺→ *mononucleosis, streptococcal pharyngitis*

Fetid breath ⁻⁺→ *streptococcal pharyngitis*

Pain worse when swallowing orange juice/carbonate beverages ⁻⁺→ *mononucleosis, streptococcal pharyngitis*

Ulcers on posterior pharynx ⁻⁺→ *HFMD*

Vesicles on palms of hands/ soles of feet ⁻⁺→ *HFMD.*

CASE 8.1
ANSWER KEY

Roby Tussin, a 68-year-old male, presents to the pharmacy 4 months after a bout of viral pneumonia. When you ask how he is feeling, he tells you that while he still gets tired occasionally, he has not been able to get rid of his cough, which is dry and hacking and worse at night.

List three possible causes for his cough. Explain your rationale.

Tuberculosis
Lung cancer
PICS
Asthma   → *All are possible causes for persistent dry hacking cough*
Drug
GERD
Heart failure (CHF)
Allergic rhinitis

List three questions you would ask Roby. Explain your rationale.

History of smoking   → *lung cancer*
Medication   → *ACEI?*
Travel to third world country/   → *TB*
  around someone with cough
History of asthma, allergic   → *allergic rhinitis/asthma*
  rhinitis, atopic dermatitis
Heartburn   → *GERD*
Weight gain/edema   → *CHF*
Timing of cough at night   → *shortly after lying down*   → *GERD, allergic rhinitis*
                                      → *2 to 3 hours after lying*   → *CHF (paroxysmal noctur-*
                                        down   *nal dyspnea)*
                                      → *–3 to 6 AM*   → *asthma*

List four diagnostic tests or physical examinations you would order or perform to help make the diagnosis. Explain your rationale.

Chest x-ray → *rule out TB, lung cancer*
Respiratory rate → *>20 breaths per minute* → *hypoxia* → *asthma, heart failure*
PPD → *rule out TB*
ENT examination → *rule out allergic rhinitis*
Auscultation and percussion of lungs   → *wheezes*   → *asthma*
                                         → *crackles* → *heart failure*
Peak flow/PFTs → *rule out asthma*

CASE 8.2
ANSWER KEY

You are introduced to TW, a famous 82-year-old golfer at a Tucson AZ golf function. He has been visiting here for the last 3 months overseeing the construction of a golf course he designed. When he finds out you are a pharmacist, he asks if there is anything stronger than promethazine with codeine for coughing spells that have been bothering him for the last 4 weeks. It seems to be worse at night. He finished a 10-day course of amoxicillin 2 weeks ago for a cough "that went to his chest." He also complains about his recent 10-lb weight gain and the shot of him on TV last night made him look "fat as a hog." "Even my feet are getting fat! Why even my favorite slippers are getting tight." An excellent historian, TW tells you about his long-standing hypertension, which is treated with carvedilol and doxazosin (also for his prostate), and coronary artery disease that resulted in a tiny heart attack that led to a four-vessel CABG 15 years ago. He also takes aspirin, tiotropium inhaler for his smoking-induced COPD, and atorvastatin. You notice that his breathing appears to somewhat rapid.

Given TW's history and his current complaints, list three possible causes for his coughing attacks. Explain your rationale.

Valley fever (coccidioidomycosis) → *dust exposure supervising golf course construction*
Lung cancer → *long history of smoking*
COPD → *exacerbation*
Heart failure → *history of hypertension, CABG, edema*
Cor pulmonale → *right-sided heart failure due to COPD, edema, slippers tight*
Whooping cough → *cough lasting more than 4 weeks*
Respiratory syncytial virus (RSV) → *cold that went to his chest, antibiotic ineffective*
Atypical pneumonia → *Amoxycillin does not cover atypical pathogens*

List six questions, examinations, or tests you would ask/order/perform to help clarify his diagnosis. Explain your rationale.

Chest x-ray → *cardiac enlargement* → *heart failure, cor pulmonale*
→ *infiltrate* → *viral (RSV), bacterial, or atypical pneumonia, cocci*
→ *shadow/cavity* → *lung cancer, cocci*
→ *clear* → *COPD, RSV, whooping cough*
→ *displaced PMI* → *heart failure*
Auscultation → *faint breath sounds* → *emphysema*
→ *crackles in lung base* → *heart failure, cor pulmonale*
→ *crackles elsewhere* → *viral/atypical/bacterial pneumonia*
→ *rhonchi* → *COPD*
→ *clear* → *lung cancer*

Shortness of breath, dyspnea on exertion → *heart failure, cor pulmonale, COPD*

Paroxysmal nocturnal dyspnea, orthopnea → *heart failure*

Productive cough → *COPD, heart failure*
Nonproductive cough → *early RSV, cocci, whooping cough, lung CA*
Coughing in spasms → *whooping cough*
CBC → *>10,000 WBC + >80% PMNs/bands* → *bacterial pneumonia*
Amount of exposure to dust → *cocci*
Cocci serology → *cocci*
Pedal edema → *heart failure, cor pulmonale*

CASE 9.1
ANSWER KEY

Ferf Barfel, a 56-year-old overweight male, is playing golf when he has a sudden onset of severe chest pain. A 911 call brings him to the ER. The only other recent history is a visit 2 days ago for various aches and pains of 3 days duration after falling off his golf cart when he forgot to set the brake and it rolled over his left lower leg. To stop it Ferf had to hang on for dear life, putting all his considerable weight behind it to keep it from rolling down the hill. He hurt his chest, back, and shoulder in the process. Examination and x-rays were negative at the time. Ferf's problem list is as follows.

1990   Obesity
2001   Hypertension
2001   Hypercholesterolemia
2008   Type 2 diabetes mellitus

List four likely causes of Ferf's chest pain. Explain your rationale.

Pulmonary embolism → golf cart ran over left leg → phlebitis/DVT → sudden onset
Angina → four risk factors (hypertension, obesity, hyperlipidemia, diabetes)
Myocardial infarction → four risk factors (hypertension, obesity, hyperlipidemia, diabetes)
   plus sudden onset
Chest wall twinge syndrome/costochondritis → trauma to chest in stopping cart
Hyperventilation syndrome → fits sudden onset
Mitral valve prolapse → unlikely
Esophagitis → not likely due to sudden onset but obesity potential for hiatal hernia

List 10 questions, diagnostic tests, or physical examinations you would ask, order, or perform to find the cause of his chest pain. Explain your rationale.

Calf pain/positive Homan sign → phlebitis/DVT → pulmonary embolus
Ultrasound of the calf → clot → DVT → pulmonary embolus
Describe chest pain → squeezing/crushing → angina or MI
                      sharp → mitral valve prolapse, PE, chest wall twinge syndrome
                      burning → esophagitis
                      dull → costochondritis
Location of chest pain → substernal/epigastric → angina, MI, esophagitis, costochondritis
                         peripheral chest → PE, chest wall twinge syndrome
What makes it better? → resting → angina
                       nothing → MI
                       antacids/H$_2$ blockers → esophagitis
                       breathing slowly into a paper bag → hyperventilation
                       splinting → chest wall twinge syndrome, costochondritis
ECG → ST-segment elevation → STEMI
      ST-segment depression → angina, NSTEMI
      Right axis deviation → pulmonary embolism
Elevated CK^{MB}, troponin levels → angina
Elevated D-dimer levels → pulmonary embolism
Spiral CT scan → + → pulmonary embolism
Palpate the area of pain → makes pain worse → costochondritis
Pain on deep breath → makes pain worse → chest wall twinge syndrome, PE

CASE 10.1
ANSWER KEY

Eddie Jones, a 78-year-old veteran, presents to clinic requesting something stronger for heartburn. A quick review of his health record reveals a history of recurrent bleeding duodenal ulcers starting 20 years ago. However, since treatment for *Helicobacter pylori* in 1989 he has been without problems. He says he first noticed this new problem about 6 weeks ago and OTC H_2 blockers have not helped very much. He has been taking ibuprofen 400 mg three to four times a day for the last year for "old age" aches and pains.

a. List three likely causes for Eddie's problem. Explain your rationale.

Recurrence of duodenal ulcer → *by history*
Gastritis/gastric ulcer → *heartburn unrelieved by H_2 blockers, taking ibuprofen*
Esophagitis/GERD → *heartburn unrelieved by H_2 blockers*
Cholecystitis → *heartburn is back*
Gastric carcinoma → *>60 years of age, H_2 blockers do not work*
Angina/myocardial infarction → *age, chest pain*

b. List four examinations, questions, or laboratory tests you would perform to differentiate between the probable causes listed above. Explain your rationale.

Timing of pain relative to meals → *1 to 2 hours after meals* → *duodenal ulcers*
        → *3 to 4 hours after fatty meal* → *cholecystitis*
        → *variable* → *gastric ulcers, gastritis,*
                gastric cancer
        → *bedtime* → *esophagitis/GERD*
        → *after ibuprofen ingestion* → *ibuprofen*
Relief by H_2 blockers/antacids/food → *variable* → *GERD, esophagitis, gastritis,*
                gastric ulcer, gastric cancer
        → *relieved* → *duodenal ulcer*
What makes it worse? → *lying down* → *esophagitis, GERD*
        ETOH, spicy food, ibuprofen → *gastritis, gastric*
                ulcer, gastric cancer
        anger, stress, exercise, cold → *angina*
Esophagogastroduodenoscopy → *ulcers, cancer, GERD*
Description of pain → *as before with ulcers* → *peptic ulcer disease, GERD*
        sharp → *cholecystitis*
        squeezing, crushing → *angina, MI*
Location → *epigastric* → *peptic ulcer disease, GERD, gastric cancer, gastritis*
        → *substernal, radiate to L arm* → *angina, MI*
        → *right upper quadrant* → *cholecystitis*
Other symptoms → *palpitations, diaphoresis, dyspnea* → *angina, MI*

c. Just as you complete your interview, Eddie mentions that he has noticed his stools are much darker than usual and is concerned about a recurrence of his bleeding ulcers. List four questions, examinations, or laboratory tests that would help determine if Eddie is bleeding from his upper gastrointestinal tract.

CBC $\rightarrow$ anemia $\rightarrow$ UGI bleed

Pale conjunctivae, frenulum of tongue, nail beds $\rightarrow$ anemia $\rightarrow$ UGI bleed

Tachycardia, tachypnea, orthostasis $\rightarrow$ severe anemia $\rightarrow$ UGI bleed

BUN/serum creatinine ratio >20:1 $\rightarrow$ UGI bleed

Hematemesis, coffee ground vomitus $\rightarrow$ UGI bleed

Fatigue, DOE, SOB $\rightarrow$ anemia $\rightarrow$ UGI bleed

Color of stool $\rightarrow$ black tarry (melena) $\rightarrow$ UGI bleed

Check stool for occult blood $\rightarrow$ UGI bleed

CASE 11.1
ANSWER KEY

Edwin Bourke, a 40-year-old Gulf War veteran presents with a 36-hour history of nausea and vomiting with intermittent abdominal pain. His past medical history is significant in that he received a penetrating abdominal wound from which he fully recovered 15 years ago. He also complains of a headache, chills, and general arthralgias and myalgias. A review of his chart reveals a dental visit 2 days ago, where he received prescriptions for erythromycin 500 mg four times a day, Vicodin one to two tablets every 4 hours for severe pain, and ibuprofen 600 mg one table, four times a day for 3 days.

a. List three possible causes for Edwin's problems. Explain your rationale.

> *Gastroenteritis → nausea and vomiting plus chills and malaise*
> *Appendicitis → nausea and vomiting plus abdominal pain*
> *Pancreatitis → nausea and vomiting plus abdominal pain*
> *Intestinal obstruction → nausea and vomiting plus abdominal pain, old abdominal wound*
> *Cholecystitis → abdominal pain, nausea*
> *Medication → erythromycin and ibuprofen (local irritants), Vicodin (central effect)*
> *Meningitis → headache plus nausea and vomiting, malaise, chills*
> *Migraine headache → headache plus nausea and vomiting*

b. List four questions, examinations, or laboratory tests you would perform to confirm the diagnosis.

> *Diarrhea → gastroenteritis*
> *Constipation → intestinal obstruction*
> *Location of the pain → periumbilical or epigastric→ pancreatitis*
> *   right upper quadrant → gall bladder*
> *   right lower quadrant → appendicitis*
> *Timing of pain/N/V → shortly after taking meds → medication*
> *   3 to 4 hours after a fatty meal → cholecystitis*
> *Auscultate abdomen → high-pitched tinkling bowel sounds → intestinal obstruction*
> *Palpate/percuss abdomen → fecal masses → intestinal obstruction*
> *   → Murphy sign → cholocystitis*
> *Examination for signs of appendicitis → Markle, rebound tenderness, psoas, obturator signs*
> *CBC → >10,000 WBCs with >80% PMNs → appendicitis, meningitis*
> *Abdominal x-ray → fecal masses, dilated bowel loops → intestinal obstruction*
> *Abdominal Ultrasound/CT → appendicitis*

CASE 12.1
ANSWER KEY

Martha Oncedaly, a 72-year-old school teacher who 2 weeks ago retired to Tucson and lives at the Desert Legacy in independent living comes into your store. She asks what is good for this constipation she has had since she arrived here. You remember her because she had complained about the food at Desert Legacy while she was waiting for several prescriptions to be filled 2 weeks ago when she arrived. They include calcium carbonate 500 mg, 3 qd, vitamin D 400 IU qd, Vicodin 2 tablets q6h severe joint pain, and piroxicam 20 mg qd.

What are the two most likely causes of her constipation?
Dehydration 2° low humidity
Decreased food intake
Calcium carbonate
Hydrocodone
Early intestinal obstruction 2° old GI surgery or Cancer

List three questions/examinations/lab tests you would ask/perform to help pinpoint the cause?
How long since last bowel movement ⟶> 7 days ⟶ constipation
Describe shape color consistency of last several BMs ⟶ looking for specific causes
    eg, iron, dehydration, etc
Changes in food volume or type?
Changes in urine color, frequency ⟶ dehydration signs
How frequently $CaCO_3$, Vicodin taken?
Nausea, vomiting, diarrhea ⟶ intestinal obstruction
Past abdominal surgery?
Abdominal examination
    Surgical/traumatic scars
    Fecal masses
    High-pitched tinkling bowel sounds
    Abdominal distention/bloating
Abdominal x-ray/CT scan for signs of obstruction

CASE 12.2
ANSWER KEY

One year later Martha returns to your pharmacy and asks for something to help her with her diarrhea. You remember that Martha got an extra refill of her medications to take on vacation about a month ago. Martha looks pale and like she is not feeling well. When you note her bending over clutching her stomach, she admits to an occasional cramping RLQ abdominal pain.

List three potential causes for Martha's symptoms.
Diarrhea
    Gastroenteritis
    Bacterial/parasitic infection
    Laxative overuse
    Early intestinal obstruction
RLQ pain
    Gynecological problems, UTI, appendix
    Early intestinal obstruction
Pale
    Anemia?

List six questions/examinations/lab tests you would ask/perform to help pinpoint the cause?
Number of BMs in the last 24 hours?
How long have you had diarrhea?
Describe the stools →*color, consistency, volume, blood?*
Black tarry stools →*melena* →*UGI bleed*
Foul smelling odor →*protozoal infection*
Third world/ tropics travel in last month →*protozoal infection*
Eat at potluck, picnic, or restaurant recently →*gastroenteritis*
Nausea, vomiting, constipation →*early intestinal obstruction*
Alternating diarrhea /constipation →*mixed irritable bowel syndrome*
Fever →*bacterial*
CBC →*bacterial, anemia*
Stool for ova and parasites, Gram stain, stool culture
Abdominal examination →*masses 2° obstruction*

Edith Coiner is a 54 year-old-patient with type 2 diabetes mellitus who you see regularly in clinic. Today, during her regular follow-up visit Edith mentions that she has had four severe headaches in the last month and is concerned.

Problem List		Medication
1988	Allergic rhinitis	Loratadine 10 mg qd
1992	Diabetes mellitus type 2	NPH 70/30 insulin
1997	Proteinuria	24 units q AM
2001	Neuropathy	12 units q PM
1992	Hypertension	Chlorthalidone 25 mg q AM
		Enalapril 20 mg bid
1992	Hyperlipidemia	Atorvastatin 40 mg q PM

List three possible causes for Edith's headaches. Explain your rationale.

Bacterial sinusitis →allergic rhinitis
Stroke (CVA) →hypertension, lipids, diabetes
Poor control of hypertension →BP >200/120
Tension headache →four new headaches
Migraine headaches →four severe headaches
Cluster headaches →four severe headaches, allergic rhinitis
Mass occupying lesion →four severe headaches
Nonketotic hyperosmolar coma →Diabetes way out of control

List six diagnostic tests, physical examinations, or questions you would order, perform, or ask to evaluate Edith's headaches. Explain your rationale.

Neurological examination →abnormalities →CVA, mass occupying lesion
Check control of diabetes and hypertension →causes for headache
CT/MRI →mass occupying lesion/CVA
ENT examination →bacterial sinusitis
Temperature →elevated →bacterial sinusitis
CBC →>10,000 WBCs with >80% PMNs →bacterial sinusitis
Careful specific history of headache symptoms →tension versus migraine versus cluster versus other
*   Unilateral →migraine, cluster*
*   Throbbing, phonophobia, photophobia →migraine*
*   Tenderness of shoulder and neck muscles →tension*
*   Dull widely distributed →tension*
*   Rhinorrhea, tearing →cluster*
*   Visual disturbances/aura →migraine*

CASE 14.1
ANSWER KEY

Rick O'Shea comes to your pharmacy to pick up a refill on his fluticasone inhaler. He also asks what is good for his bloodshot eyes. Pertinent history includes his love of dirt biking in the desert, which he does every evening after work, plus his nightly swim at the YMCA. He also complains of a recent onset of joint pain in his hands. Upon observation you notice mild diffuse inflammation of both conjunctivae, no discharge, and small yellowish patches at the 3- and 9-o'clock positions in both eyes.

1. List two possible causes for Rick's bloodshot eyes. Explain your rationale.

   Pinguecula/pterygium → yellow patches at 3 and 9 o'clock, dirt bike riding
   Allergic conjunctivitis → allergic rhinitis, outside exposure to allergens
   Irritative conjunctivitis → dirt bike riding, dust, chlorine
   Acute iritis? → autoimmune arthritis → hand joint pain

2. List three questions that you would ask to help determine the cause of Rick's inflamed eyes. Explain your rationale.

   Other signs of allergic rhinitis → allergic shiners, eyelid atopic dermatitis → AKC
   Specific information about amount of dirt bike riding, use of goggles → pinguecula, pterygium irritative conjunctivitis
   Specific information about amount of swimming, use of goggles → irritative conjunctivitis
   Does he wear contact lens? → potential for GPC and referral
   Is there a discharge from the eye? Nature of the discharge?
      clear watery discharge → allergic conjunctivitis
      purulent discharge → bacterial conjunctivitis
   Viral cold symptoms or anyone else with similar eye or cold symptoms → viral conjunctivitis
   How bad do they itch? → lots → allergic conjunctivitis
   Sensation of grit in the eye? → allergic/viral/bacterial conjunctivitis
   Where is the joint pain? → metacarpal, metacarpal phalangeal joints, bilateral? → rheumatoid arthritis → uveitis/iritis

3. List three questions you would ask to make sure this was not a vision-threatening condition that would require immediate referral.

   True eyeball pain?
   Photophobia?
   Decreased visual acuity?
   Severe foreign body sensation?
   Trauma?
   Swelling around eyes?
   Herpetic vesicular cutaneous lesions on the face or around eye?

CASE 15.1
ANSWER KEY

You are on rotation at Posada Del Diablo Convalescent Center. All new patients have their records reviewed and are interviewed by the pharmacy student to evaluate potential drug-related problems and make any recommendations for changes in the therapeutic regimen. Samantha Roanhorse, a 58-year-old Native American, was admitted last night and it is your job to review her records and interview her.

Problem List	*Medication*
1960 Gran mal epilepsy d/t severe head trauma	Phenytoin 400 mg q hs
	Phenobarbital 120 mg q hs
1972 Alcoholism	
1980 Schizophrenia	Risperidone 4 mg q hs
2001 Diabetes mellitus type 2	Metformin 500 mg bid
ALLERGIES: milk, penicillin, aspirin	

Sam's chart has not caught up with her, but the discharge summary from the psychiatric hospital reveals she was admitted for exacerbation of her schizophrenia. During her stay she was switched to risperidone with good results. The nurse tells you that her counterpart at the hospital called to tell her that the hydrocortisone cream that was sent back with the patient is for a rash on her face, neck, and elbows. During your interview, Sam's biggest complaint is about pains in her arms and legs that are poorly relieved by acetaminophen. When asked, she complains of pains in her hands, wrists, forearms, shins, knees, and toes. She also makes a vague reference to a recent fall that upon further questioning she denies. Given her medical history, list three likely causes of Sam's aches and pains. Explain your rationale.

Psoriatic arthritis → *pains in hands/wrists/plus rash on face, neck, and elbow*
Systemic lupus erythematosus (SLE) → *pains in joints and bones and rash on face*
Osteoporosis → *postmenopausal and ? ?fall* → *fracture*
Osteoarthritis → *pains in knees and toes*
Osteomalacia → *on phenytoin/phenobarbital, little sun since in nursing home, lactase deficiency d/t Native American ethnicity*

List six questions you would ask, examinations you would perform, and/or diagnostic tests that you would order to better determine the cause of her pain. Explain your rationale.
Careful history of pain as to which sites, onset, timing relative to trauma
Past history of trauma → *old fractures* → *osteoarthritis*
Examine all painful joints and locations by palpation, observation, and range of motion
X-rays of affected area → *fractures joint erosion*
Examine skin rash → *butterfly* → *SLE*
    raised plaque → *psoriatic arthritis*
LE Prep/ANA ⟶ *SLE*
RF/ACPA ⟶ *psoriatic arthritis*
ESR/ CRP ⟶ *autoimmune arthritis*
Serum creatinine/microalbuminuria ⟶ *SLE nephritis*
Previous stable history of control of schizophrenia ⟶ *SLE CNS vasculitis*
Vitamin D level → *<20 ng/ml* → *osteomalacia*
Bone scan → *Looser's lines* → *osteomalacia*

CASE 16.1
ANSWER KEY

Doris Daye, a 52 year-old patient, presents to clinic with a chief complaint of dysuria and vaginal discharge. She also has a nonspecific rash over a large area around her groin. She takes Lo-Ovral, an oral contraceptive. Her recent medical history includes type 2 diabetes mellitus, and since she was divorced last year, she has had multiple sexual encounters with different partners.

a. List three potential causes for her dysuria and vaginal discharge. Explain your rationale.

STD → multiple partners/encounters, dysuria, and vaginal discharge
UTI → DM, dysuria, active sexually
VVC → DM, vaginal discharge, rash on groin
Other vaginitis → dysuria, vaginal discharge

b. List six questions/examinations or lab tests you would ask/conduct/run to determine the cause of her symptoms. Explain your rationale.

Is dysuria external or internal? → internal → UTI/STD
→ external → vaginitis
Dyspareunia? → UTI/STD/vaginitis
Frequency/urgency/suprapubic pain → UTI
Fever → Acute pyelonephritis/PID
Flank tenderness → UTI (acute pyelonephritis)
MSCCUA w/ C&S → ≥ 10² CFU/ml of single organism → UTI
Spun urine microscopy → ≥ 10 WBCs/hpf or ≥ 5 RBCs/hpf + symptoms → UTI
Leukocyte esterase/nitrite test → positive → UTI
Unspun urine microscopy → any bacteria → UTI
Last sexual partner → new/recent → STD
NAATs for gonorrhea/chlamydia ⁺→ STD
Gram stain and culture of discharge ⁺→ gonorrhea
Cervicitis on vaginal examination → STD
Wet prep → clue cells → bacterial vaginosis (BV)
→ motile flagellates → trichomonas
KOH prep → fishy odor → BV
→ hyphae → candida (VVC)
Discharge on vaginal examination → white cottage cheesy → VVC
Gray, off-white, clinging to vaginal walls → BV
Thin frothy whitish → trichomoniasis
Itching → VVC
Fishy odor → BV
Satellite lesions on groin → VVC
NAATs for trichomoniasis ⁺→ trichomoniasis
Sialidase test for BV ⁺→ BV

c. You ordered several tests for which results have now returned. Interpret the test results. Explain your rationale. How does this change your original a Susceptibility ssessment?

Microscopic UA

Epi	1 to 2/hpf
WBC	TNTC
Glucose	4+
Protein	2+

Culture and Susceptibility of Urine

>10^2 *Staphylococcus saprophyticus*

Vaginal Discharge
   Wet mount—negative for clue cells/motile flagellates
   KOH prep—multiple hyphae present

1 to 2 epithelial cells/hpf means that the MSCCUA procedures were followed.

TNTC WBC and ≥10^2 CFU/ml pure culture indicates UTI.

Glucosuria and hyphae in KOH prep indicates VVC.

4+ glucosuria indicates poor control of diabetes.

2+ proteinuria indicates potential diabetic nephropathy. Could also be due to asymptomatic acute pyelonephritis. Check old records for evidence of previous proteinuria. If none, do microalbuminuria test in 2 weeks.

Need to do NAATs for chlamydia and gonorrhea because Doris is a high-risk patient. If either is positive then need to test for syphilis, HIV, and hepatitis B.

CASE 16.2
ANSWER KEY

"All the way" Mae Ilovtuparti, a 24 year-old fourth-year student pharmacist, presents with a chief complaint of dysuria.

a.   List three likely causes of her complaint.

STD → sexually active 24 year-old
UTI → sexually active 24 year-old
Vaginitis → sexually active 24 year-old

b.   List six initial lab tests/physical examinations and/or questions you would *most* like to ask Mae to evaluate the nature of her complaint. Explain your rationale.

Vaginal discharge? → vaginitis/STD
Sexual history → high risk → STD
*   → low risk → UTI*
Same as for Doris Day in case #1 depending on response to initial questions

c.   Mae's urine report comes back as follows:

UA	Culture
Epi –neg	>10^3 E. coli
WBC – 10 to 12/hpf	
RBC - neg	
Glucose - neg	
Ketones	

What is the likely diagnosis? Explain your rationale.

No epithelial cells means it is a good MSCCUA.
≥10^2 CFU/ml pure culture single organism indicates UTI.
10 to 12 WBC/hpf probable UTI. Would indicate UTI if patient had frequency/urgency.

d.   Interpret the following urinalysis/urine culture report if it was Mae's. Explain your rationale.

UA	Culture
Epi – many	>10^2 E. Coli
WBC – TNTC	>10^2 Serratia marscesens
RBC – TNTC	>10^2 Staphylococcus epidermiditis
Glucose- 3+	

Many epithelial cells indicates poor MSCCUA technique.
Many epithelial cells plus three different organisms indicate contaminated specimen.
RBC and WBC—TNTC (too numerous to count) indicates contaminated specimen plus
*   potential menstruation (RBCs) and potential vaginitis (WBCs). Need follow-up*
*   questions and potential pelvic examination plus additional lab work to rule out other*
*   causes.*

CASE 17.1
ANSWER KEY

Helen Autry brings in her 7-year-old son Gene and asks you to take a look at his left arm. You note that there is a red, hot, tender, and swollen area starting at the wrist and ending in his cubital fossa. Helen says it started at his elbow and has spread toward the wrist. There you also note severely excoriated and lichenified skin. The right cubital fossa reveals typical eczematous lesions with mild excoriation and lichenification. Helen and her husband Roy are regular customers in your asthma disease management program. Helen says that she has tried everything to keep him from scratching the itching areas without success. Gene's past medical history is unremarkable except that his patient profile reveals several prescriptions for antihistamine/decongestant combinations for URIs and a single albuterol syrup prescription for a viral chest infection.

a. List the most probable cause for the acute problem and the most likely cause for the chronic problems. Explain your rationale.

Acute problem
Cellulitis—broken skin, with red, hot, tender, swollen area, that spreads. Caused by
        scratching (excoriation) of atopic dermatitis of left arm.
Chronic problem
Atopic dermatitis—typical itching eczematous lesions in cubital fossa. Family history
        of asthma, prescriptions for antihistamines = allergic rhinitis?? Lichenification indicates
        long-standing atopic dermatitis.

b. List four questions/examinations or lab tests you would ask/conduct/run to determine the cause of Gene's symptoms. Explain your rationale.

Gently palpate cellulitis for tenderness and heat.
Observe for redness, pus, and swelling.
Mark borders of red swollen area with ink. If cellulitis moves past ink lines confirms cellulitis.
CBC—if bacterial cellulitis it will reveal >10,000 WBCs with >80% PMNs/bands
Runny nose with watery discharge, swollen, pale boggy nasal mucosa on nasal examination,
        allergic shiners, nasal crease, and Dennie lines all confirm allergic rhinitis, which helps confirm
        atopic dermatitis diagnosis
Check other areas (popliteal fossa) for atopic dermatitis
CBC in >80% of patients will show eosinophilia (>600 absolute count)

CASE 17.2
ANSWER KEY

One month later, you dispense a 7-day supply of trimethoprim-sulfamethoxazole suspension for Gene's ear infection. About 2 weeks later, Helen calls and is concerned that Gene's skin has just broken out with a red bumpy rash all over his chest, stomach, and back. In addition, on both hands and forearms, there are different lesions that do not itch and look like overlapping pink and red circles. Her son calls them "bull's-eyes." At first, she thought it might be the antibiotic but he has been off that for almost a week! What is Helen most likely describing? What other questions/examinations/lab tests could you use to help confirm diagnosis? Explain your rationale.

Truncal maculopapular rash plus "target lesions" on hands and forearms indicate erythema multiforme.

Check oral cavity, eyes for signs of Stevens-Johnson syndrome, and skin exfoliation for TENS.

Was this Gene's first exposure to sulfonamides?—If so, it would explain delayed reaction. If multiple recent exposures to sulfonamides, then less likely sulfa is the cause.

Other recent autoimmune disease, bacterial or viral infection besides AOM, and medication that could be the cause of EM?

CASE 18.1
ANSWER KEY

RJ, a 42-year-old male recently diagnosed with mild hypertension, comes to your pharmacy clinic for initiation of antihypertensive therapy. He had four blood pressure readings in the clinic over the last 6 months; all of which were greater than 140/90: 150/100, 150/90, 148/100, and 142/96, all R arm sitting. He also has a strong family history of hypertension on his father's side of the family. Today's reading by the medical aide is 150/90 with a pulse of 92. He had home blood pressure readings twice a day for the last 2 weeks, taken by his wife who is a registered nurse. They range from 120-138/82-88. He had a complete physical examination by his primary care provider 2 weeks ago along with appropriate laboratory tests. All findings and results were normal or unremarkable. What should be your next steps?

1. *Given the rounded off blood pressure readings in clinic, there is strong evidence of rounding off bias by the medical aide. The pulse of 92 plus normal to high normal home blood pressure readings indicate the potential for white coat hypertension, so the diagnosis of hypertension is in doubt.*

   Using appropriate technique, take RJ's blood pressure yourself.

   Have RJ's wife continue to take blood pressure readings twice daily for a week.

   Return to your clinic in 1 week, bringing in the sphygmomanometer used at home to compare your office readings with clinic equipment versus his home device to confirm potential assessment of white coat hypertension.

2. *Time permitting, with his family history and since his readings may indicate high normal blood pressure, it might be appropriate to assess his current lifestyle (smoking, caffeine, salt intake, etc.) to judge the potential benefits of any lifestyle changes on his long-term cardiovascular health regardless of whether or not he is currently hypertensive.*

CASE 18.2
ANSWER KEY

LK is a 68-year-old female with hypertension previously seen in the pharmacy clinic by a colleague (now on maternity leave) for the last 2 years. Chart review reveals that LK is under good control (120s over 70s) and has been steadily losing weight at the rate of 5 lb per year. She is on chlorthalidone 25 mg q AM, lisinopril 20 mg q AM, and carvedilol 6.25 mg bid. Her home blood pressure readings are excellent over the last 6 months with a slight downward trend in evening and bedtime readings (as low as 100/66). In taking her history, she denies any problems except for occasional dizziness that occurs most frequently after getting up from the dinner table, especially after a big meal (about one to two times/week). The other change is that she has begun to walk 2 miles a day with her new next-door neighbor, with whom she is becoming fast friends. Her sitting blood pressure reading by you today at 11 AM is 110/68 with a pulse of 72. What should you do next?

1. *With her steady weight loss and new increase in exercise, combined with the existing medication regimen the potential exists for orthostasis. Have her stand up quickly. Does that cause dizziness? Check her blood pressure for orthostasis. Also get more detail about the dizziness. Does she feel like she is going to faint when it happens?*

2. *Given her age and the occurrence of the dizziness after a big dinner, postprandial drop in blood pressure may be a factor. Ask what time she takes her evening dose of carvedilol. If she takes it before dinner, her dizziness could be due to orthostasis due to a combination of postprandial hypotension, peak effect of the predinner carvedilol, and the lifestyle changes.*

3. *Have her take her blood pressure at 30 and 60 minutes after eating each meal for the next week. She is to call if any of the readings are below 100/70. If she has a dizzy spell, sit down and take her blood pressure immediately.*

4. *If these blood pressure readings continue to be in the 100s/60s range on subsequent visits or she has clear postprandial hypotension, then consideration should be given to lowering the dose of either lisinopril or carvedilol and having the patient measure BP more frequently during the transition to allow small changes without loss of control.*

5 *Using LOQQSAM evaluate the potential for CVA or angina.*

CASE 18.3
ANSWER KEY

MS is a 54-year-old male who is regularly seen in your clinic for his hypertension, diabetes, and hyperlipidemia. He has been stable on enalapril 20 mg bid, HCTZ 25 mg q AM, and amlodipine 5 mg q AM for the last 3 years. He is returning today, 2 weeks since his last visit because his systolic blood pressure readings have been consistently over 140 when he awakens in recent weeks. Two weeks ago he was asked to increase the frequency of his blood pressure readings to several times a day, then return today. His blood pressure taken by you today is 144/88 and pulse of 92 with your cuff and 146/90 with his home device. MS typically exhibits white coat hypertension. About 70% of his home readings indicate a systolic pressure between 130 and 140, with the diastolic blood pressure readings typically in the mid- to high 70s. Almost all of the high readings are in the morning before he takes his medication or in the evening before he takes his second enalapril dose. Where do we go from here?

1. *Because the readings were the same today with both yours and his home device, his home readings are probably accurate.*

2. *Carefully check his refill records and question him carefully about his medication adherence, changes in daily schedule/medication administration time, etc. Check pharmacy records to make sure the manufacturer of his generic medications has not recently changed. Order liver function tests and/or question him about any changes in his ETOH ingestion (could be minihangover with release of sympathomimetic amines is due to markedly increased consumption). Also check for any changes in his diet and exercise regimen.*

3. *Assuming there are no adherence problems, changes in manufacturer, changes in diet and exercise, or ethanol consumption, it is clear that one or both of his once-a-day medications are not lasting the full 24 hours. It is fairly well established that HCTZs antihypertensive effects do not last 24 hours as compared to chlorthalidone or his amlodipine's effects have ceased to last the full 24 hours.*

4. *There are several options here. Since his readings are only slightly above target, continued intensified blood pressure surveillance for 2 to 4 weeks would confirm the consistency of the change. Second, HCTZ could be stopped and chlorthalidone 25 mg q AM started and have him return to clinic in 1 month. Finally, continue the diuretic, but switch the amlodipine dose to bedtime or at the same time as the evening enalapril dose for one month. Intensified blood pressure surveillance would continue for the next 30 days regardless of what option was chosen.*

Age: 58

Sex: Female

Medical Conditions: Diabetes, BP = 130/80

Family Hx: Mother died of heart attack at age 47

Smoking Status: Nonsmoker

Meds: Glyburide, metformin, HCTZ, lisinopril

Goal LDL: _____

Results: TC: 212   LDL: 126   HDL: 42   Trig: 180

What is the LDL-C goal? What would you tell the patient? Explain your rationale.

- *Goal LDL <100 (since patient has diabetes)*
- *LDL above goal of <100*
- *HDL should be >50 since she is a woman with diabetes*
- *Trig above goal of <150*
- *TC above goal of <200*
- *TC/HDL ratio = 5, LDL/HDL = 3 (both exactly at goal ... but better to be below these numbers)*
- *Diet/exercise modifications may be worth a try before initiating medications since a 20% drop of LDL may get the patient to the goal*

CASE 19.2
ANSWER KEY

Age:	35
Sex:	Male
Medical Conditions:	None, BP usually runs approx 130/80
Family Hx:	Unremarkable
Smoking Status:	Just quit … last cigarette was last weekend
Meds:	None

Goal LDL: _____

Results: TC: 190   LDL: 145   HDL: 22   Trig: 170

What is the LDL-C goal? What would you tell the patient? Explain your rationale.

- *Goal LDL <130 (since patient has two risk factors: has smoked within last 30 days and HDL < 40)*

- *You would do the Framingham risk assessment on the patient as well since he has two or more risk factors … –4 for age, +4 for TC, +8 for smoking (will be 0 after 1 month with no smoking), 2 for HDL, 1 pt for BP … total 11 pts confer 8% risk … LDL goal does not change*

- *LDL above goal of <130*

- *HDL below goal of >40*

- *Trig above goal of <150*

- *TC OK*

- *TC/HDL ratio = 8.6 (greater than 5), LDL/HDL = 6.6 (greater than 3)*

- *If patient stays quit for three more weeks, he will no longer have a positive risk factor of smoking … thus he will only have one risk factor (HDL <40) and his goal LDL will change to <160. Also, quitting smoking may cause a considerable increase in HDL … so he may not even have an HDL <40 after a while … thus reducing his risk factors to zero. Therefore, it would be prudent to praise the patient for quitting smoking, encourage him to stay quit, and tell him to recheck his cholesterol panel after a few more weeks.*

- *You may also discuss diet and exercise with this patient. Triglycerides are slightly elevated and this may be due to fats and/or carbohydrates in his diet. This patient along with his smoking cessation may be interested in exercising … his HDL may further improve with 30 minutes of aerobic exercise at least three times per week.*

CASE 19.3
ANSWER KEY

Age:	75
Sex:	Male
Medical Conditions:	Emphysema
Family Hx:	Mother died of a heart attack at age 80
Smoking Status:	Quit smoking in 1985 (had smoked for 40 years)
Meds:	Albuterol, ipratropium
Goal LDL: _____	
Results:	TC: 185 LDL: 125 HDL: 65 Trig: 165

What is the LDL-C goal? What would you tell the patient? Explain your rationale.

- *Goal LDL <160 (since patient has a net of zero risk factors: his age is a positive risk factor but his HDL >60 is a negative risk factor)*
- *LDL OK*
- *HDL great*
- *Trig above goal of <150*
- *TC OK*
- *TC/HDL ratio = 2.8 (less than 5), LDL/HDL = 1.92 (less than 3)*
- *Overall, panel looks great ... praise the patient! Advise that triglycerides are slightly above goal ... ask about patient's diet (too many carbohydrates?/fats?).*

CASE 19.4
ANSWER KEY

Age:	56
Sex:	Female
Medical Conditions:	Allergies, BP usually 120s/80s
Family Hx:	Sister had MI at age 62
Smoking Status:	Nonsmoker
Meds:	Claritin
Goal LDL: _____	
Results:	TC: 225 LDL: 122 HDL: 55 Trig: 230

What is the LDL-C goal? What would you tell the patient? Explain your rationale.

- *Goal LDL <130 (since the patient has two risk factors: female ≥55 and sister had MI at age < 65)*

- *You would do the Framingham risk assessment on the patient as well since she has two or more risk factors … 8 pts for age, 4 for TC, 0 for smoking, 0 for HDL, 1 pt for BP … total 13 pts confer 2% risk … LDL goal does not change*

- *LDL OK*

- *HDL OK*

- *Trig above goal of <150*

- *TC above goal of <200*

- *TC/HDL ratio = 4 (less than 5), LDL/HDL = 2.2 (less than 3)*

- *Ask the patient if she has ever had a high (or borderline high) blood sugar … excess blood sugar can be converted to triglycerides. Patients with high blood sugars need to control their blood sugars to lower their triglycerides before initiating triglyceride-lowering therapy.*

- *May also discuss fat/carbohydrate intake in her current diet and offer potential modifications that may improve triglycerides.*

- *Even though TC is high, would not necessarily recommend medications at this point because ratios look good and LDL below goal.*

CASE 20.1
ANSWER KEY

You are working in the VA refill clinic and Kyle Maloney, a 67-year-old Korean War veteran, comes to the pharmacy to get refills on all his chronic medications for diabetes, cholesterol, and blood pressure. He missed his doctor's appointment this week because they could not get his old 1956 Thunderbird "Betsy" started. He needs enough to last until his next physician visit in 6 weeks. A review of his computerized medical record reveals the following medications and the results of the lab tests he had drawn last week for the missed appointment.

Medications	*Lab Test Results*	
Metformin 500 mg bid	A1C	7.2%
Atorvastatin 20 mg q hs	Microalbuminuria	70 mg/L
	Creat	1.1
	Tot Chol	232
	LDL	148
	HDL	46
	TG	126

HCTZ 25 mg q AM
Enalapril 20 mg q AM 10 mg q PM

The clinic nurse vital signs are as follows:
BP: 170/98   Weight: 210 (up 10 lb)   T/P/R: 98.6/80/14

a.   Based on this information evaluate the level of control for all three disorders. Explain your rationale.

Diabetes Mellitus
A1C should be less than 7%. However, it is close to target A1C goal and at this time there is no need to add medication.
Weight gain is not good for control of diabetes mellitus. If the patient has just been started on insulin or a sulfonylurea some weight gain would be expected, but shouldn't happen with metformin alone. This 10-lb weight is in all likelihood due to suboptimal adherence to diet, exercise, and/or medication regimen. Careful questioning about what has recently changed in their diet and/or exercise and checking refill records is appropriate. Whatever the cause, correcting that is the best therapeutic approach in this patient rather than without investigation altering the medication regimen.
This patient has early diabetic nephropathy (>30 mg/L). Therapy such as ACE Inhibitor usually is not started until >300 mg/mL. However, the patient is already on an ACE inhibitor.

Hypertension
First depending on who took the blood pressure, it should be repeated using proper technique, then compared with home blood pressure readings done with an accurate automated arm BP cuff. If they differ, have patient return with their BP cuff and take BP with proper technique in the office with both BP cuffs. If they agree, then use home BP monitor to adjust therapy.
If this BP is accurate, then it is above the target goal of 130-140/90 and therapy needs to be adjusted. Raising the enalapril to 20 bid or switching HCTZ to chlorthalidone with its longer duration of antihypertensive action would be alternatives.

Cholesterol
Target LDL for patients with Type 2 diabetes is <100 mg/dL in the 2002 guidelines so both total cholesterol and LDL cholesterol are above target. The total cholesterol/ HDL and LDL/HDL are both above their targets so after confirming appropriate adherence with existing regimen an increase in dose is indicated. Under the 2013 guidelines Kyle should have his atorvastatin dose raised to 80 mg.
Triglycerides are <150 mg/dL, which is consistent with good control of diabetes.

b. For each of the three diseases list three questions or physical examinations you would conduct to evaluate the level of disease control and/or the presence of disease complications.

DM
How many times do you urinate at night? (nocturia)
Skin rash with satellite lesions? (candida)
Infected cuts, sores? (bacterial infection)
Diabetic foot examination? (early detection of diabetic foot)
Numbness, tingling, or pain in feet? (neuropathy)
Visual changes? (retinopathy)
Check for pedal edema? (nephropathy d/t 10-lb weight gain)

BP
Number of pillows sleep on? (orthopnea)
Awakes in middle of night? (PND)
Ankle swelling? (CHF)
Check for pedal edema? (CHF)
Shortness of breath? (CHF)
Auscultation/percussion of the lungs? (CHF)
Point of maximal impulse? (CHF)

LIPID
Chest pain? (angina)
Headache? (CVA)
Forgetfulness? (CVA)
Neurological examination? (CVA)
Leg cramps while exercising? (PAD)
Trouble chewing/talking? (CVA)
Auscultation of abdomen for bruits? (abdominal aortic aneurysm)

Howkani Stopwhesin, a 32-year-old asthmatic, comes to your pharmacy for his third visit in your asthma disease management program. Howkani has a peak flow meter, and an asthma action plan. He is on fluticasone inhaler 110 µg/spray, 3 puffs q AM and albuterol, 2 puffs per action plan up to four times a day.

List four questions you would ask and four objective parameters you would check to evaluate the level of control of Howie's asthma. Explain your rationale.

Subjective

How many times per week have you had symptoms?
How many days have you used your rescue inhaler since the last visit?
How many times per month do you awaken between 2-6 AM due to cough or dyspnea?
How many asthma attacks have you had since your last visit?
How many visits to the ER/urgent have you had since your last visit?
What have your PEFR readings been since your last visit?
How many times have your PEFR readings been in the yellow or red zone since your last visit?
How is your medication working?
What kind of changes have there been in your exposure to potential triggers at home and at work?

Closed-ended questions regarding symptoms

Have you had any of the following since your last visit?

Wheezing?	*Chest tightness?*	*Shortness of breath?*
Coughing?	*Coughing at night?*	*Coughing with exercise?*
Runny/stuffy nose?	*Itching skin/rash?*	*Awaken at night?*
Decreased ability to do normal activities?		*Heartburn?*
Exposure to animals/dust/pollens/other triggers?		

Objective

Auscultate lungs → wheezes → poor control
Respiratory rate → >20 → poor control
Inability to speak in complete sentences → poor control
Ancillary muscle use during breathing → poor control
Cough rate/type → dry hacking worse between 2 and 6 AM → poor control
Peak flow/other PFT → yellow zone → poor control
Oxygenation (blood gases or pulse oximetry) <92% on room air → poor control
Improvement in peak flow after bronchodilator → poor control

CASE 22.1
ANSWER KEY

Ralph Malph, a 62-year-old retired Chief Petty Officer who recently moved to your city, presents to your clinic for assistance in controlling his hypertension, type 2 diabetes mellitus, and dyslipidemia. Ralph has had high blood pressure for 15 years and was diagnosed with diabetes and dyslipidemia 8 years ago at the time of his *mild heart attack* (NSTEMI). Both his diabetes and LDL cholesterol are near target goals (A1C = 7.2, LDL = 104). Because of his relocation he has not seen his primary physician in 4 months. His blood pressure has been problematic ever since diagnosis with his readings consistently between 155 and 170/94-104. Today, his first visit to your facility, the intake nurse noted a BP of 178/102. He takes lisinopril 10 mg q AM, chlorthalidone 25 mg q AM, atorvastatin 40 mg q AM and metformin 500 mg bid, but with limited success. He needs refills primarily of his BP medication to last until he sees his new physician at your facility in 3 weeks. Because his records have still not arrived, the intake nurse sends him to you to authorize his refills.

During your interview of Ralph, when you ask him closed-ended questions about potential complications of his chronic diseases, he mentions some difficulty sleeping and some shortness of breath. Further probing reveals he wakes up several times a week about 3 to 4 hours after falling asleep with palpitations and mild breathlessness. Sitting up or going to get a glass of water relieves the problem. He says the episodes are like the dreams he used to have after coming back from Iraq, but without the nightmares, which he has not had in 4 or 5 years. In addition, walking up the slight grade from the mailbox to the house occasionally leaves him winded, which he attributes to old age.

List six additional questions, laboratory tests, or physical examinations you would ask/order or conduct to confirm your suspicion of heart failure.

How many pillows do you sleep on at night?..orthopnea

Swelling in your ankles?..edema

Respiratory rate/pulse.. tachypnea, tachycardia

Apical impulse/PMI............................... lateral/inferior displacement indicating enlarged heart

Auscultation and percussion of the lungs................................areas of dullness, crackles in bases

Auscultation of heart...S3 gallop

Chest x-ray .... cardiac/left ventricular enlargement

Check ankles for edema...CHF

Check for jugular vein distention/hepatojugular reflux...CHF

Liver function tests ....elevated in CHF-induced liver engorgement

Renal function tests..decreased renal perfusion

Serum BNP ➞ *>100 pg/mL* ➞*CHF*

CASE 23.1
ANSWER KEY

JT, a 23-year-old male graduate student with a 3-year history of complex partial seizures with occasional secondary generalization, presents to your pharmacy disease management clinic for adjustment of his antiseizure regimen. Initially controlled on valproate, a 25-kg weight gain over 28 months prompted a change to lamotrigine. Lamotrigine was slowly titrated upward over several months. A week ago, just as he reached a maintenance dose of 200 mg bid, he developed erythema multiforme and was hospitalized temporarily because it appeared as if it was progressing to Stevens-Johnson syndrome. The drug was discontinued and high-dose corticosteroids started. No mucous membrane lesions developed and he was discharged 9 days ago on carbamazepine 100 mg bid. The neurologist recommended a slow upward titration to approximately 8 to 10/mg/kg or a serum level of about 8 µg/mL. Carbamazepine serum level drawn yesterday was 1.1 µg/mL (target range 5 to 12 µg/ml).

a. List six questions you would ask/laboratory tests you would order or physical examinations you would perform to evaluate the efficacy and potential adverse effects of carbamazepine in JT?

How many seizures/spells have you had since your last visit?
What kind of problems have you had remembering to take your medicine?
How are things going with your life?
What kind of changes/problems have you had since starting the carbamazepine?
Yes/No Questions

   Memory problems, fatigue, drowsiness, problems with walking or balance, stomach problems, skin rashes
Complete cerebellar examination
Folstein mental status examination
Make sure baseline labs were done in the hospital (CBC, LFTs, RFTs)

b. During the visit, JT revealed that he had had no generalized seizures. However, his mother thought he might have had a brief spell 2 days after leaving the hospital consisting of just some walking around in a daze. He claims it was the carbamazepine that made him "spaced out." JT says that spaced out feeling has gotten better the last 2 days. JT's cerebellar examination as well as a complete neurological screening examination were normal. Discuss the impact of your findings and your plan.

By history, JT has had CNS side effects that normally occur with these medications upon initiation, and they also seem to have gotten better over time, which is typical. Want to check about interferences with work/school/driving, etc., because problems in those areas become causes for adherence problems. In spite of subjective problems, his cerebellar examination was normal, indicating no excessive CNS effects.

Efficacy
His serum levels as expected are subtherapeutic because of the slow titration and only starting on the medicine 9 days ago. Somewhat worrisome is what could be a witnessed complex partial seizure "walking around in a daze." Further questioning about its similarity to previous episodes is warranted. However, carbamazepine could have accounted for what was witnessed by his mother. With subtherapeutic serum levels breakthrough seizures are possible.

Plan
Increase the dose of carbamazepine by 100 mg/day. Discuss with the patient his ability to tolerate a repeat of what happened after hospital discharge (since you are increasing the dose). If it potentially interferes with normal activity, maybe just add

100 mg in the evening to minimize effects on daytime activity. Based on CNS side effects slowly titrate dose to a target between 600 and 800 mg/day. Reeducate the patient regarding the high likelihood of CNS effects returning with the increased dose. If he has any suspected seizures/spells or the CNS effects are worse than postdischarge, have him call you as soon as possible. Order a carbamazepine serum level just prior to next visit 7 to 10 days from now.

CASE 24.1
INTERPRETING LIVER FUNCTION TESTS
ANSWER KEY

Total Protein 8.2 g/L
Albumin 5.0 g/L
ALT 600 units/L*
AST 390 units/L*
Alk Phos 54 units/L
INR 1.0
Bilirubin 4.0 mg/dL*
* abnormal lab test values

Patient has markedly elevated AST and ALT (>300 units/L), which is consistent with acute hepatocellular damage seen in hepatitis A, B, or C. Since patient has a bilirubin >3.0, check conjunctivae, nail beds, and frenulum of the tongue for jaundice.

CASE 24.2
INTERPRETING LIVER FUNCTION TESTS
ANSWER KEY

Total Protein 5.6 g/L*
Albumin 2.7 g/L*
ALT 60 units/L*
AST 39 units/L*
Alk Phos 104 units/L
INR 2.0*
Bilirubin 4.0 mg/dL*
BUN 2 mg/dL*
Serum Creatinine 1.0 mg/dL
eGFR >60 mL/min

* abnormal lab test values

1. *Protein synthesis is obviously impaired. The total protein and albumin levels are low. Total protein minus the albumin yields a globulin level of 2.9. A/G ratio is 2.7/2.9, which is less than 1, probably indicating cirrhosis. The INR is >1; therefore, prothrombin synthesis and activity are reduced, increasing the risk of bleeding. The value probably indicates that the patient has cirrhosis of the liver. Physical examination should reveal ascites, pedal edema, jaundice, markedly enlarged hard liver, and probably several of the following: spider angiomata, splenomegaly, caput medusa, gynecomastia, and testicular atrophy.*

2. *The AST/ALT levels are slightly above the upper limits of normal, which is typical of cirrhosis. The levels are not higher because there are very few functional hepatocytes remaining. Blood urea nitrogen is well below normal, indicating some combination of poor nutrition and more likely terminal liver function, because so much of the liver is damaged, it cannot convert amino acids to urea through the arginine-ornithine cycle. Both the creatinine and eGFR are near upper limits of normal so renal function is near normal.*

3. *Bilirubin is markedly elevated (≥3.0 mg/dL) so one would expect that the conjunctivae, frenulum of the tongue, and nail beds would be yellow, indicating the patient is jaundiced.*

CASE 24.3
INTERPRETING LIVER FUNCTION TESTS
ANSWER KEY

Total Protein 8.1 g/L
Albumin 5.0 g/L
ALT 200 units/L*
AST 194 units/L*
Alk Phos 640 units/L*
INR 1.0
Bilirubin 4.0 mg/dL*
Direct Bilirubin 2.4 mg/dL*
BUN 45 mg/dL*
Serum Creatinine 3.0*
eGFR 38 mL/min*
Urine Albumin/Creatinine 2000 mg/g
* abnormal lab test values

1. *This is clearly a pattern for obstructive or cholestatic liver disease. There is no impairment of protein synthesis and the elevations of AST/ALT are modest (<300 units/L). The alkaline phosphatase is greater than five times the upper limit of normal, which is the hallmark of biliary obstruction.*

2. *Bilirubin is markedly elevated (≥3.0 mg/dL), so one would expect that the conjunctivae, frenulum of the tongue, and nail beds would be yellow, indicating the patient is jaundiced. The direct bilirubin, which is normally less than 10% of the total bilirubin, makes up about 60% of all the bilirubin in the blood stream. This means that the liver is still efficiently conjugating bilirubin, but the normal route of excretion through the intra- and extrahepatic bile ducts is obstructed. Obstruction is likely caused by gallbladder disease (the patient would have history of symptoms) or by a medication, like chlorpromazine, that causes a cholestatic pattern of liver dysfunction.*

3. *All four renal function tests are abnormal. The BUN/creatinine ratio is 15:1 so these represent actual decreased renal function, along with the eGFR. An ACR of 2000 mg/g also indicates significant renal damage. Without a history, it is unclear whether or not this is acute or chronic. If urinalysis showed RBC, RBC casts, or epithelial casts, then acute damage might be involved.*

CASE 24.4
INTERPRETING LIVER FUNCTION TESTS
ANSWER KEY

Total Protein 8.2 g/L
Albumin 5.0 g/L
ALT 65 units/L*
AST 52 units/L*
Alk Phos 94 units/L
INR 1.0
Bilirubin 0.1 mg/dL
BUN 11 mg/dL
Serum Creatinine 0.8 mg/dL
* abnormal lab test values

Everything is normal except for the mildly elevated AST/ALT. The value could be the normal value for the patient. If they have the metabolic syndrome or type 2 diabetes, then NAFLD could be the likely cause. Order blood tests to screen for chronic hepatitis B/C. (HBsAg, anti-HCV antibodies). Finally, a careful history regarding ethanol intake in the days before the LFTs were drawn as well as daily level of ethanol intake are needed.
Patient's renal function is normal.

INTERPRETING LIVER FUNCTION TESTS
ANSWER KEY

Total Protein 6.1 g/L*
Albumin 3.0 g/L*
ALT 650 units/L*
AST 520 units/L*
Alk Phos 94 units/L
INR 2.5*
Bilirubin 3.0 mg/dL*
BUN 64 mg/dL*
eGFR >60
Serum Creatinine 1.0 mg/dL
* abnormal lab test values

1. *This patient has both cirrhosis and acute hepatocellular damage!*

2. *Protein synthesis is obviously impaired. The total protein and albumin levels are low. Total protein minus the albumin yields a globulin level of 3.1. A/G ratio is 3.0/3.1, which is less than 1, indicating cirrhosis. The INR is >1; therefore, prothrombin synthesis and activity are reduced, increasing the risk of bleeding. The values indicate that the patient has cirrhosis of the liver. Physical examination should reveal ascites, pedal edema, jaundice, markedly enlarged hard liver, and probably several of the following: spider angiomata, splenomegaly, caput medusa, gynecomastia, and testicular atrophy.*

3. *The AST/ALT levels are >300 units, which is typical of acute hepatocellular damage. The elevation of AST/ALT values could be hepatitis due to ethanol or other hepatotoxic drug- like acetaminophen plus ethanol.*

4. *The BUN is well above normal while the serum creatinine and eGFR are normal. The BUN/ creatinine ratio is 64:1, which indicates excess protein intake probably due to an upper gastrointestinal bleed given his cirrhosis, possibly due to bleeding esophageal varices. Bilirubin is markedly elevated (≥3.0 mg/dL) so one would expect that the conjunctivae, frenulum of the tongue, and nail beds would be yellow, indicating the patient is jaundiced.*

Harvey Wallbanger, a <u>rotund</u> 68-year-old <u>Native American</u> Korean war veteran, who supplements his veteran's pension by <u>bartending</u> at the Arizona Inn, presents to clinic complaining
of a week long history of <u>fatigue, malaise, and nausea without vomiting</u>. He came in because
he noticed his <u>urine had gotten dark brown</u>. Harvey's only health problems are severe
osteoarthritis of both knees and hips for which he takes <u>4 to 6 g/day of acetaminophen</u> and
the <u>recent onset of hemorrhoids</u> for which he was given Anusol HC about 6 weeks ago. His
only other pertinent medical history is a recent trip to <u>rural Costa Rica</u> as chaperone for a
group of teens who were part of a church-sponsored community help program, <u>where he
lived with local people</u>.

a. List two probable causes for his problem. Explain your rationale.

Cirrhosis of the liver → *rotund = ascites?, recent hemorrhoids = portal
hypertension, bartender, chronic high-dose acetaminophen*

Hepatitis A → *nausea, fatigue, malaise for 1 week, had local food and water
in poor sanitation conditions in rural Costa Rica*

Cholecystitis → *Native American (high incidence of gallbladder disease), dark
brown urine, due to bilirubin*

Acetaminophen hepatotoxicity → *4 gm/day*

b. List four questions you would ask or examinations you would perform to help confirm
your diagnosis. Explain your rationale.

Status for hepatitis A/B vaccination → *if positive, would decrease chance of
hepatitis A/B*

Exposure to food and water in Costa Rica → *hepatitis A*
Others in party have similar symptoms? → *hepatitis A*
ETOH intake? How much for how long? → *cirrhosis*
Fever → *hepatitis A*
Check conjunctivae, frenulum, nail beds → *jaundice*
Palpate/percuss abdomen → *hard, enlarged liver → cirrhosis →
tender liver → hepatitis A*

LFTs
Rectal examination to confirm hemorrhoids

c. Below are results of lab tests ordered. What is your assessment of Harvey's complaints?
Explain your rationale.

Total Bilirubin	10.0*	Total Protein	5.2 g/L*	Alk Phos	102 units/L
AST units/L	310*	Albumin	2.5 g/L*	BUN	12 mg/dL
ALT units/L	540*	INR	2.0/L*	Serum Creatinine	0.8 mg/dL

* abnormal lab test values

AST/ALT both greater than 300 units/L → *acute hepatocellular damage 2°
hepatitis A or hepatitis 2°
acetaminophen + ETOH*

Low albumin, A/G Ratio <1, INR >1 → *cirrhosis of the liver 2°
acetaminophen + ETOH*

Total Bilirubin >3 → *patient will be jaundiced*
Renal function normal

CASE 25.1
ANSWER KEY

CJ is a 27-year-old female who presents with the primary complaint of fatigue. Other pertinent medical history includes long-standing menorrhagia and perennial allergic rhinitis. Interpret the CBC and relevant lab tests.

HCT	27%*		TOTAL WBC	7200
HGB	8*		PMN	60%
MCV	75*		BANDS	–0–
MCH	23*		LYMPH	25%
MCHC	30*		MONOS	4%
RETIC	0.3%		BASO	2%
			EOS	9%*
Platelets	400,000			
Ferritin	6 ng/mL*			

* abnormal lab test values

Because the HCT is less than 36%, CJ is anemic. The MCV, MCH, and MCHC are low. The serum ferritin is below 10 ng/mL. All of these values indicate a hypochromic, microcytic anemia due to iron deficiency. Given her history of heavy bleeding during her menses, the cause is most likely chronic blood loss due to menorrhagia.

The white cell count is normal except for the eosinophil count. To calculate the absolute eosinophil count, multiply the total WBC count (7200) by the decimal value of the percentage of eosinophils (9% = 0.09). 7200 x 0.09 = an absolute eosinophil count of 648. Since that value exceeds the threshold of 600, CJ has eosinophilia, most likely due to her perennial allergic rhinitis.

CASE 25.2
ANSWER KEY

AB is a 66-year-old male, who has been on phenytoin and phenobarbital for 50 years for a seizure disorder, presents because his wife thinks he does not look well. When asked, he admits to fatigue and tiring easily. Interpret the CBC and relevant lab tests.

HCT	28%*	TOTAL WBC	5400
HGB	12.4*	PMN	50%
MCV	119*	BAND	0%
MCH	28	LYMPHS	44%
MCHC	34	MONOS	4%
RETIC	0.4%	BASO	–0–
		EOS	2%
RDW	20%*		
Platelets	150,000	Hypersegmented PMNs*	

Anisocytosis and poikilocytosis*

B_{12} and folate serum levels are both normal. So a Castle test is ordered.
After 5 days of 1 µg IM of folic acid/day, reticulocyte count = 17%
* abnormal lab test values

AB is anemic due to hematocrit less than 41 and HGB<13.5. The MCV>100 indicates a macrocytic anemia due to either a B_{12} or folate deficiency. Anisocytosis and poikilocytosis are consistent with the high RDW (>15%). Hypersegmented neutrophils are also consistent with a macrocytic anemia. However, the B_{12} and folate serum levels are normal!!! Given the accuracy of serum levels of these vitamins, further testing is warranted. RBC folate levels are more accurate than serum levels. Also not available are homocysteine and MMA levels, which could help differentiate between folate and B_{12} deficiencies. They should be ordered. Instead, the Castle test was ordered, which consists of 5 days IM injection of 10 µg folic acid followed by 5 days IM injection of 1 µg of B_{12}. On days 5 and 10 the reticulocyte count is measured. A reticulocyte count of double digits on day 5 is consistent with folate deficiency. Minidoses of each agent prevent "masking" the deficiency by either drug.

Folate deficiency would be expected in long-term users of conventional anticonvulsants like phenytoin and phenobarbital. Folate is an essential coenzyme to induction of CYP 450 and is used up by the long-term self-induction process.

CASE 25.3
ANSWER KEY

KJ is a 53-year-old female with a 25-year history of rheumatoid arthritis, who was admitted June 1 with a 6-day history of severe cough and fever. The patient was diagnosed with bacterial pneumonia, based on bilateral consolidated infiltrates in both lower lobes, and antibiotics were started the same day. Interpret the CBC and relevant lab tests.

				June 1	June 8
HCT	32%*	TOTAL WBC		12,400*	8500
HGB	11.5*	PMN		68%	63%
MCV	88	BANDS		17%*	6%
MCH	32	LYMPHS		13%	21%
MCHC	34	MONO		2%	5%
RETIC	0.8%	BASO		0%	1%
		EOS		0%	4%

Ferritin = 100 ng/ml,   folate/B_{12} = wnl

* abnormal lab test values

KJ is anemic based on her hematocrit of less than 36% and her HGB is <12.0. The red cell indices (MCV, MCH, MCHC) indicate a normochromic, normocytic anemia, which could be due to acute blood loss, hemolysis, or anemia of chronic disease. Patients like CJ with long-standing autoimmune diseases like rheumatoid arthritis, many times have the anemia of chronic disease. Obviously, acute blood loss (orthostasis, hypotension, tachycardia, tachypnea, etc.) and hemolytic anemia (elevated bilirubin levels, which are breakdown products of hemoglobin) would have to be ruled out.

KJ's white count and differential are consistent with the diagnosis of bacterial pneumonia. On June 1, the day of admission, KJ's total WBC count of >10,000 (12,400) plus >80% PMNs and bands (85%) indicate a bacterial infection. In addition, >10% bands indicates a left shift, which is consistent of her 6 days of illness prior to diagnosis. The lymphocyte percentage is below normal because their absolute count was unchanged, but the absolute count of mature and immature neutrophils went way up. The CBC on June 8 shows resolution of the infection with the total WBC count falling below 10,000 and the significant fall in both PMNs and bands. Note the percentage of lymphocytes now returns to normal range even though the absolute count is unchanged.

Is this patient, having an IgE-mediated allergic reaction to the antibiotic? (9800 x 0.04 = 392 eosinophils, which is below the threshold of 600 eosinophils, so it is not likely). Alternatively, if the eosinophil percentage were 7% (9800 x 0.07 = 686), the absolute count would exceed the threshold for eosinophilia (>600 eosinophils) and would be consistent with an IgE-mediated allergic reaction to the antibiotic such as urticaria, angioedema, or anaphylaxis.

INDEX

Note: Page references followed by *f* indicate figures; those followed by *t* indicate tables.

A

A/G ratio, 306*t*, 307, 310
ABCD classification system, 277
Abdominal architecture, 117*f*
Abdominal distention, 141
Abdominal pain. *See* Heartburn and abdominal pain
Absence seizure, 295
Acarbose, 139
ACC/AHA cholesterol guidelines, 245, 245*t*
ACCORD studies, 49
ACD. *See* Allergic contact dermatitis (ACD)
ACEI. *See* Angiotensin-converting enzyme (ACEI) inhibitors
Acetaminophen, 92
ACL injury, 177
Aclidinium, 283*t*
Acne, 207
Acne rosacea, 208–209, 210*f*
Acne vulgaris, 207–208, 208*f*
ACPA. *See* Anticyclic citrullinated peptide antibodies (ACPA)
ACQ. *See* Asthma Control Questionnaire (ACQ)
ACR. *See* Albumin to creatinine ratio (ACR)
ACS. *See* Acute coronary syndrome (ACS)
ACT. *See* Asthma Control Test (ACT)
Active problems, 33
Active TB, 96
Acute asthma attacks, 278, 278*t*
Acute bacterial sinusitis, 71–72*t*, 73–74
Acute biliary pancreatitis, 123
Acute bronchitis, 91*t*, 93
Acute cerebrovascular events, 154
Acute coronary syndrome (ACS), 107*t*, 109–111
Acute cough, 90
Acute diarrhea, 136
Acute epiglottitis, 84
Acute hepatocellular damage, 308, 309*t*, 383
Acute neurovascular syndrome, 155
Acute onset headache, 148
Acute otitis media (AOM), 74, 75–76*t*, 77, 348
Acute pyelonephritis, 124, 186, 194

Adenovirus, 137
Adherence, 48. *See also* Patient adherence
Adherence aids, 53, 56
Administration technique (inhalers, eye drops, etc.), 55
ADO index, 279
AEDs. *See* Antiepileptic drugs (AEDs)
AER. *See* Albumin excretion rate (AER)
Afterload, 288
Agranulocytosis, 331
AKC. *See* Atopic keratoconjunctivitis (AKC)
Alanine aminotransferase (ALT), 306, 306*t*, 312
Albumin, 306*t*, 307, 310, 315
Albumin excretion rate (AER), 315
Albumin to creatinine ratio (ACR), 315
Albumin to globulin ratio (A/G) ratio, 306*t*, 307, 310
Albuminuria, 315
Albuterol, 283*t*
Aldosterone agonists, 290
Aliskiren, 234*t*
Alkaline phosphatase (AP), 306*t*, 307
Allergic conjunctivitis, 165*t*, 166, 167*f*, 359
Allergic contact dermatitis (ACD), 190, 199–202
Allergic rhinitis (AR), 70, 71–72*t*, 73
ALT. *See* Alanine aminotransferase (ALT)
Amebiasis, 137
Aminotransferases, 306–307
Amoxicillin/clavulanic acid, 139
Ampicillin rash, 221
Anabolic steroids, 309
Analytic diagnostic process, 9–10, 10*t*
Anaphylaxis, 218
Anemia, bleeding, and infection, 325–337
　anemia, defined, 326
　anticoagulants, 332–334
　aplastic anemia, 299, 331
　bacterial infections, 330
　bleeding complications of anticoagulants, 332*t*, 333–334
　cases, 335–337, 385–387

classification of anemias, 327, 327*t*
drug-induced red/white blood cell reduction, 331
hemolytic anemia, 309*t*
iron deficiency anemia, 328
leukocytosis, 330, 331
macrocytic anemia, 327*t*, 328, 329
megaloblastic anemia, 328
pernicious anemia, 328
platelets, 331
red blood cells, 326–328
signs/symptoms of significant anemia, 326*t*
white blood cells, 329–330
Angina pectoris, 107*t*, 109
Angioedema, 216, 218, 218*f*
Angioneurotic edema, 216, 218, 218*f*
Angiotensin-converting enzyme inhibitors (ACEI)
angioedema, 218
bleeding complications, 333
CHF, 290, 291*t*
cough, 94–95*t*, 97
hypertension, 234*t*, 235*t*
Angiotensin receptor blockers (ARBs)
CHF, 290, 291*t*
hypertension, 234*t*, 235*t*
Anisocytosis, 328
Ankle sprain, 176
Ankylosing spondylitis, 181
Answer key, 339–387. *See also* Cases
Antacids, 139
Anterior cruciate ligament (ACL) injury, 177
Anti-Smith antibodies, 181
Anticoagulants, 332–334
Anticonvulsant hypersensitivity syndrome, 221
Anticyclic citrullinated peptide antibodies (ACPA), 179
Antiepileptic drugs (AEDs), 297*t*, 298*t*, 299
Antiplatelet medications, 331
Antistreptolysin O (ASO) test, 82
AOM. *See* Acute otitis media (AOM)
AP. *See* Alkaline phosphatase (AP)
Aplastic anemia, 299, 331
Apley test, 177
ApoB/ApoA1 ratio, 246*t*, 247
Appendicitis, 118–119*t*, 123–124
AR. *See* Allergic rhinitis (AR)
ARBs. *See* Angiotensin receptor blockers (ARBs)
Arformoterol, 283*t*
Arthritides, 178–181
Arthrocentesis, 178
Ascites, 310, 310*f*, 311*f*
ASCVD, 244. *See also* Dyslipidemia
Aseptic meningitis, 152
Ask, Listen, and Summarize, 56

Ask, Provide, Ask, 56
ASO test, 82
Aspartate aminotransferase (AST), 306, 306*t*, 312
Aspirin, 153, 331
Assessment, 35
Associated symptoms questions, 18*t*, 19
AST. *See* Aspartate aminotransferase (AST)
Asthma, 273–285
action plans, 281
acute asthma attacks, 278, 278*t*
case, 285, 375
classification, 277
complications, 278, 281*t*
COPD, compared, 274*t*
cough, 93, 94–95*t*, 96
diagnosis, 275, 276
etiology, 274–275
follow-up visits, 279–282
green zone/yellow zone/red zone, 281
initial visit, 279
overview, 274*t*
rule of 2s, 279
self-assessment, 279
Asthma action plans, 281
Asthma Control Questionnaire (ACQ), 279
Asthma Control Test (ACT), 279
Asthma Therapy Assessment Questionnaire (ATAQ), 279
Asymptomatic chronic diseases, 44, 49, 50
Asymptomatic pyelonephritis, 191
ATAQ. *See* Asthma Therapy Assessment Questionnaire (ATAQ)
Atherosclerosis, 244, 249
Atherosclerotic cardiovascular disease (ASCVD), 244, 331. *See also* Dyslipidemia
Athlete's foot, 212
Atopic dermatitis, 198–199, 199*f*, 200*f*, 364
Atopic eczema, 198
Atopic keratoconjunctivitis (AKC), 165*t*, 166
Atopic triad, 93
Atorvastatin, 252
Atrophic vaginitis, 190
Atrophy, 223
Atypical pneumonia, 99–100*t*, 101

B
Back injuries, 177–178
Bacterial conjunctivitis, 165*t*, 169–171
Bacterial diarrhea, 136
Bacterial gastroenteritis, 137, 138*t*
Bacterial infections, 330
Bacterial meningitis, 152
Bacterial pneumonia, 91*t*, 92
Bacterial sinusitis, 71–72*t*, 73–74
Bacterial skin infections, 203–209
Bacterial vaginosis (BV), 187–188, 188*t*
Bands, 329

Barrett's esophagitis, 122
Basophils, 329
BCG vaccine, 96
Benign meningioma, 152
Benzocaine, 202
Beta-adrenergic bronchodilators, 281*t*
Beta-blockers
    CHF, 290, 291*t*
    hypertension, 234*t*, 235*t*
Biliary tree abnormalities, 316
Bilirubin, 306*t*, 307–308, 316
Bleeding. *See* Anemia, bleeding, and infection
Bleeding complications of anticoagulants,
    332*t*, 333–334
Blepharitis, 171
Bloating/abdominal distention, 141
Blood pressure measurement, 231. *See also*
    Essential hypertension (EHT)
Blood urea nitrogen (BUN), 311, 313–314
Blumberg sign, 123
BNP. *See* Brain natriuretic peptide (BNP)
BODE index, 279
Boil, 205
Bone diseases, 181–182
Bordetella pertussis, 97
Bowel disorders, 124
Bowel movements, 142
Brain natriuretic peptide (BNP), 290
Brain tumor, 152
Brudzinski, sign, 152
Bruxism, 151
Bulbar conjunctiva, 160
Bullae, 198
Bullous impetigo, 205, 206*f*
BUN. *See* Blood urea nitrogen (BUN)
BUN/serum creatinine ratio, 314
Butalbital, 151
BV. *See* Bacterial vaginosis (BV)

C

C. diff., 137
C-reactive protein high-sensitivity assay
    (hs-CRP), 246*t*, 247
CAD. *See* Coronary artery disease (CAD)
Calcitonin gene-related peptide (CGRP), 150
Calcium channel blockers, 142
Calcium salts, 142
Cancer chemotherapy
    diarrhea, 140
    nausea and vomiting, 130
Candida, 188–189, 188*t*
Candida albicans, 189
Candida glabrata, 189
Candidal skin infection, 214–216
CAP. *See* Community-acquired pneumonia
    (CAP)
Capricious nonadherence, 48*t*

Carbamazepine
    anemia, 329
    seizure disorders, 297*t*, 298*t*, 377
Carbuncle, 206–207
Cardiac sphincter of the stomach, 122
Carpal tunnel syndrome, 177
Carvedilol, 234*t*, 235*t*
Cases
    anemia, bleeding, and infection, 335–337,
        385–387
    answer key, 339–387
    asthma and COPD, 285, 375
    chest pain, 114, 352
    cough, 103, 104, 350, 351
    diabetes mellitus, 271, 373–374
    diarrhea and constipation, 144, 145,
        356, 357
    dyslipidemia, 254–257, 369–372
    dysuria and vaginal discharge, 195, 196,
        361–363
    ears, nose, and throat, 85–88, 346–349
    headache, 157, 358
    heart failure, 292, 376
    heartburn and abdominal pain, 126,
        353–354
    hypertension, 239–241, 366–368
    inflamed red eye, 173, 359
    liver and renal disease, 318–323, 379–384
    musculoskeletal disorders, 183, 360
    nausea and vomiting, 134, 355
    patient script (chief complaint history-
        taking), 23–26
    patient script (chronic visit history-
        taking), 27–29
    problem list, 36–38, 341–343
    seizure disorders, 301, 377–378
    skin disorders, 224, 225, 364, 365
    SOAP note (permanent problems),
        40, 345
    SOAP note (temporary problems),
        39, 344
Castle test, 328
Casts, 316
CAT. *See* COPD Assessment Test (CAT)
CBC. *See* Complete blood count (CBC)
Celiac disease, 124, 140–141
Celiac sprue, 140
Cellulitis, 203, 204*f*, 205, 206, 364
Cerebral edema, 151
Cerebrospinal fluid (CSF), 152, 153*t*
Cerebrovascular accident (CVA), 154–155
Cervicitis, 187
CGRP. *See* Calcitonin gene-related peptide
    (CGRP)
Chalazion, 171
Cheerleader approach, 49
Chemosis, 170

Chemotherapy
    diarrhea, 140
    nausea and vomiting, 130
Chest cold, 93
Chest pain, 105–114
    ACS, 107*t*, 109–111
    angina pectoris, 107*t*, 109
    CAD, 106–111
    cardiac causes, 106–111
    case, 114, 352
    chest wall twinge syndrome, 108*t*, 112
    costochondritis, 108*t*, 112–113
    diagnosis, 106
    esophagitis, 108*t*, 113
    etiology, 106
    gastrointestinal causes, 113
    hyperventilation syndrome, 107*t*, 112
    mitral valve prolapse, 108*t*, 111
    musculoskeletal causes, 112–113
    NSTEMI, 107*t*, 110
    overview, 107–108*t*
    pericarditis, 108*t*, 111
    pleurisy, 108*t*, 112
    pulmonary embolism, 107*t*, 111–112
    respiratory causes, 111–112
    STEMI, 107*t*, 110–111
    trauma/rib fracture, 112
    unstable angina, 107*t*, 110
Chest wall twinge syndrome, 108*t*, 112
CHF. *See* Congestive heart failure (CHF)
Chicken pox, 211
Chief complaint history, 17–19
    Associated symptoms questions, 18*t*, 19
    Location questions, 18–19, 18*t*
    Modifying factors questions, 18*t*, 19
    Onset questions, 18*t*, 19
    patient scripts (cases), 27–29
    Quality questions, 18*t*, 19
    Quantity questions, 18*t*, 19
    Setting questions, 18*t*, 19
    Summary/Close, 18*t*, 19
    "What do you think caused this
        problem?" question, 18*t*, 19
    "What medications are you currently
        taking?" question, 18*t*, 19
Chlamydia, 188*t*, 190
Chlamydia trachomatis, 190
Chlamydial conjunctivitis, 165*t*
Chlamydophila pneumoniae, 101
Cholecystitis
    abdominal pain/discomfort, 122–123
    liver disease, 384
    nausea and vomiting, 132
Cholestatic jaundice, 309
Cholestatic liver disease, 309–310, 309*t*, 381
Cholesterol, 244. *See also* Dyslipidemia
Chronic asymptomatic diseases, 44, 49, 50

Chronic cough, 90
Chronic disease follow-up visit history,
    19–21
    Compliance questions, 20, 20*t*
    Complications questions, 20–21, 20*t*
    Concern questions, 21
    Control questions, 20, 20*t*
    patient scripts (cases), 27–29
Chronic esophagitis, 122
Chronic hepatocellular damage, 309*t*,
    310–311
Chronic kidney disease epidemiology
    collaborative equation (CKD-EPI), 314,
    314*t*
Chronic obstructive pulmonary disease
    (COPD), 273–285
    asthma, compared, 274*t*
    case, 285, 375
    classification, 277–278
    complications, 278–279, 283*t*
    cough, 91*t*, 93
    diagnosis, 275, 276–277
    etiology, 275
    follow-up visit, 282–283
    functional dyspnea severity, 277
    initial visit, 279
    overview, 274*t*
Chronic or recurrent headaches, 148
Chronic/recurrent mild hepatocellular
    damage, 309*t*, 311–313
Chronic suppurative otitis media (CSOM),
    75–76*t*, 78, 348
Ciliary flush, 162–163, 163*f*
Cimetidine, 313
Cirrhosis, 309*t*, 310–311, 383, 384
CK serum levels, 249, 250
CKD-EPI, 314, 314*t*
CK^{MB}, 110
Classic erythema multiforme, 218, 219*f*
Classical pyelonephritis, 191
Clavulanic acid, 139
Clonic phase, 295
Clonidine, 234*t*, 235*t*
Clopidogrel, 153, 331
Closed-ended questions, 16
Clostridium difficile, 137
Closure statement, 22
Clot formation, 106
Cluster headache, 149*t*, 150
CMV. *See* Cytomegalic virus (CMV)
Coccidioidomycosis, 152, 216
Cockcroft-Gault equation, 314, 314*t*, 315
Common cold, 70, 71–72*t*, 73*t*
Common warts, 209, 210*f*
Communication with health care
    professionals, 44–46
Community-acquired pneumonia (CAP), 92

Complete blood count (CBC)
platelets, 331
red blood cells, 326–328
white blood cells, 329–330
Complete medical history, 17
Complex medical regimen, 51, 54–55
Compliance, 11, 13*t*, 48. *See also* Patient
adherence
Compliance questions, 20, 20*t*
Complications (disease), 11, 13*t*
Complications (drug), 11, 13*t*
Complications questions, 20–21, 20*t*
Computerized prescription lid, 53
Concern questions, 21
Concordance, 48
Congestive heart failure (CHF), 287–292
BNP, 290
case, 292, 376
classification, 289*t*
complications, 291*t*
cough, 98, 99–100*t*, 101
diagnosis, 289–290
DOE, 289
etiology, 288
follow-up visits, 290–291, 291*t*
Framington criteria, 290, 290*t*
PND, 289
preload/afterload, 288
SOB, 289
systolic/diastolic cardiac dysfunction, 288
Conjunctiva, 160
Conjunctivitis, 165*t*. *See also* Inflamed (red) eye
Constipation, 142–143. *See also* Diarrhea and
constipation
Contact dermatitis
allergic, 199–202
irritant, 199, 200*f*
Contact lenses, 163–164
Control questions, 20, 20*t*
COPD. *See* Chronic obstructive pulmonary
disease (COPD)
COPD Assessment Test (CAT), 277
Cornea, 160
Coronary artery disease (CAD), 106–111
Corrected reticulocyte count, 328
Corticosteroids
asthma, 281*t*
bleeding complications, 333
COPD, 283*t*
skin disorders, 222–223
Cost of medication, 51, 55
Costochondritis, 108*t*, 112–113
Cough, 89–104
ACE inhibitors, 94–95*t*, 97
acute bronchitis, 91*t*, 93
asthma, 93, 94–95*t*, 96
atypical pneumonia, 99–100*t*, 101

bacterial pneumonia, 91*t*, 92
CAP, 92
cases, 103, 104, 350, 351
CHF, 98, 99–100*t*, 101
classification, 90
COPD, 91*t*, 93
diagnosis, 90
dry, 90, 93–98
etiology, 90
functions, 90
GERD, 94–95*t*, 97
influenza, 98, 99–100*t*
lung cancer, 94–95*t*, 97
mixed, 90, 98–101
overview, 91*t*, 94–95*t*, 99–100*t*
pertussis, 94–95*t*, 97–98
PICS, 98, 99–100*t*
productive, 90, 91*t*, 92–93
TB, 94–95*t*, 96–97
UACS, 98, 99–100*t*
viral pneumonia, 98, 99–100*t*
Creatine kinase (CK), 249, 250
Creatine phosphate, 313
Creatinine, 313
Crohn disease, 124, 140
Croup, 84
Crust, 198
Cryptosporidiosis (crypto), 139
Cryptosporidium hominis, 137
CSF. *See* Cerebrospinal fluid (CSF)
CSOM. *See* Chronic suppurative otitis media
(CSOM)
CVA. *See* Cerebrovascular accident (CVA)
Cyclosporine, 309
Cylindruria, 316
Cystitis, 191–193
Cytomegalicvirus (CMV), 141

D

D-dimer, 112
dabl Education Trust web site, 231
Dacryocystitis, 163
Dandruff, 202
DAP, 32
Deep vein thrombosis (DVT), 111
Degenerative joint disease (DJD), 178–179
Dehydration, 142
Dennie lines, 276
Depression, 298–299
Dermatological problems. *See* Skin disorders
DEXA. *See* Dual energy x-ray absorptiometry
(DEXA)
DHS. *See* Drug hypersensitivity syndrome
(DHS)
Diabetes mellitus, 259–271
A1C, 262, 268, 268*t*
case, 271, 373–374

classification/etiology, 260–261
complications, 262–265, 267t
dental care, 270
diabetic foot, 262, 264t
diabetic foot examination, 263, 264t, 269
diagnosis, 261–262
diarrhea, 139
dyslipidemia, 252
ESRD, 263
follow-up visits, 266–270
hypoglycemia, 269, 269t
infection, 265
initial visit, 265–266, 266t
macroangiopathy, 265
metabolic syndrome, 261, 261t
nausea and vomiting, 133
nephropathy, 263
neuropathy, 263–265
prediabetes, 262
retinopathy, 262
SBGM, 269
type 1/type 2, 260, 260t
Diabetic foot, 262, 264t
Diabetic foot examination, 263, 264t, 269
Diabetic gastroparesis, 141, 263
Diabetic ketoacidosis, 262, 316
Diabetic neuropathy, 263–265
Diabetic retinopathy, 262
Diagnosis, 7–13
analytic vs. nonanalytic approaches, 9–11
elements needed to assess illness, 8, 9t
textbook organization, 11
Diagnostic/evaluative criteria, 8, 9t
Diagnostic schemata, 10
Diaper rash, 199
Diarrhea and constipation, 135–145
amebiasis, 139
bloating/abdominal distention, 141
cases, 144, 145, 356, 357
celiac disease, 140–141
constipation, 142–143
cryptosporidiosis, 139
diabetic gastroparesis, 141
diagnosis, 136–137
dietary causes, 138t, 139
etiology, 136
giardiasis, 139
HIV, 141
inflammatory bowel disease, 140
irritable bowel syndrome, 141
medication, 138t, 139–140
overview, 138t
parasitic diarrhea, 137, 138t, 139
toxigenic bacterial gastroenteritis, 137, 138t
usually self-limiting gastroenteritis, 137, 138t
viral gastroenteritis, 137, 138t

Diastolic blood pressure, 230
Differential diagnosis. *See also* Diagnosis
chest pain, 107–108t
cough, 91t, 94–95t, 99–100t
diarrhea and constipation, 138t
ear pain/discharge, 75–76t
headache, 149t
heartburn and abdominal pain, 118–120t
inflamed (red) eye, 165t
musculoskeletal disorders, 179t
nausea and vomiting, 128t, 129t
sore throat, 80–81t
stuffy/runny nose, 71–72t
vaginal discharge, 188t
Differential white count, 329
Diffusion weighted imaging MRI (MRI-DWI), 155
Digoxin, 290, 291t
Diphenhydramine, 202
Dipstick tests, 192t, 194
Direct bilirubin, 308
Disease control, 11, 13t
Disease-specific structured provider checklist, 63, 64–65t
Disease-specific tables, 13t, 22
Diseases, overview. *See* Differential diagnosis
Dishpan hands, 199
Diuretics
CHF, 288, 291t
hypertension, 234t, 235t
photosensitivity reactions, 221
DJD. *See* Degenerative joint disease (DJD)
Documentation, 31–40
free-flowing narrative, 32
POMR, 32–33
problem list, 32–33, 36–38
SOAP notes, 33–35, 39, 40
structured approach, 32
DOE. *See* Dyspnea on exertion (DOE)
Drawer tests, 177
DRESS. *See* Drug reaction with eosinophilia and systemic symptoms (DRESS)
Drug hypersensitivity syndrome (DHS), 221, 299
Drug-induced cholestasis, 309
Drug-induced hepatitis, 299
Drug-induced nausea and vomiting, 130
Drug-induced red/white blood cell reduction, 331
Drug-induced skin reactions, 216–221
Drug reaction with eosinophilia and systemic symptoms (DRESS), 221, 299
Drug-related problems, 11, 13t
Dry cough, 90, 93–98
Dual energy x-ray absorptiometry (DEXA), 181
Duodenal ulcer, 117, 118–119t
DVT. *See* Deep vein thrombosis (DVT)

Dysentery, 136
Dyslipidemia, 243–257
  ACC/AHA cholesterol guidelines, 245, 245*t*
  ApoB/ApoA1 ratio, 246*t*, 247
  cases, 254–257, 369–372
  cognitive dysfunction, 251–252
  diabetes, 252
  disease complications, 249, 250*t*
  drug complications, 249–252
  follow-up visit check list, 250*t*
  Framingham Study ratios, 246–247, 246*t*
  good/bad cholesterol, 244
  hepatotoxicity, 251
  hs-CRP, 246*t*, 247
  monitoring treatment efficiency, 248–249
  musculoskeletal system, 249–251
  NCEP ATP III guidelines, 244, 245*t*
  Non-HDL Cholesterol, 246*t*, 247
  types of lipids, 244
Dyspnea on exertion (DOE), 289
Dysuria and vaginal discharge, 185–196
  allergic or irritant contact dermatitis, 190
  bacterial vaginosis, 187–188, 188*t*
  candida, 188–189, 188*t*
  cases, 195, 196, 361–363
  Chlamydia, 188*t*, 190
  differential diagnosis, 188*t*
  gonorrhea, 188*t*, 190
  initial questions, 186*t*
  leukorrhea, 190
  testing vaginal/urethral discharge
    samples, 189*t*
  trichomoniasis, 188*t*, 189–190
  urine testing, 192*t*
  UTI, 190–194

E

Ear pain/discharge, 74–79
  acute otitis media, 74, 75–76*t*, 77
  chronic suppurative otitis media, 75–76*t*, 78
  ear pain with a normal otoscopic
    examination, 78–79
  otitis externa (swimmer's ear), 75–76*t*, 78
  otitis media with effusion, 75–76*t*, 77–78
  TMJ pain dysfunction syndrome, 75–76*t*, 79
Ears, nose, and throat, 69–88
  cases, 85–88, 346–349
  ear pain/discharge, 74–79
  overview, 75–76*t*
  runny/stuffy nose, 70–74
  sore throat/hoarseness, 79–84
EBV. *See* Epstein-Barr virus (EBV)
ECG. *See* Electrocardiogram (ECG)
Ectopic pregnancy, 124
Ectropion, 171

Eczema, 198
Eczematous disorders, 198–202
Educating the patient, 43–44
EEG. *See* Electroencephalogram (EEG)
EF. *See* Ejection fraction (EF)
EGD. *See* Esophagogastroduodenoscopy (EGD)
eGFR. *See* Estimated glomerular filtration rate (eGFR)
EHR. *See* Electronic health record (EHR)
EHT. *See* Essential hypertension (EHT)
EIA. *See* Enzyme immunoassay (EIA)
Ejection fraction (EF), 288
Electrocardiogram (ECG), 106
Electroencephalogram (EEG), 294, 295
Electronic health record (EHR), 33
EM. *See* Erythema multiforme (EM)
Embolic stroke, 154
Emphysema, 93
End-stage renal disease (ESRD), 263
Enlisting the support of others, 56
ENT. *See* Ears, nose, and throat
Entamoeba histolytica, 139
Entropion, 171
Enzyme immunoassay (EIA), 312
Eosinophilia, 221
Eosinophilic folliculitis, 206
Eosinophils, 329
Epicondylitis, 176–177
Epiglottitis, 84
Epilepsy. *See* Seizure disorders
Epstein-Barr virus (EBV), 79, 83
Ergotamine, 151
Ergots, 151
Erysipelas, 207
Erythema multiforme (EM), 218–219, 219*f*, 220*f*
Erythema multiforme major, 218
Erythema multiforme minor, 218, 219*f*
Erythema nodosum, 221
Erythrocytes, 326
Erythromycin
  diarrhea, 139
  liver damage, 309
Escherichia coli, 191
Esophageal varices, 311
Esophagitis, 108*t*, 113, 118–119*t*, 122
Esophagogastroduodenoscopy (EGD), 117, 121
ESR. *See* Erythrocyte sedimentation rate (ESR)
ESRD. *See* End-stage renal disease (ESRD)
Essential hypertension (EHT), 229–241
  blood pressure measurement, 231
  blood pressure technique, 232*t*
  blood pressure values below target values, 236
  cases, 239–241, 366–368
  common errors in measurement, 233*t*
  compliance, 234*t*, 237

complications, 231, 234–235*t*, 237–238
control, 234–237, 234*t*
decrease the blood pressure slowly, 236
diagnosis, 230
etiology, 230
follow-up visits, 234–238
headache, 151
home blood pressure techniques, 235
idiopathic intracranial hypertension, 153
initial visit/workup, 231–232
J-curve, 236
lab tests, 232
patient's willingness to make lifestyle
    modifications, 232
portal hypertension, 310–311, 311*f*
significant drop in blood pressure, 235
white coat hypertension, 230
Estimated glomerular filtration rate (eGFR),
    314–315, 314*t*
Estrogen, 130, 309
Ethanol ingestion, 312
Evaluative or diagnostic criteria, 8, 9*t*
Excoriation, 198
Exenatide, 267*t*
Expert Panel, Report 3 (EPR-3) Guidelines
    for the Diagnosis and Management of
    Asthma, 277
External locus of control, 50
Eye conditions, 171. *See also* Inflamed (red)
    eye
Eye contact, 21
"Eyeball" method (refill record), 53

F

Facial expression, 21
Family history, 17
FAST, 155
Fasting plasma glucose, 262
FDA MedWatch program, 251
Febrile seizure, 296
Fecal matter, 142
Fecal volume, 142
Felbamate, 297*t*, 298*t*
Felty's syndrome, 180
FE_{NO}, 276
FEV_1, 275–277
Fixed drug eruptions, 221
Flesh-eating bacteria, 207
Fluorinated, high-potency topical
    corticosteroids, 222–223
Folate blood levels, 328
Folliculitis, 205, 206*f*
Follow-up visits, 61
Forced expiratory volume (FEV_1), 275–277
Forced vital capacity (FVC), 275, 281
Formed elements, 316
Formoterol, 283*t*

Fornix, 160
Framingham criteria (CHF), 290, 290*t*
Framingham Study ratios, 246–247, 246*t*
Free-flowing narrative, 32
Frequency of contact with patient, 55–56
Friedewald formula, 247
Functional dyspepsia, 121
Functional dyspnea severity, 277
Fungal meningitis, 152
Fungal skin infections, 212–216
Furuncle, 205, 207*f*
FVC. *See* Forced vital capacity (FVC)

G

Gabapentin, 297*t*, 298*t*
GABHS. *See* Group A β-hemolytic strep
    (GABHS)
Gallbladder disease, 118–119*t*, 122–123, 309
Gallstones, 123
γ-glutamyl transpeptidase (GGTP), 306*t*,
    307, 309
Giardia lamblia, 139
Gardnerella vaginalis, 187
Gastric carcinoma, 121
Gastric ulcer, 118–119*t*, 121
Gastritis, 121
Gastroenteritis, 128, 129*t*, 137, 138*t*
Gastroesophageal reflux disease (GERD),
    94–95*t*, 97, 118–119*t*, 122
Gastroparesis, 141, 263
Generalized tonic-clonic seizures, 295
Genitourinary system, 186. *See also* Dysuria
    and vaginal discharge
GERD. *See* Gastroesophageal reflux disease
    (GERD)
Geriatric patients, 44
GFR. *See* Glomerular filtration rate (GFR)
GGTP. *See* γ-glutamyl transpeptidase (GGTP)
GI cocktail, 113
Giant papillary conjunctivitis (GPC), 165*t*, 166
Giardiasis, 139
Gliadin, 140
Gliptins, 267*t*
Glitazones, 267*t*
Global Strategy for the Diagnosis,
    Management and Prevention of Chronic
    Obstructive Pulmonary Disease: GOLD
    Executive Summary, 278
Globulin, 307, 315
Glomerular filtration rate (GFR), 314
GLP-agonists, 267*t*
Gluten peptides, 140
Gluten-sensitive enteropathy, 140
Glycosylated hemoglobin (A1C), 262, 268, 268*t*
Golfer elbow, 177
Gonococcal/chlamydial conjunctivitis, 165*t*
Gonorrhea, 170, 188*t*, 190

GPC. *See* Giant papillary conjunctivitis (GPC)
Granulocytes, 329, 331
Granulocytopenia, 299, 331
Granuloma, 96
Group A β-hemolytic strep (GABHS)
　　erysipelas, 207
　　impetigo, 79
　　sore throat, 79

H

H. pylori, 116, 121
HAART. *See* Highly active antiretroviral
　　therapy (HAART)
Haemophilus influenzae, 74, 77, 92
Hand, foot, and hand disease (HFMD),
　　80–81*t*, 83
HBsAg. *See* Hepatitis B surface antigen
　　(HBsAg)
hCG. *See* Human chorionic gonadotropin
　　(hCG)
HCT. *See* Hematocrit (HCT)
HCV-RNA, 312
HDL-C, 244
Headache, 147–157
　　acute trauma/post-trauma, 153
　　case, 157, 358
　　cluster, 149*t*, 150
　　diagnosis, 148
　　differential diagnosis, 149*t*
　　etiology, 148
　　hypertensive emergency, 151
　　medication overuse, 151
　　meningitis, 152–153, 153*t*
　　migraine, 149–150, 149*t*
　　primary, 148–150
　　pseudotumor cerebri, 153
　　secondary, 150–155
　　SNOOP 4, 150–151
　　stroke, 154–155
　　temporomandibular joint pain
　　　dysfunction syndrome, 151
　　tension, 148–149, 149*t*
　　tumor/mass occupying lesion, 152
Health literacy, 44
Health summary, 17
Heart failure (HF). *See* Congestive heart
　　failure (CHF)
Heart failure with preserved ejection fraction
　　(HFPEF), 288
Heart failure with reduced ejection fraction
　　(HFREF), 288
Heartburn and abdominal pain, 115–126
　　abdominal architecture, 117*f*
　　appendicitis, 118–119*t*, 123–124
　　bowel disorders, 124
　　case, 126, 353–354
　　diagnosis, 116

duodenal ulcer, 117, 118–119*t*
esophagitis, 118–119*t*, 122
etiology, 116
gallbladder disease, 118–119*t*, 122–123
gastric ulcer, 118–119*t*, 121
GERD, 118–119*t*, 122
gynecological, 119–120*t*
hiatal hernia, 122
intestinal obstruction, 119–120*t*, 124
MI/angina, 119–120*t*
overview, 118–120*t*
pancreatitis, 119–120*t*, 123
PID, 124
renal calculus, 119–120*t*, 124
upper gastrointestinal bleeding, 121
UTI, 119–120*t*, 124
Heel drop test, 123
Helicobacter pylori, 116, 121
Hematemesis, 121
Hematocrit (HCT), 326, 327
Hematuria, 316, 333
Hemoglobin (HGB), 326
Hemoglobin A1C, 262, 268, 268*t*
Hemolytic anemia, 309*t*
Hemorrhagic complications of
　　anticoagulants, 332*t*, 333–334
Hemorrhagic stroke, 154–155
Hemorrhoids, 311
Hepatitis
　　AEDs, 299
　　liver damage, 309*t*, 311–313, 379, 384
　　viral, 132
Hepatitis B surface antigen (HBsAg), 312
Hepatojugular reflux (HJR), 289
Herpangina, 80–81*t*, 83
Herpes simplex, 209, 211*f*
Herpes simplex keratitis, 162*f*
Herpes simplex keratoconjunctivitis, 165*t*,
　　169
Herpes zoster, 211–212, 212*f*
Herpes zoster ophthalmicus (HZO), 165*t*, 169
HF. *See* Congestive heart failure (CHF)
HFMD. *See* Hand, foot, and mouth disease
　　(HFMD)
HFPEF. *See* Heart failure with preserved
　　ejection fraction (HFPEF)
HFREF. *See* Heart failure with reduced
　　ejection fraction (HFREF)
HGB. *See* Hemoglobin (HGB)
HHNS. *See* Hyperosmolar, hyperglycemic,
　　non-ketotic syndrome (HHNS)
Hiatal hernia, 122
High-density lipoprotein (HDL-C), 244
High-potency fluorinated topical
　　corticosteroids, 222–223
High-sensitivity C-reactive protein (hs-CRP),
　　179

Highly active antiretroviral therapy (HAART), 141
History of present illness (HPI), 17. *See also* Chief complaint history
History taking. *See* Patient history
HIV, 141
Hives, 216, 217*f*
HJR. *See* Hepatojugular reflux (HJR)
HLA. *See* Human lymphocyte antigen (HLA)
HOAP, 32
Hoarseness, 84
Homan sign, 111
Home blood pressure techniques, 235
Homeless patients, 51
Hordeolum, 171
Hospital-acquired bacterial pneumonia, 92
HPI, 17
hs-CRP, 246*t*, 247. *See* High-sensitivity C-reactive protein (hs-CRP)
Human chorionic gonadotropin (hCG), 130
Human lymphocyte antigen (HLA), 140
Hyaline casts, 316
Hydralazine, 234*t*, 235*t*
Hyperammonemia, 299
Hyperemesis gravidarum, 130
Hyperosmolar non-ketotic coma, 262
Hyperpurulent or hyperacute conjunctivitis, 170
Hyperosmolar, hyperglycemic, non-ketotic syndrome (HHNS), 262
Hypertension. *See* Essential hypertension (EHT)
Hypertensive encephalopathy, 151
Hyperventilation syndrome, 107*t*, 112
Hyphema, 163
Hypochromic, microcytic anemia, 327
Hypoglycemia, 269, 269*t*
Hypopyon, 163, 164*f*
Hypotension, 290
HZO. *See* Herpes zoster ophthalmicus (HZO)

I

"I" message, 45
IBD. *See* Inflammatory bowel disease (IBD)
IBS. *See* Irritable bowel syndrome (IBS)
ICHD-2, 148, 149
Idiopathic intracranial hypertension, 153
IgA-anti-tTG antibodies, 141
IgE-mediated reactions, 216–218
Immature neutrophils, 329
Impetigo, 205, 205*f*
Inactive problems, 33
Inclusion conjunctivitis, 171
Indacaterol, 283*t*
Indian Health Service counseling technique, 43
Indirect bilirubin, 308

Inflamed (red) eye, 159–173
    allergic conjunctivitis, 165*t*, 166, 167*f*
    anatomy, 160
    bacterial conjunctivitis, 165*t*, 169–171
    case, 173, 359
    contact lenses, 163–164
    gonococcal/chlamydial conjunctivitis, 165*t*
    hyphema/hypopyon, 163, 164*f*
    irritant conjunctivitis, 164
    limbal or ciliary flush, 162–163, 163*f*
    miscellaneous eye conditions, 171
    overview, 165*t*
    photophobia, 161
    severe foreign body sensation, 161–162
    viral conjunctivitis, 165*t*, 166–169
    when to refer, 160–164
Inflammatory bowel disease (IBD), 140
Influenza, 70, 71–72*t*, 73*t*, 98, 99–100*t*
Inhaled corticosteroids
    asthma, 281*t*
    COPD, 283*t*
Initial visit, 61
INR. *See* International normalized ratio (INR)
Insulin, 267*t*
Intelligent nonadherence, 48*t*
Intentional nonadherence, 48*t*
Interferon-γ release assay, 96
Internal jugular vein distention (JVD), 289
Internal locus of control, 50
International Headache Society classification system (ICHD-2), 148, 149
International normalized ratio (INR), 306*t*, 307, 310
Intestinal obstruction, 119–120*t*, 124
Intrinsic factor, 328
Ipratropium, 283*t*
Iritis, 164*f*, 359
Iron deficiency anemia, 328
Irritable bowel syndrome (IBS), 124, 141
Irritant conjunctivitis, 164, 359
Irritant contact dermatitis, 190, 199, 200*f*
Ischemic events, 154
Ischemic heart disease, 109
Isospora belli, 141
Isotretinoin, 153
"Itch that rashes," 198

J

J-curve, 236
Jaw clenching, 151
Job or family stress, 51
Joint pain, 178–181
Jugular vein distention (JVD), 289
JUPITER study, 247
JVD. *See* Jugular vein distention (JVD)

K

Keratitis, 160, 162
Keratoconjunctivitis, 160
Keratosis pilaris, 202
Kernig sign, 152
Ketones, 316
Ketotifen, 168
Kidney stone, 124
Kissing disease, 83
Klebsiella pneumoniae, 92
Knee injuries, 177
Knowledge, 8, 9*t*

L

Laboratory tests, 8
Lachman test, 177
Lamotrigine, 297*t*, 298*t*
Latent TB infection (LTBI), 96
Lateral cruciate ligament (LCL) injury, 177
Latex, 201
LCL injury, 177
LDL-C, 244
LE Prep, 181
Leather, 201
Left lower quadrant (LLQ), 117*f*
Left shift, 330
Left upper quadrant (LUQ), 117*f*
Legionella infection, 101
Lennox-Gastaut syndrome, 296
LES. *See* Lower esophageal sphincter (LES)
Leukocyte esterase (LE), 192*t*, 193
Leukocytosis, 330, 331. *See* Post-infectious cough syndrome (PICS)
Leukorrhea, 190
Levetiracetam, 297*t*, 298*t*
LFTs. *See* Liver function tests (LFTs)
Lichenification, 198
Limbal or ciliary flush, 162-163, 163*f*
Limbus, 160
Lipids, 244. *See also* Dyslipidemia
Listening skills, 16
Liver and renal disease, 305-323
  acute hepatocellular damage, 308, 309*t*, 383
  alkaline phosphatase, 307
  aminotransferases, 306-307
  BUN, 313-314
  cases, 318-323, 379-384
  causes of abnormal renal function tests, 316-317
  cholestatic or obstructive damage, 309-310, 309*t*
  chronic hepatocellular damage, 309*t*, 310-311
  chronic/recurrent mild hepatocellular damage, 309*t*, 311-313
  cirrhosis, 309*t*, 310-311, 383, 384
  eGFR, 314-315, 314*t*
  formed elements, 316
  GGTP, 307
  hemolytic anemia, 309*t*
  hepatitis, 309*t*, 311-313, 379, 384
  lab tests, 306*t*
  LFTs, 306-308
  miscellaneous diagnostic tests, 316
  NAFLD, 312
  NASH, 312
  RFTs, 313-316
  serum bilirubin, 307-308
  serum creatinine, 313
  serum proteins, 307
  serum renal function tests, 313-315
  urine protein/albumin, 315-316
  urine renal function tests, 315-316
Liver function tests (LFTs), 251, 306-308
LLQ. *See* Left lower quadrant (LLQ)
Local tissue hypoxia, 106
Location questions, 18-19, 18*t*
Locus of control, 50
Looser lines, 181
LOQQSAM, 17-19, 45*t*
Loss of voice/hoarseness, 84
Low-density lipoprotein (LDL-C), 244
Low serum drug levels, 53
Lower esophageal sphincter (LES), 122
Lower tract UTI, 190
LTBI. *See* Latent TB infection (LTBI)
Lung cancer, 94-95*t*, 97
LUQ. *See* Left upper quadrant (LUQ)
Lymphocytes, 329
Lymphocytosis, 221

M

MAC. *See* Myobacterium avium complex (MAC)
Macroalbuminuria, 315
Macroangiopathy, 262, 265
Macrocytic anemia, 327*t*, 328, 329
Macrolide antibiotics, 130
Macrolides, 139
Macrophages, 96, 329
Macule, 198
Maculopapular skin rash, 221
Magnesium, 139
Malassezia furfur, 202
Malignant hypertension, 151
Mantoux test, 96
Markle test, 123
MB fraction of creatine kinase (CK^MB), 110
MCH. *See* Mean corpuscular hemoglobin (MCH)
MCHC. *See* Mean corpuscular hemoglobin content (MCHC)
MCL injury, 177
McMurray test, 177

MCV. *See* Mean corpuscular volume (MCV)
MDRD. *See* Modified diet in renal disease equation (MDRD)
Mean corpuscular hemoglobin (MCH), 327
Mean corpuscular hemoglobin content (MCHC), 327
Mean corpuscular volume (MCV), 327
Measles, 221
Mechanical and chemical cough receptors, 90
Medial cruciate ligament (MCL) injury, 177
Medical jargon, 44
Medication nonadherence, 48. *See also* Patient adherence
Medication overuse headache, 151
Medication possession ratio (MPR), 53
Megaloblastic anemia, 328
Meglitinides, 267*t*
Melena, 121
Meningitis, 152–153, 153*t*
Meniscus damage, 177
Mentally ill patients, 51
Metabolic syndrome, 252, 261, 261*t*
Metformin, 11, 267*t*
Metformin-induced lactic acidosis, 11
Methylmalonic acid (MMA), 328
MI. *See* Motivational interviewing or myocardial infarction
Microalbuminuria, 315
Microangiopathy, 262, 263
Microcolitis, 140
Midstream clean catch urinalysis (MSCCUA), 124, 191–194
Miglitol, 139
Migraine headache, 149–150, 149*t*
Mild chronic hepatocellular damage, 311–313
Minerals, 139
Mini-mental status examination (MMSE), 299
Ministroke, 154
Minocycline, 153
Mitral valve prolapse (MVP), 108*t*, 111
Mixed cough, 90, 98–101
Mixed drug-induced liver disease, 309
MMA. *See* Methylmalonic acid (MMA)
mMRC, 277
MMSE. *See* Mini-mental status examination (MMSE)
Modified diet in renal disease equation (MDRD), 314, 314*t*
Modified Medical Research Council scale (mMRC), 277
Modifying factors questions, 18*t*, 19
Monocytes, 329
Mononucleosis, 80–81*t*, 83
Monospot test, 83
Moraxella catarrhalis, 74, 77
Morning sickness, 130
Motilin agonists, 139

Motion sickness, 129*t*, 130
Motivation (self-motivation), 57
Motivational interviewing (MI), 56
MPR. *See* Medication possession ratio (MPR)
MRI-DWI, 155
MSCCUA. *See* Midstream clean catch urinalysis (MSCCUA)
Mumps, 152
Murphy sign, 309
Musculoskeletal disorders, 175–183
   ankle sprain, 176
   ankylosing spondylitis, 181
   back injuries, 177–178
   bone diseases, 181–182
   carpal tunnel syndrome, 177
   case, 183, 360
   common arthritides, 178–181
   diagnosis, 176
   differential diagnosis, 179*t*
   etiology, 176
   Felty's syndrome, 180
   golfer elbow, 177
   knee injuries, 177
   osteoarthritis, 178–179, 179*t*
   osteomalacia, 181
   osteoporosis, 181–182
   plantar fasciitis, 176
   psoriatic arthritis, 180
   rheumatoid arthritis, 179–180, 179*t*, 180*t*
   scleroderma, 181
   Sjögren syndrome, 180
   systemic lupus erythematosus (SLE), 179*t*, 180–181
   tennis elbow, 176–177
MVP. *See* Mitral valve prolapse (MVP)
Mycobacterial meningitis, 152
Mycobacterium tuberculosis, 96
Mycoplasma pneumoniae, 101
Myobacterium avium complex (MAC), 141
Myocardial infarction, 109–111
Myoglobin, 110

N
NAAT. *See* Nucleic acid amplification test (NAAT)
NAFLD, 312
NALD. *See* Nonalcoholic liver disease (NALD)
NASH. *See* Nonalcoholic steatohepatitis (NASH)
National Cholesterol Eduction Program Adult Treatment Panel III guidelines, 244, 245*t*
National Jewish Health, 282
Nausea and vomiting, 127–134
   appendicitis, 132
   case, 134, 355
   cholecystitis, 132
   diabetes mellitus, 133

Nausea and vomiting (*Cont.*)
  diagnosis, 128
  differential diagnosis, 128*t*, 129*t*
  etiology, 128
  gastroenteritis, 128, 129*t*
  medication, 129*t*, 130
  meningitis, 131
  migraine headache, 131
  motion sickness, 129*t*, 130
  myocardial infarction, 131
  pancreatitis, 132
  pelvic inflammatory disease, 132
  peptic ulcer disease, 131–132
  pregnancy, 129*t*, 130
  serious causes, 131*t*
  trauma/stroke (CVA), 131
  uremia, 132
  urinary tract infection, 132, 194
  viral hepatitis, 132
NCEP ATP III guidelines, 244, 245*t*
NDDI-E. *See* Neurological Disorders
  Depression Inventory for Epilepsy
  (NDDI-E)
Necrotizing fasciitis, 207
Neisseria gonorrhoeae, 190
Neomycin, 202
NERD. *See* Nonerosive chronic reflux disease
  (NERD)
Neurological Disorders Depression Inventory
  for Epilepsy (NDDI-E), 299
Neutropenia, 331
Neutrophils, 329
Nickel, 200–201
Nitric oxide (NO), 150
Nitrite, 192*t*, 193
Nitrofurantoin, 130
NO. *See* Nitric oxide (NO)
Nocturia, 261
Nodding, 21
Nodule, 198
Non-HDL Cholesterol, 246*t*, 247
Non-small cell lung cancer (NSCLC), 97
Non-ST-segment-elevation myocardial
  infarction (NSTEMI), 107*t*, 110
Nonalcoholic liver disease (NALD), 251, 312
Nonalcoholic steatohepatitis (NASH), 312
Nonanalytic diagnostic process, 10*t*, 11
Nonerosive chronic reflux disease (NERD), 122
Nonsteroidal anti-inflammatory drugs
  (NSAIDs)
  bacterial pneumonia, 92
  bleeding complications, 333
  headache, 153
  nausea and vomiting, 130
  osteomalacia, 181
Nonverbal clues, 16
Nonverbal encouragement, 21

Normochromic, macrocytic anemia, 327
Normochromic, normocytic anemia, 327, 327*t*
Norovirus, 137
NSAIDs. *See* Nonsteroidal anti-inflammatory
  drugs (NSAIDs)
NSCLC. *See* Non-small cell lung cancer
  (NSCLC)
NSTEMI. *See* Non-ST-segment-elevation
  myocardial infarction (NSTEMI)
Nucleic acid amplification test (NAAT)
  meningitis, 153
  trichomoniasis, 190

O

OA. *See* Osteoarthritis (OA)
Oat-cell lung cancer, 97
Objective data, 8, 9*t*, 10, 16, 35
Obstructive liver disease, 309–310, 309*t*, 381
Occupational irritant contact dermatitis, 200*f*
Ocular conjunctiva, 160
OE. *See* Otitis externa (OE)
OME. *See* Otitis media with effusion (OME)
Onset questions, 18*t*, 19
Open-ended questions, 16
Opiates, 142
Opioid analgesics, 151
Opioids
  headache, 151
  nausea and vomiting, 130
Orbital cellulitis, 163
Orolabial herpes simplex virus, 211*f*
Orthopnea, 101, 289
Orthostasis, 234*t*, 235, 290
Orthostatic hypotension, 290
Osteoarthritis (OA), 178–179, 179*t*
Osteomalacia, 181, 309
Osteopenia, 181
Osteoporosis, 181–182
Otitis externa (OE), 75–76*t*, 78, 348
Otitis media with effusion (OME), 75–76*t*,
  77–78
Overview of diseases. *See* Differential
  diagnosis
Oxcarbazepine, 297*t*, 298*t*

P

PAC. *See* Perennial allergic conjunctivitis
  (PAC)
PACAP. *See* Pituitary adenylate cyclase
  activating peptide (PACAP)
Paget's disease, 309
Palpebral conjunctiva, 160
Pancreatitis, 119–120*t*, 123
Pancytopenia, 331
Papule, 198
Parasitic diarrhea, 137, 138*t*, 139
Paronychia, 206

Paroxysmal nocturnal dyspnea (PND), 101, 289
Past medical history, 17
Patch, 198
Patient adherence, 47-57
    cheerleader approach, 49
    cost of medication, 51, 55
    extent of problem, 48
    guiding principles, 56-57
    helping patient improve adherence, 54-57
    homelessness, 51
    interviewing patient about adherence problems, 52-53
    locus of control, 50
    mental illness, 51
    objective measures of adherence, 53-54
    physical handicap, 52
    provider misconceptions, 48-49
    requirements for medication adherence, 49-50
    risk factors for suboptimal adherence, 50-52
    setting the stage, 52, 52t
    supportive adherence probe, 54
    terminology, 48
    threatening, chastising approach, 49, 52
    types of nonadherence, 48t
    white coat compliance, 53
Patient attitudes, 42
Patient education, 43-44
Patient history, 15-29
    cases (patient scripts), 23-29
    chief complaint history, 17-19
    chronic disease follow-up visit history, 19-21
    closure statement, 22
    complete medical history, 17
    importance, 8
    LOQQSAM, 17-19
    patient comfort, 21
    private environment, 21
    process to obtain history, 16
    reflecting or empathetic responses, 21
    summarization, 18t, 19, 21
    types of histories, 16
    verbal and nonverbal encouragement, 21
Patient-oriented history, 16
Patient-provider relationship, 42
Patient scripts
    chief complaint history-taking, 23-26
    chronic visit history-taking, 27-29
Patient visits, 59-65
    follow-up visits, 61
    functions, 60, 60t
    initial visit, 61
    introduction, 62-63

organizing the flow of the visit, 63
    pre-visit planning, 61-62, 62t
Patient workup of drug therapy (PWDT), 9
PCL injury, 177
PCR assay. *See* Polymerase chain reaction (PCR) assay
PDC. *See* Proportion of days covered (PDC)
PE. *See* Pulmonary embolism (PE)
Peak expiratory flow rate (PEFR) monitoring, 278, 279, 281
Pedal edema, 289
PEFR. *See* Peak expiratory flow rate (PEFR)
Pelvic inflammatory disease (PID), 124, 132
Peptic ulcer disease (PUD), 131-132
Perennial allergic conjunctivitis (PAC), 166
Pericarditis, 108t, 111
Permanent problems, 33
Pernicious anemia, 328
Persistence, 48
Pertussis, 94-95t, 97-98
PFT. *See* Pulmonary function test (PFT)
Pharmacist
    communication with health care professionals, 44-46
    documentation. *See* Documentation
    educating the patient, 43-44
    frequency of contact with patient, 55-56
    patient-provider relationship, 42
    skill requirements, 42-43
Pharmacist-physician communication, 44-46
Pharmacist skill requirements, 42-43
Pharyngitis
    post-nasal drip, 80-81t, 83
    streptococcal, 79, 80-81t, 82
    viral, 80-81t, 82-83
Phenobarbital, 297t, 298t
Phenothiazines, 309
Phenytoin
    anemia, 329
    epilepsy, 297t, 298t
    headache, 153
PHN. *See* Postherpetic neuralgia (PHN)
Photoallergic reactions, 222
Photophobia, 161
Photosensitivity reactions, 221-222
Phototoxic reactions, 221-222
PICS. *See* Post-infectious cough syndrome (PICS)
PID. *See* Pelvic inflammatory disease (PID)
Pill organizer, 56
Pink eye, 160. *See also* Inflamed (red) eye
Pink flags, 57
Pituitary adenylate cyclase activating peptide (PACAP), 150
Pityrosporum ovale, 202
Plan, 35

Plantar fasciitis, 176
Plantar warts, 209, 211*f*
Plaque, 198
Plaque buildup, 106
Plaque psoriasis, 204*f*
Platelets, 331
Pleurisy, 108*t*, 112
PMNs. *See* Polymorphonuclear cells (PMNs)
PND. *See* Paroxysmal nocturnal dyspnea
    (PND); Post-nasal drip (PND)
Poikilocytosis, 328
Poison oak, 202*f*
Polyarthritis, 178
Polymerase chain reaction (PCR) assay
    liver disease, 312
    meningitis, 153
Polymorphonuclear cells (PMNs), 329
Polyols, 263
Polys, 329
Polyuria, 261
POMR. *See* Problem-oriented medical record
    (POMR)
Portal hypertension, 310–311, 311*f*
Post-concussion headache, 153
Post-ictal phase, 295
Post-infectious cough syndrome (PICS), 98,
    99–100*t*
Post-nasal drip (PND), 80–81*t*, 83
Posterior cruciate ligament (PCL) injury, 177
Postherpetic neuralgia (PHN), 212
PPD skin test, 96
Practice examples. *See* Cases
Prasugrel, 331
Pravastatin, 251, 252
Pre-visit planning, 61–62, 62*t*
Precordial catch, 112
Prediabetes, 262
Pregnancy
    constipation, 142
    meningitis, 152
    nausea and vomiting, 129*t*, 130
    UTI, 191
Preload, 288
Preseptal cellulitis, 163
Primary headaches, 148–150
Primary patient education, 43–44
Primary progressive TB infection, 96
Primidone, 297*t*, 298*t*
Principle of self-efficacy, 43
Problem identification. *See* Diagnosis
Problem list, 17
Problem-oriented medical record (POMR),
    32–33
Procalcitonin, 92
Productive cough, 90, 91*t*, 92–93
Proportion of days covered (PDC), 53
Protein synthesis, 380

Proteinuria, 315
Prothrombin, 307, 310
Provider-centered patient history, 16
Pseudogout, 178
Pseudomonas aeruginosa, 78, 92
Pseudotumor cerebri, 153
Psoas sign, 123
Psoriasis, 202, 204*f*
Psoriatic arthritis, 180, 202
Pterygium, 171, 172*f*, 359
PUD. *See* Peptic ulcer disease (PUD)
"Pull-down menu," 10, 11
Pulmonary edema, 101
Pulmonary embolism (PE), 107*t*, 111–112
Pulmonary function test (PFT), 275
Purified protein derivative (PPD), 96
Pustule, 198
PWDT. *See* Patient workup of drug therapy
    (PWDT)
Pyelonephritis, 124, 186, 191, 194
Pyuria, 316

Q

Q-wave myocardial infarction, 110
Quality questions, 18*t*, 19
QuantiFERON-TB Gold Test, 96
Quantity questions, 18*t*, 19

R

RA. *See* Rheumatoid arthritis (RA)
Radioimmunoblot assay (RIBA), 312
Rapid antigen detection test (RADT), 82
Raynaud's phenomenon, 181
RBC casts, 316
RBCs. *See* Red blood cells (RBCs)
RDW. *See* Red blood cell distribution widths
    (RDW)
Recurrent mild hepatocellular damage, 309*t*,
    311–313
Recurrent UTI, 191
Red blood cell distribution widths (RDW), 327
Red blood cells (RBCs), 326–328
Refill record, 53
Reflecting or empathetic responses, 21
Reflux disease, 97
Renal calculus, 119–120*t*, 124
Renal disease. *See* Liver and renal disease
Renal function tests (RFTs), 313–316
Resolved problems, 33
Reticulocyte, 328
Reticulocyte count, 328
Reticulocyte index (RI), 328
Reticulocytosis, 328
Reversible ischemic neurological deficit
    (RIND), 154
Review of systems (ROS), 17, 332
Rewarding patient successes, 55

RF. *See* Rheumatoid factor (RF)
RFTs. *See* Renal function tests (RFTs)
Rhabdomyolysis, 248, 249, 251
Rheumatoid arthritis (RA), 179–180, 179*t*,
  180*t*
Rheumatoid factor (RF), 179
Rhinophymatous rosacea, 210*f*
RI. *See* Reticulocyte index (RI)
Rib fracture, 112
RIBA. *See* Radioimmunoblot assay (RIBA)
Right lower quadrant (RLQ), 117*f*
Right upper quadrant (RUQ), 117*f*
RIND. *See* Reversible ischemic neurological
  deficit (RIND)
Ringworm, 212
RLQ. *See* Right lower quadrant (RLQ)
ROS. *See* Review of systems (ROS)
Rosacea, 208–209, 210*f*
Rosuvastatin, 247, 251, 252
Rotavirus, 137
Routine, 54, 57
Rovsing sign, 123
Rule of 2*s*, 279
Runny/stuffy nose, 70–74
  allergic rhinitis, 70, 71–72*t*, 73
  bacterial sinusitis, 71–72*t*, 73–74
  common cold, 70, 71–72*t*, 73*t*
  flu/common cold, compared, 73*t*
  influenza, 70, 71–72*t*, 73*t*
  overview, 71–72*t*
  vasomotor rhinitis, 71–72*t*, 73
RUQ. *See* Right upper quadrant (RUQ)

S

S3 gallop rhythm, 289
SABA. *See* Short-acting beta-adrenergic
  agonist inhalers (SABA)
SAC. *See* Seasonal allergic conjunctivitis
  (SAC)
Salmeterol, 283*t*
SBAR technique, 45, 46*t*
Scale, 198
Scaly dermatoses, 202
Scarlatina, 82
Scarlet fever, 82
Schachter, Steven, 298
SCLC. *See* Small cell lung cancer (SCLC)
Sclera, 160
Scleroderma, 181
Seasonal allergic conjunctivitis (SAC), 166
Seborrhea/seborrheic dermatitis, 202, 203*f*
Secondary education, 43
Secondary headaches, 150–155
Segs, 329
Seizure disorders, 293–301
  AEDs, 297*t*, 298*t*, 299
  case, 301, 377–378

classification, 295
compliance, 296, 297*t*, 298
complications, 297*t*, 298–299, 298*t*
control, 296, 297*t*
depression/suicide, 298–299
diagnosis, 294–295
EEG, 294, 295
etiology, 294
follow-up visits, 296–299
initial visit, 296
medication holiday, 298
Self-efficacy, 43
Self-motivation, 57
Semi-Fowler position, 289
Serous otitis media (SOM), 75–76*t*, 77–78
Serum bilirubin, 307–308, 309, 311
Serum creatinine, 313
Serum drug levels, 53
Serum folate levels, 328
Serum renal function tests, 313–315
Setting questions, 18*t*, 19
Setting the stage, 52, 52*t*
Sexually transmitted diseases (STDs), 186.
  See also Dysuria and vaginal discharge
  chlamydia, 188*t*, 190
  gonorrhea, 188*t*, 190
Shingles, 211–212
Short-acting beta-adrenergic agonist
  inhalers (SABA), 277
Shortness of breath (SOB), 289
SIBO. *See* Small intestine bacterial
  overgrowth (SIBO)
Silence, 21
Silent infarction, 154
Silent pyelonephritis, 191
Simplify the treatment regimen, 54–55
Simvastatin, 252
6-minute walk test, 279
Sjögren syndrome, 180
Skin disorders, 197–225
  acne rosacea, 208–209, 210*f*
  acne vulgaris, 207–208, 208*f*
  allergic contact dermatitis (ACD),
    199–202
  anaphylaxis, 218
  angioneurotic edema, 216, 218, 218*f*
  atopic dermatitis, 198–199, 199*f*, 200*f*
  bacterial infections, 203–209
  bullous impetigo, 205, 206*f*
  candida, 214–216
  carbuncle, 206–207
  cases, 224, 225, 364, 365
  corticosteroids, 222–223
  drug hypersensitivity syndrome
    (DHS), 221
  drug-induced skin reactions, 216–221
  eczematous disorders, 198–202

Skin disorders (*Cont.*)
erythema multiforme, 218–219,
219*f,* 220*f*
erythema nodosum, 221
fixed drug eruptions, 221
folliculitis, 205, 206*f*
fungal infections, 212–216
furuncle, 205, 207*f*
glossary, 198
herpes simplex, 209, 211*f*
herpes zoster, 211–212, 212*f*
IgE-mediated reactions, 216–218
impetigo, 205, 205*f*
irritant contact dermatitis, 199, 200*f*
maculopapular skin rash, 221
necrotizing fasciitis, 207
photosensitivity reactions, 221–222
psoriasis, 202, 204*f*
scaly dermatoses, 202
seborrhea/seborrheic dermatitis, 202,
203*f*
sunburn, 221–222
T-lymphocyte-mediated reactions,
218–221
tineas, 212–214
urticaria, 216, 217*f*
verrucae (warts), 209, 210*f,* 211*f*
viral infections, 209–212
SLE. *See* Systemic lupus erythematosus
(SLE)
Small cell lung cancer (SCLC), 97
Small intestine bacterial overgrowth (SIBO),
141
SNOOP4, 150–151
SOAP notes
assessment (A), 35
example (permanent problem), 40
example (temporary problem), 39
labeling, 33–34
objective data (O), 35
plan (P), 35
signing the SOAP, 34–35
subjective data (S), 35
titling entries (permanent problems), 34*f*
titling entries (temporary problems), 34*f*
SOAPIER, 32
SOB. *See* Shortness of breath (SOB)
SOM. *See* Serous otitis media (SOM)
Sore throat/hoarseness, 79–84
hand, foot, and mouth disease,
80–81*t,* 83
herpangina, 80–81*t,* 83
loss of voice/hoarseness, 84
mononucleosis, 80–81*t,* 83
overview, 80–81*t*
pharyngitis due to post-nasal drip,
80–81*t,* 83

streptococcal pharyngitis, 79, 80–81*t,* 82
viral pharyngitis, 80–81*t,* 82–83
Spirometry, 275
Spironolactone
CHF, 290, 291*t*
hypertension, 235*t*
ST-segment-elevation myocardial infarction
(STEMI), 107*t,* 110
Stabs, 329
Staphylococcus aureus, 92, 205
Staphylococcus saprophyticus, 191
Staphylococcus species, 78
Statin-induced cognitive dysfunction, 251–252
Statin-induced rhabdomyolysis, 249
Statin muscle side effects, 249–251
Statin therapy. *See* Dyslipidemia
Status asthmaticus, 93
STDs. *See* Sexually transmitted diseases
(STDs)
STEMI. *See* ST-segment-elevation myocardial
infarction (STEMI)
Sternocleidomastoid muscles, 283
Stevens-Johnson syndrome, 218, 220*f,* 299
Strand, Linda, 9
Strand/ASHP diagnostic process, 9
Strep throat, 79
Streptococcal pharyngitis, 79, 80–81*t,* 82
Streptococcus pneumoniae, 74, 77, 92
Streptococcus pyogenes, 79
Stress, 51
Stretch marks, 223
Striae, 223
Stroke, 154–155
Structured documentation systems, 32–35
Student exercises. *See* Cases
Stuffy/runny nose. *See* Runny/stuffy nose
Stye, 171
Subacute cough, 90
Subconjunctival hemorrhage, 171
Subjective data, 16, 35
Suicide, 298–299
Sulfonamides, 221
Sulfonylureas
diabetes mellitus, 267*t*
photosensitivity reactions, 221
Summarization, 18*t,* 19, 21
Sunburn, 221–222
Super virus (influenza), 70, 71–72*t,* 73*t*
Supportive adherence probe, 54
Swimmer's ear, 75–76*t,* 78
Symptom-specific diagnostic schemata
tables, 22
Syncope, 235
Synovial fluid, 178
Systemic lupus erythematosus (SLE), 179*t,*
180–181
Systolic blood pressure, 230

T

T-lymphocyte-mediated reactions, 218–221
T-Spot TB test, 96
Tailor the regimen, 55
Target lab values, 57
Tarsal conjunctiva, 160
TB. *See* Tuberculosis (TB)
Teach-back, 43, 50
"Telling people" educational approaches, 50
Temporary problems, 33
Temporomandibular joint (TMJ) disorders, 74, 75–76*t*, 79, 151
Temporomandibular joint pain dysfunction syndrome, 75–76*t*, 79, 151
Tennis elbow, 176–177
TENS. *See* Toxic epidermal necrolysis (TENS)
Tension headache, 148–149, 149*t*
Terazosin, 234*t*, 235*t*
Tetracyclines
    headache, 153
    nausea and vomiting, 130
    photosensitivity reactions, 221
Textbook organization, 11
Threatening, chastising approach, 49, 52
3 Cs schemata, 11, 13*t*, 63*t*
Thrombocytopenia, 331
Thrombocytosis, 331
Thyroid-stimulating-hormone (TSH), 251
TIA. *See* Transient ischemic attack (TIA)
Tiagabine, 297*t*, 298*t*
Ticagrelor, 331
Tinea corporis, 212, 213*f*
Tinea faciei, 212
Tinea pedis, 212, 213*f*
Tinea versicolor, 214, 214*f*, 215*f*
Tiotropium, 283*t*
TM. *See* Tympanic membrane (TM)
TMJ disorders, 74, 75–76*t*, 79, 151
TMJ pain dysfunction syndrome, 75–76*t*, 79, 151
Tonic phase, 295
Topiramate, 297*t*, 298*t*
Toxic epidermal necrolysis (TENS), 218–219, 220*f*
Toxigenic bacterial gastroenteritis, 137, 138*t*
Tracheostomy, 84
Transglutaminase, 140
Transient ischemic attack (TIA), 154
Transtheoretical model, 50–51
Trichomonas vaginalis, 189, 190
Trichomonas vaginitis (TV), 188*t*, 189–190
Trichomoniasis, 189–190, 188S
Triglycerides, 244
Trimethoprim, 313
Triptans, 151
Troponin I and T, 110
TSH. *See* Thyroid-stimulating-hormone (TSH)

Tuberculin skin test, 96
Tuberculosis (TB), 94–95*t*, 96–97
TV. *See* Trichomonas vaginitis (TV)
24-hour stomach flu, 137
Tympanic membrane (TM), 77, 78
Type 1 diabetes, 260, 260*t*
Type 2 diabetes, 260, 260*t*

U

UA. *See* Unstable angina (UA)
UACS. *See* Upper airway cough syndrome (UACS)
Ulcerative colitis, 124, 140
Uncomplicated UTI, 191
Unintentional nonadherence, 48*t*
Universal statement, 54
Unstable angina (UA), 107*t*, 110
Upper airway cough syndrome (UACS), 98, 99–100*t*
Upper gastrointestinal bleeding, 121
Upper respiratory infection (URI)
    common cold, 70, 71–72*t*, 73*t*
    influenza, 70, 71–72*t*, 73*t*
Upper tract UTI, 190
Uremia, 132
URI. *See* Upper respiratory infection (URI)
Urinary tract infection (UTI), 190–194
    diagnosis, 191–182
    heartburn and abdominal pain, 119–120*t*, 124
    lower tract UTI, 190
    nausea and vomiting, 132, 194
    pregnancy, 191
    recurrent UTI, 191
    uncomplicated UTI, 191
    upper tract UTI, 190
    urine culture, 193
    urine tests, 191–193
Urine culture, 193
Urine dipsticks, 193
Urine renal function tests, 315–316
Urine testing, 192*t*
Urticaria, 216, 217*f*
Usually self-limiting gastroenteritis, 137, 138*t*
UTI. *See* Urinary tract infection (UTI)
Uveal tract, 161

V

V/Q scan, 111–112
Vaginal discharge. *See also* Dysuria and vaginal discharge
Valley fever, 216
Valproate, 297*t*, 298*t*
Variable medication possession ratio (VMPR), 53
Vasomotor rhinitis, 71–72*t*, 73
Verbal and nonverbal encouragement, 21

Verbal rewards, 55
Vernal keratoconjunctivitis (VKC), 165*t*, 166
Verrucae (warts), 209, 210*f*, 211*f*
Vertigo, 130
Very-low-density lipoprotein (VLDL-C), 244
Vesicle, 198
Veterans Administration study, 49
Vignettes. *See* Cases
Viral conjunctivitis, 165*t*, 166–169
Viral diarrhea, 136
Viral gastroenteritis, 137, 138*t*
Viral hepatitis, 132
Viral laryngotracheobronchitis, 84
Viral meningitis, 152
Viral pharyngitis, 80–81*t*, 82–83
Viral pneumonia, 98, 99–100*t*
Viral skin infections, 209–212
Vitamin B$_{12}$ deficiency, 328, 329
Vitamin D deficiency, 181, 251
VKC. *See* Vernal keratoconjunctivitis (VKC)
VLDL-C, 244
VMPR. *See* Variable medication possession ratio (VMPR)
Vomiting. *See* Nausea and vomiting

Vulvovaginal candidiasis (VVC), 188–189, 188*t*
VVC. *See* Vulvovaginal candidiasis

W

Walking pneumonia, 101
Warfarin, 153
Warts, 209, 210*f*, 211*f*
WBC casts, 316
WBCs. *See* White blood cells (WBCs)
Weed, Lawrence, 32
Wet cough, 90
"What do you think caused this problem?" question, 18*t*, 19
"What medications are you currently taking?" question, 18*t*, 19
Wheals, 216, 217*f*
Whiff test, 187
White blood cells (WBCs), 329–330
White coat compliance, 53
White coat hypertension, 230
Whooping cough, 97

X

Xerosis, 202

www.ingramcontent.com/pod-product-compliance
Lightning Source LLC
Chambersburg PA
CBHW060749220326
41598CB00022B/2376